D0562402

TION

CASE FILES
Internal Medicine

Eugene C. Toy, MD

The John S. Dunn, Senior Academic Chair and Program Director
The Methodist Hospital Ob/Gyn Residency Program
Houston, Texas

Vice Chair of Academic Affairs
Department of Obstetrics and Gynecology
The Methodist Hospital
Houston, Texas

Associate Clinical Professor and Clerkship Director
Department of Obstetrics and Gynecology
University of Texas Medical School at Houston
Houston, Texas

Associate Clinical Professor
Weill Cornell College of Medicine

John T. Patlan, Jr., MD

Assistant Professor of Medicine
Department of General Internal Medicine
MD Anderson Cancer Center
Houston, Texas

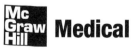 **Medical**

New York   Chicago   San Francisco   Lisbon   London   Madrid   Mexico City
Milan   New Delhi   San Juan   Seoul   Singapore   Sydney   Toronto

The McGraw·Hill Companies

Case Files®: Internal Medicine, Third Edition

Copyright © 2009 by The McGraw-Hill Companies, Inc. All rights reserved. Printed in the United States of America. Except a permitted under the United States Copyright Act of 1976, no part of this publication may be reproduced or distributed in any form or by any means, or stored in a data base or retrieval system, without the prior written permission of the publisher. Previous editions Copyright © 2007, 2004 by the McGraw-Hill Companies, Inc.

Case Files® is a registered trademark of The McGraw-Hill Companies, Inc. All rights reserved.

3 4 5 6 7 8 9 0   DOC/DOC   12 11 10

ISBN 978-0-07-161364-4
MHID 0-07-161364-1

Notice

Medicine is an ever-changing science. As new research and clinical experience broaden our knowledge, changes in treatment and drug therapy are required. The authors and the publisher of this work have checked with sources believed to be reliable in their efforts to provide information that is complete and generally in accord with the standard accepted at the time of publication. However, in view of the possibility of human error or changes in medical sciences, neither the editors nor the publisher nor any other party who has been involved in the preparation or publication of this work warrants that the information contained herein is in every respect accurate or complete, and they disclaim all responsibility for any errors or omissions or for the results obtained from use of the information contained in this work. Readers are encouraged to confirm the information contained herein with other sources. For example and in particular, readers are advised to check the product information sheet included in the package of each drug they plan to administer to be certain that the information contained in this work is accurate and that changes have not been made in the recommended dose or in the contraindications for administration. This recommendation is of particular importance in connection with new or infrequently used drugs.

This book was set in Goudy by International Typesetting and Composition.
The editors were Catherine A. Johnson and Christie Naglieri.
The production supervisor was Catherine H. Saggese.
Project management was provided by Gita Raman, International Typesetting and Composition.
The designer was Janice Bielawa; the cover designer was Aimee Nordin.
RR Donnelley was printer and binder.

This book is printed on acid-free paper.

Library of Congress Cataloging-in-Publication Data

Toy, Eugene C.
Case files. Internal medicine / Eugene C. Toy, John T. Patlan Jr. — 3rd ed.
    p. ; cm.
    Rev. ed. of: Case files. Internal medicine / [edited by] Eugene C. Toy ... [et al.]. 2nd ed. c2006.
    Includes bibliographical references and index.
    ISBN-13: 978-0-07-161364-4 (pbk. : alk. paper)
    ISBN-10: 0-07-161364-1 (pbk. : alk. paper)   1. Internal medicine—Case studies.
    I. Patlan, John T.   II. Case files. Internal medicine.   III. Title.   IV. Title: Internal medicine.
    [DNLM: 1. Internal Medicine—Case Reports.   2. Internal Medicine—Problems and Exercises.
3. Diagnosis, Differential—Case Reports.   4. Diagnosis, Differential—Problems and
Exercises.   5. Physical Examination—Case Reports.   6. Physical Examination—Problems and
Exercises.   WB18.2 T756c 2009]
    RC66.C36 2009
    616—dc22

                                                                              2009002173

McGraw-Hill books are available at special quantity discounts to use as premiums and sales promotions, or for use in corporate training programs. To contact a representative please e-mail us at bulksales@mcgraw-hill.com.

International Edition ISBN 978-0-07-163905-7; MHID 0-07-163905-5
Copyright © 2009. Exclusive rights by The McGraw-Hill Companies, Inc., for manufacture and export. This book cannot be re-exported from the country to which it is consigned by McGraw-Hill. The International Edition is not available in North America.

To our coach Victor, and our father–son teammates Bob & Jackson, Steve & Weston, Ron & Wesley, and Dan & Joel. At the inspirational JH Ranch Father–Son Retreat, all of us, including my loving son Andy, arrived as strangers, but in 6 days, we left as lifelong friends.

— ECT

To my parents who instilled an early love of learning and of the written word, and who continue to serve as role models for life.

To my beautiful wife Elsa and children Sarah and Sean, for their patience and understanding, as precious family time was devoted to the completion of "the book."

To all my teachers, particularly Drs. Carlos Pestaña, Robert Nolan, Herbert Fred, and Cheves Smythe, who make the complex understandable, and who have dedicated their lives to the education of physicians, and served as role models of healers.

To the medical students and residents at the University of Texas–Houston Medical School whose enthusiasm, curiosity, and pursuit of excellent and compassionate care provide a constant source of stimulation, joy, and pride.

To all readers of this book everywhere in the hopes that it might help them to grow in wisdom and understanding, and to provide better care for their patients who look to them for comfort and relief of suffering.

And to the Creator of all things, Who is the source of all knowledge and healing power, may this book serve as an instrument of His will.

— JTP

CONTENTS

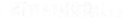

Molly Dudley Class of 2009
University of Texas Health Science Center at San Antonio
San Antonio, Texas

Approach to congestive heart failure
Approach to HIV and pneumocystits pneumonia
Approach to hypertension
Approach to Arthritis
Approach to low back pain
Approach to endocarditis
Approach to lung disease
Approach to lung cancer
Approach to health maintenance

ACKNOWLEDGMENTS

The curriculum that evolved into the ideas for this series was inspired by Philbert Yau and Chuck Rosipal, two talented and forthright students, who have since graduated from medical school. It has been a tremendous joy to work with my excellent coauthors, especially Dr. John Patlan, who exemplifies the qualities of the ideal physician—caring, empathetic, and avid teacher, and who is intellectually unparalleled. I am greatly indebted to my editor, Catherine Johnson, whose exuberance, experience, and vision helped to shape this series. I appreciate McGraw-Hill's believing in the concept of teaching through clinical cases. I am also grateful to Catherine Saggese for her excellent production expertise, and Cindy Yoo for her wonderful editing. I cherish the ever-organized and precise Gita Raman, senior project manager, whose friendship and talent I greatly value; she keeps me focused, and nurtures each of my books from manuscript to print. It has been a privilege and honor to work with one of the brightest medical students I have encountered, Molly Dudley who was the principal student reviewer of this book. She enthusiastically provided feedback and helped to emphasize the right material. I appreciate Dorothy Mersinger and Jo McMains for their sage advice and support. At Methodist, I appreciate Drs. Judy Paukert, Dirk Sostman, Marc Boom and Alan Kaplan who have welcomed our residents; John N. Lyle VII, a brilliant administrator and Barbara Hagemeister, who holds the department together. Without my dear colleagues, Drs. Weilie Tjoa, Juan Franco, Waverly Peakes, Nicolas Stephanou, and Vincente Zapata, this book could not have been written. Most of all, I appreciate my ever-loving wife Terri, and our four wonderful children, Andy, Michael, Allison, and Christina, for their patience and understanding.

Eugene C. Toy

Mastering the cognitive knowledge within a field such as internal medicine is a formidable task. It is even more difficult to draw on that knowledge, procure and filter through the clinical and laboratory data, develop a differential diagnosis, and, finally, to make a rational treatment plan. To gain these skills, the student learns best at the bedside, guided and instructed by experienced teachers, and inspired toward self-directed, diligent reading. Clearly, there is no replacement for education at the bedside. Unfortunately, clinical situations usually do not encompass the breadth of the specialty. Perhaps the best alternative is a carefully crafted patient case designed to stimulate the clinical approach and the decision-making process. In an attempt to achieve that goal, we have constructed a collection of clinical vignettes to teach diagnostic or therapeutic approaches relevant to internal medicine.

Most importantly, the explanations for the cases emphasize the mechanisms and underlying principles, rather than merely rote questions and answers. This book is organized for versatility: it allows the student "in a rush" to go quickly through the scenarios and check the corresponding answers, and it allows the student who wants thought-provoking explanations to obtain them. The answers are arranged from simple to complex: the bare answers, an analysis of the case, an approach to the pertinent topic, a comprehension test at the end, clinical pearls for emphasis, and a list of references for further reading. The clinical vignettes are purposely placed in random order to simulate the way that real patients present to the practitioner. A listing of cases is included in Section III to aid the student who desires to test his/her knowledge of a certain area, or to review a topic, including basic definitions. Finally, we intentionally did not use a multiple choice question format in the case scenarios, because clues (or distractions) are not available in the real world.

How to Approach Clinical Problems

Part 1. Approach to the Patient

The transition from the textbook or journal article to the clinical situation is one of the most challenging tasks in medicine. Retention of information is difficult; organization of the facts and recall of a myriad of data in precise application to the patient is crucial. The purpose of this text is to facilitate in this process. The first step is gathering information, also known as establishing the database. This includes taking the history (asking questions), performing the physical examination, and obtaining selective laboratory and/or imaging tests. Of these, the historical examination is the most important and useful. Sensitivity and respect should always be exercised during the interview of patients.

Clinical Pearl

▶ The history is the single most important tool in obtaining a diagnosis. All physical findings and laboratory and imaging studies are first obtained and then interpreted in the light of the pertinent history.

HISTORY

1. Basic information: Age, gender, and ethnicity must be recorded because some conditions are more common at certain ages; for instance, pain on defecation and rectal bleeding in a 20-year-old may indicate inflammatory bowel disease, whereas the same symptoms in a 60-year-old would more likely suggest colon cancer.
2. Chief complaint: What is it that brought the patient into the hospital or office? Is it a scheduled appointment, or an unexpected symptom? The patient's own words should be used if possible, such as, "I feel like a ton of bricks are on my chest." The chief complaint, or real reason for seeking medical attention, may not be the first subject the patient talks about (in fact, it may be the last thing), particularly if the subject is embarrassing, such as a sexually transmitted disease, or highly emotional, such as depression. It is often useful to clarify exactly what the patient's concern is, for example, they may fear their headaches represent an underlying brain tumor.
3. History of present illness: This is the most crucial part of the entire database. The questions one asks are guided by the differential diagnosis one begins to consider the moment the patient identifies the chief complaint, as well as the clinician's knowledge of typical disease patterns and their natural history. The duration and character of the primary complaint, associated symptoms, and exacerbating/relieving factors should be recorded. Sometimes, the history will be convoluted and lengthy, with multiple diagnostic or therapeutic interventions at different locations. For patients

with chronic illnesses, obtaining prior medical records is invaluable. For example, when extensive evaluation of a complicated medical problem has been done elsewhere, it is usually better to first obtain those results than to repeat a "million-dollar workup." When reviewing prior records, it is often useful to review the primary data (eg, biopsy reports, echocardiograms, serologic evaluations) rather than to rely upon a diagnostic label applied by someone else, which then gets replicated in medical records and by repetition, acquires the aura of truth, when it may not be fully supported by data. Some patients will be poor historians because of dementia, confusion, or language barriers; recognition of these situations and querying of family members is useful. When little or no history is available to guide a focused investigation, more extensive objective studies are often necessary to exclude potentially serious diagnoses.

4. Past history
    a. Any illnesses such as hypertension, hepatitis, diabetes mellitus, cancer, heart disease, pulmonary disease, and thyroid disease should be elicited. If an existing or prior diagnosis is not obvious, it is useful to ask exactly how it was diagnosed; that is, what investigations were performed. Duration, severity, and therapies should be included.
    b. Any hospitalizations and emergency room visits should be listed with the reason(s) for admission, the intervention, and the location of the hospital.
    c. Transfusions with any blood products should be listed, including any adverse reactions.
    d. Surgeries: The year and type of surgery should be elucidated and any complications documented. The type of incision and any untoward effects of the anesthesia or the surgery should be noted.

5. Allergies: Reactions to medications should be recorded, including severity and temporal relationship to the medication. An adverse effect (such as nausea) should be differentiated from a true allergic reaction.

6. Medications: Current and previous medications should be listed, including dosage, route, frequency, and duration of use. Prescription, over-the-counter, and herbal medications are all relevant. Patients often forget their complete medication list; thus, asking each patient to bring in all their medications—both prescribed and nonprescribed—allows for a complete inventory.

7. Family history: Many conditions are inherited, or are predisposed in family members. The age and health of siblings, parents, grandparents, and others can provide diagnostic clues. For instance, an individual with first-degree family members with early onset coronary heart disease is at risk for cardiovascular disease.

8. Social history: This is one of the most important parts of the history in that the patient's functional status at home, social and economic circumstances, and goals and aspirations for the future are often the critical determinant in what the best way to manage a patient's medical problem is. Living arrangements, economic situations, and religious affiliations may provide important clues for puzzling diagnostic cases, or suggest the acceptability of various

diagnostic or therapeutic options. Marital status and habits such as alcohol, tobacco, or illicit drug use may be relevant as risk factors for disease.

9. Review of systems: A few questions about each major body system ensures that problems will not be overlooked. The clinician should avoid the mechanical "rapid-fire" questioning technique that discourages patients from answering truthfully because of fear of "annoying the doctor."

PHYSICAL EXAMINATION

The physical examination begins as one is taking the history, by observing the patient and beginning to consider a differential diagnosis. When performing the physical examination, one focuses on body systems suggested by the differential diagnosis, and performs tests or maneuvers with specific questions in mind; for example, does the patient with jaundice have ascites? When the physical examination is performed with potential diagnoses and expected physical findings in mind ("one sees what one looks for"), the utility of the examination in adding to diagnostic yield is greatly increased, as opposed to an unfocused "head-to-toe" physical.

1. General appearance: A great deal of information is gathered by observation, as one notes the patient's body habitus, state of grooming, nutritional status, level of anxiety (or perhaps inappropriate indifference), degree of pain or comfort, mental status, speech patterns, and use of language. This forms your impression of "who this patient is."

2. Vital signs: Temperature, blood pressure, heart rate, and respiratory rate. Height and weight are often placed here. Blood pressure can sometimes be different in the two arms; initially, it should be measured in both arms. In patients with suspected hypovolemia, pulse and blood pressure should be taken in lying and standing positions to look for orthostatic hypotension. It is quite useful to take the vital signs oneself, rather than relying upon numbers gathered by ancillary personnel using automated equipment, because important decisions regarding patient care are often made using the vital signs as an important determining factor.

3. Head and neck examination: Facial or periorbital edema and pupillary responses should be noted. Funduscopic examination provides a way to visualize the effects of diseases such as diabetes on the microvasculature; papilledema can signify increased intracranial pressure. Estimation of jugular venous pressure is very useful to estimate volume status. The thyroid should be palpated for a goiter or nodule, and carotid arteries auscultated for bruits. Cervical (common) and supraclavicular (pathologic) nodes should be palpated.

4. Breast examination: Inspect for symmetry, skin or nipple retraction with the patient's hands on her hips (to accentuate the pectoral muscles), and also with arms raised. With the patient sitting and supine, the breasts should then be palpated systematically to assess for masses. The nipple should be assessed for discharge and the axillary and supraclavicular regions should be examined for adenopathy.

5. Cardiac examination: The point of maximal impulse (PMI) should be ascertained for size and location, and the heart auscultated at the apex of the heart as well as at the base. Heart sounds, murmurs, and clicks should be characterized. Murmurs should be classified according to intensity, duration, timing in the cardiac cycle, and changes with various maneuvers. Systolic murmurs are very common and often physiologic; diastolic murmurs are uncommon and usually pathologic.

6. Pulmonary examination: The lung fields should be examined systematically and thoroughly. Wheezes, rales, rhonchi, and bronchial breath sounds should be recorded. Percussion of the lung fields may be helpful in identifying the hyperresonance of tension pneumothorax, or the dullness of consolidated pneumonia or a pleural effusion.

7. Abdominal examination: The abdomen should be inspected for scars, distension, or discoloration (such as the Grey Turner sign of discoloration at the flank areas indicating intra-abdominal or retroperitoneal hemorrhage). Auscultation of bowel sounds to identify normal versus high-pitched and hyperactive versus hypoactive. Percussion of the abdomen can be utilized to assess the size of the liver and spleen, and to detect ascites by noting shifting dullness. Careful palpation should begin initially away from the area of pain, involving one hand on top of the other, to assess for masses, tenderness, and peritoneal signs. Tenderness should be recorded on a scale (eg, 1 to 4 where 4 is the most severe pain). Guarding, and whether it is voluntary or involuntary, should be noted.

8. Back and spine examination: The back should be assessed for symmetry, tenderness, and masses. The flank regions are particularly important to assess for pain on percussion, which might indicate renal disease.

9. Genitalia
   a. Females: The pelvic examination should include an inspection of the external genitalia, and with the speculum, evaluation of the vagina and cervix. A pap smear and/or cervical cultures may be obtained. A bimanual examination to assess the size, shape, and tenderness of the uterus and adnexa is important.
   b. Males: An inspection of the penis and testes is performed. Evaluation for masses, tenderness, and lesions is important. Palpation for hernias in the inguinal region with the patient coughing to increase intra-abdominal pressure is useful.

10. Rectal examination: A digital rectal examination is generally performed for those individuals with possible colorectal disease, or gastrointestinal bleeding. Masses should be assessed, and stool for occult blood should be tested. In men, the prostate gland can be assessed for enlargement and for nodules.

11. Extremities: An examination for joint effusions, tenderness, edema, and cyanosis may be helpful. Clubbing of the nails might indicate pulmonary diseases such as lung cancer or chronic cyanotic heart disease.

12. Neurological examination: Patients who present with neurological complaints usually require a thorough assessment, including the mental status, cranial nerves, motor strength, sensation, and reflexes.

13. The skin should be carefully examined for evidence of pigmented lesions (melanoma), cyanosis, or rashes that may indicate systemic disease (malar rash of systemic lupus erythematosus).

LABORATORY AND IMAGING ASSESSMENT

1. Laboratory
   a. CBC (complete blood count) to assess for anemia and thrombocytopenia.
   b. Chemistry panel is most commonly used to evaluate renal and liver function.
   c. Lipid panel is particularly relevant in cardiovascular diseases.
   d. Urinalysis is often referred to as a "liquid renal biopsy," because the presence of cells, casts, protein, or bacteria provides clues about underlying glomerular or tubular diseases.
   e. Gram stain and culture of urine, sputum, and cerebrospinal fluid, as well as blood cultures, are frequently useful to isolate the cause of infection.
2. Imaging procedures
   a. Chest radiography is extremely useful in assessing cardiac size and contour, chamber enlargement, pulmonary vasculature and infiltrates, and the presence of pleural effusions.
   b. Ultrasonographic examination is useful for identifying fluid-solid interfaces, and for characterizing masses as cystic, solid, or complex. It is also very helpful in evaluating the biliary tree, kidney size, and evidence of

Clinical Pearl

➤ Ultrasonography is helpful in evaluating the biliary tree, looking for ureteral obstruction, and evaluating vascular structures, but has limited utility in obese patients.

ureteral obstruction, and can be combined with Doppler flow to identify deep venous thrombosis. Ultrasonography is noninvasive and has no radiation risk, but cannot be used to penetrate through bone or air, and is less useful in obese patients.
   c. Computed tomography (CT) is helpful in possible intracranial bleeding, abdominal and/or pelvic masses, and pulmonary processes, and may help to delineate the lymph nodes and retroperitoneal disorders. CT exposes the patient to radiation and requires the patient to be immobilized during the procedure. Generally, CT requires administration of a radiocontrast dye, which can be nephrotoxic.

    d. Magnetic resonance imaging (MRI) identifies soft-tissue planes very well and provides the best imaging of the brain parenchyma. When used with gadolinium contrast (which is not nephrotoxic), MR angiography (MRA) is useful for delineating vascular structures. MRI does not use radiation, but the powerful magnetic field prohibits its use in patients with ferromagnetic metal in their bodies, for example, many prosthetic devices.

    e. Cardiac procedures

        i. Echocardiography: Uses ultrasonography to delineate the cardiac size, function, ejection fraction, and presence of valvular dysfunction.

        ii. Angiography: Radiopaque dye is injected into various vessels and radiographs or fluoroscopic images are used to determine the vascular occlusion, cardiac function, or valvular integrity.

        iii. Stress treadmill tests: Individuals at risk for coronary heart disease are monitored for blood pressure, heart rate, chest pain, and electrocardiogram (ECG) while increasing oxygen demands on the heart, such as running on a treadmill. Nuclear medicine imaging of the heart can be added to increase the sensitivity and specificity of the test. Individuals who cannot run on the treadmill (such as those with severe arthritis), may be given medications such as adenosine or dobutamine to "stress" the heart.

INTERPRETATION OF TEST RESULTS: USING PRETEST PROBABILITY AND LIKELIHOOD RATIO

Because no test is 100% accurate, it is essential when ordering them to have some knowledge of the test's characteristics, as well as how to apply the test results to an **individual patient's clinical situation**. Let us use the example of a patient with chest pain. The first diagnostic concern of most patients and physicians regarding chest pain is **angina pectoris**, that is, the pain of myocardial ischemia caused by coronary insufficiency. Distinguishing angina pectoris from other causes of chest pain relies upon two important factors: the clinical history, and an understanding of how to use objective testing. In making the diagnosis of angina pectoris, the clinician must establish whether the pain satisfies the **three criteria for typical anginal pain**: (1) retrosternal in location, (2) precipitated by exertion, and (3) relieved within minutes by rest or nitroglycerin. Then, the clinician considers other factors, such as patient age and other risk factors, to determine a **pretest probability** for angina pectoris.

After a pretest probability is estimated by applying some combination of statistical data, epidemiology of the disease, and clinical experience, the next decision is whether and how to use an objective test. **A test should only be ordered** if the results would change the posttest probability high enough or low enough in either direction that it will affect the decision-making process. For example, a 21-year-old woman with chest pain that is not exertional and not relieved by rest or nitroglycerin has a very low pretest probability of coronary artery disease, and any positive results on a cardiac stress test are very likely to be false positive. Any test result is unlikely to change her management; thus, the test should not be obtained. Similarly, a 69-year-old diabetic smoker with a recent coronary angioplasty who now has recurrent episodes of typical angina has a very high pretest probability that the pain is a result of myocardial ischemia. One could argue that a negative cardiac stress test is likely to be a falsely negative, and that the clinician should proceed directly to a coronary angiography to assess for a repeat angioplasty. **Diagnostic tests, therefore, are usually most useful for those patients in the midranges of pretest probabilities in whom a positive or negative test will move the clinician past some decision threshold.**

In the case of diagnosing a patient with atherosclerotic coronary artery disease (CAD), one test that is frequently used is the exercise treadmill test. Patients are monitored on an electrocardiogram, while they perform graded exercise on a treadmill. A positive test is the development of ST-segment depression during the test; the greater the degree of ST depression, the more useful the test becomes in raising the posttest probability of CAD. In the example illustrated by Figure I-1, if a patient has a pretest probability of CAD of 50%, then the test result of 2mm of ST-segment depression raises the post-test probability to 90%.

If one knows the sensitivity and specificity of the test used, one can calculate the **likelihood ratio** of the positive test as **sensitivity/(1– specificity)**. Posttest probability is calculated by multiplying the positive likelihood ratio by the pretest probability, or plot the probabilities using a nomogram (see Figure I–1).

Thus, knowing something about the characteristics of the test you are employing, and how to apply them to the patient at hand is essential in reaching a correct diagnosis and avoid falling into the common trap of "positive test = disease" and "negative test = no disease." Stated another way, **tests do not make diagnoses; doctors do, considering test results quantitatively in the context of their clinical assessment.**

Clinical Pearl

> ➤ If test result is positive,
> ➤ Posttest Probability = Pretest Probability × Likelihood Ratio
> ➤ Likelihood Ratio = Sensitivity/(1 – Specificity)

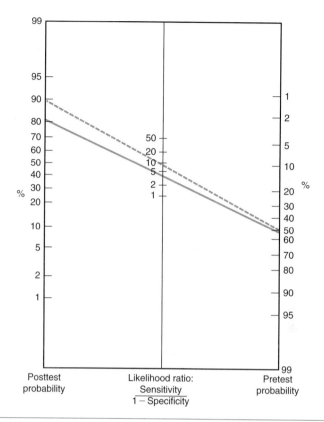

Figure I–1. Nomogram illustrating the relationship between pretest probability, posttest probability, and likelihood ratio. *Reproduced with permission from Braunwald E, Fauci AS, Kasper KL, et al. Harrison's Principles of Internal Medicine. 16th ed. New York, NY: McGraw-Hill; 2005:10.*

Part 2. Approach to Clinical Problem Solving

There are typically four distinct steps to the systematic solving of clinical problems:

1. Making the diagnosis
2. Assessing the severity of the disease (stage)
3. Rendering a treatment based on the stage of the disease
4. Following the patient's response to the treatment

MAKING THE DIAGNOSIS

There are two ways to make a diagnosis. Experienced clinicians often make a diagnosis very quickly using **pattern recognition**, that is, the features of the patient's illness match a scenario the physician has seen before. If it does not fit a readily recognized pattern, then one has to undertake several steps in diagnostic reasoning:

1. The first step is to **gather information with a differential diagnosis in mind**. The clinician should start considering diagnostic possibilities with initial contact with the patient which are continually refined as information is gathered. Historical questions and physical examination tests and findings are all pursued tailored to the potential diagnoses one is considering. This is the principle that "you find what you are looking for." When one is trying to perform a thorough head-to-toe examination, for instance, without looking for anything in particular, one is much more likely to miss findings.

2. The next step is to try to move from subjective complaints or nonspecific symptoms to focus on objective abnormalities in an effort to **conceptualize the patient's objective problem with the greatest specificity one can achieve.** For example, a patient may come to the physician complaining of pedal edema, a relatively common and nonspecific finding. Laboratory testing may reveal that the patient has renal failure, a more specific cause of the many causes of edema. Examination of the urine may then reveal red blood cell casts, indicating glomerulonephritis, which is even more specific as the cause of the renal failure. The patient's problem, then, described with the greatest degree of specificity, is glomerulonephritis. The clinician's task at this point is to consider the differential diagnosis of glomerulonephritis rather than that of pedal edema.

3. The last step is to **look for discriminating features** of the patient's illness. This means the features of the illness, which by their presence or their absence narrow the differential diagnosis. This is often difficult for junior learners because it requires a well-developed knowledge base of the typical features of disease, so the diagnostician can judge how much weight to assign to the various clinical clues present. For example, in the diagnosis of a patient with a fever and productive cough, the finding by chest x-ray of bilateral apical infiltrates with cavitation is highly discriminatory. There are few illnesses besides tuberculosis that are likely to produce that radiographic pattern. A negatively predictive example is a patient with exudative pharyngitis who also has rhinorrhea and cough. The presence of these features makes the diagnosis of streptococcal infection unlikely as the cause of the pharyngitis. Once the differential diagnosis has been constructed, the clinician uses the presence of discriminating features, knowledge of patient risk factors, and the epidemiology of diseases to decide which potential diagnoses are most likely.

> **Clinical Pearl**

> ➤ There are three steps in diagnostic reasoning:
>   1. Gathering information with a differential diagnosis in mind
>   2. Identifying the objective abnormalities with the greatest specificity
>   3. Looking for discriminating features to narrow the differential diagnosis

Once the most specific problem has been identified, and a differential diagnosis of that problem is considered using discriminating features to order the possibilities, the next step is to consider using diagnostic testing, such as laboratory, radiologic, or pathologic data, to confirm the diagnosis. Quantitative reasoning in the use and interpretation of tests were discussed in Part 1. Clinically, the timing and effort with which one pursues a definitive diagnosis using objective data depends on several factors: the potential gravity of the diagnosis in question, the clinical state of the patient, the potential risks of diagnostic testing, and the potential benefits or harms of empiric treatment. For example, if a young man is admitted to the hospital with bilateral pulmonary nodules on chest X-ray, there are many possibilities including metastatic malignancy, and aggressive pursuit of a diagnosis is necessary, perhaps including a thoracotomy with an open-lung biopsy. The same radiographic findings in an elderly bed-bound woman with advanced Alzheimer dementia who would not be a good candidate for chemotherapy might be best left alone without any diagnostic testing. Decisions like this are difficult, require solid medical knowledge, as well as a thorough understanding of one's patient and the patient's background and inclinations, and constitute the art of medicine.

ASSESSING THE SEVERITY OF THE DISEASE

After ascertaining the diagnosis, the next step is to characterize the severity of the disease process; in other words, it is describing "how bad" a disease is. There is usually prognostic or treatment significance based on the stage. With malignancy, this is done formally by cancer staging. Most cancers are categorized from stage I (localized) to stage IV (widely metastatic). Some diseases, such as congestive heart failure, may be designated as mild, moderate, or severe based on the patient's functional status, that is, their ability to exercise before becoming dyspneic. With some infections, such as syphilis, the staging depends on the duration and extent of the infection, and follows along the natural history of the infection (ie, primary syphilis, secondary, latent period, and tertiary/neurosyphilis).

TREATING BASED ON STAGE

Many illnesses are stratified according to severity because prognosis and treatment often vary based on the severity. If neither the prognosis nor the treatment was affected by the stage of the disease process, there would not be a reason to subcategorize as mild or severe. As an example, a man with mild chronic obstructive pulmonary disease (COPD) may be treated with inhaled bronchodilators as needed and advice for smoking cessation. However, an individual with severe COPD may need round-the-clock oxygen supplementation, scheduled bronchodilators, and possibly oral corticosteroid therapy.

The treatment should be tailored to the extent or "stage" of the disease. In making decisions regarding treatment, it is also essential that the clinician identify the therapeutic objectives. When patients seek medical attention, it is generally because they are bothered by a symptom and want it to go away. When physicians institute therapy, they often have several other goals besides symptom relief, such as prevention of short- or long-term complications or a reduction in mortality. For example, patients with congestive heart failure are bothered by the symptoms of edema and dyspnea. Salt restriction, loop diuretics, and bed rest are effective at reducing these symptoms. However, heart failure is a progressive disease with a high mortality, so other treatments such as angiotensin-converting enzyme (ACE) inhibitors and some beta-blockers are also used to reduce mortality in this condition. It is essential that the clinician know what the therapeutic objective is, so that one can monitor and guide therapy.

> ### Clinical Pearl
>
> ➤ The clinician needs to identify the objectives of therapy: symptom relief, prevention of complications, or reduction in mortality.

FOLLOWING THE RESPONSE TO TREATMENT

The final step in the approach to disease is to follow the patient's response to the therapy. The "measure" of response should be recorded and monitored. Some responses are clinical, such as the patient's abdominal pain, or temperature, or pulmonary examination. Obviously, the student must work on being more skilled in eliciting the data in an unbiased and standardized manner. Other responses may be followed by imaging tests, such as CT scan of a retroperitoneal node size in a patient receiving chemotherapy, or a tumor marker such as the prostate-specific antigen (PSA) level in a man receiving chemotherapy for prostatic cancer. For syphilis, it may be the nonspecific treponemal antibody test rapid plasma reagent (RPR) titer over time. The student must be prepared to know what to do if the measured marker does not respond according to what is expected. Is the next step to retreat, or to repeat the metastatic workup, or to follow up with another more specific test?

Part 3. Approach to Reading

The clinical problem–oriented approach to reading is different from the classic "systematic" research of a disease. Patients rarely present with a clear diagnosis; hence, the student must become skilled in applying the textbook information to the clinical setting. Furthermore, one retains more information when one reads with a purpose. In other words, the student should read with the goal of answering specific questions. There are several fundamental questions that facilitate **clinical thinking**. These questions are:

1. What is the most likely diagnosis?
2. What should be your next step?
3. What is the most likely mechanism for this process?
4. What are the risk factors for this condition?
5. What are the complications associated with the disease process?
6. What is the best therapy?
7. How would you confirm the diagnosis?

Clinical Pearl

> ➤ Reading with the purpose of answering the seven fundamental clinical questions improves retention of information and facilitates the application of "book knowledge" to "clinical knowledge."

WHAT IS THE MOST LIKELY DIAGNOSIS?

The method of establishing the diagnosis was discussed in the previous section. One way of attacking this problem is to develop standard "approaches" to common clinical problems. It is helpful to understand the most common causes of various presentations, such as "the most common causes of pancreatitis are gallstones and alcohol." (See the **Clinical Pearls** at end of each case.)

The clinical scenario would entail something such as:

A 28-year-old pregnant woman complains of severe epigastric pain radiating the back, nausea and vomiting, and an elevated serum amylase level. What is the most likely diagnosis?

With no other information to go on, the student would note that this woman has a clinical diagnosis of pancreatitis. Using the "most common cause" information, the student would make an educated guess that the patient has gallstones, because being female and pregnant are risk factors. If, instead, cholelithiasis is removed from the equation of this scenario, a phrase may be added such as:

"The ultrasonogram of the gallbladder shows no stones."

> ## Clinical Pearl

> ➤ The two most common causes of pancreatitis are gallstones and alcohol abuse.

Now, the student would use the phrase "patients without gallstones who have pancreatitis most likely abuse alcohol." Aside from these two causes, there are many other etiologies of pancreatitis.

WHAT SHOULD BE YOUR NEXT STEP?

This question is difficult because the next step may be more diagnostic information, or staging, or therapy. It may be more challenging than "the most likely diagnosis," because there may be insufficient information to make a diagnosis and the next step may be to pursue more diagnostic information. Another possibility is that there is enough information for a probable diagnosis, and the next step is to stage the disease. Finally, the most appropriate action may be to treat. Hence, from clinical data, a judgment needs to be rendered regarding how far along one is on the road of:

Make a Dx → Stage the disease → Treat based on stage → Follow response

Frequently, the student is "taught" to regurgitate the same information that someone has written about a particular disease, but is not skilled at giving the next step. This talent is learned optimally at the bedside, in a supportive environment, with freedom to make educated guesses, and with constructive feedback. A sample scenario may describe a student's thought process as follows.

1. Make the diagnosis: "Based on the information I have, I believe that Mr. Smith has stable angina *because* he has retrosternal chest pain when he walks three blocks, but it is relieved within minutes by rest and with sublingual nitroglycerin."
2. Stage the disease: "I don't believe that this is severe disease because he does not have pain lasting for more than 5 minutes, angina at rest, or congestive heart failure."
3. Treat based on stage: "Therefore, my next step is to treat with aspirin, beta-blockers, and sublingual nitroglycerin as needed, as well as lifestyle changes."
4. Follow response: "I want to follow the treatment by assessing his pain (I will ask him about the degree of exercise he is able to perform without chest pain), performing a cardiac stress test, and reassessing him after the test is done."

In a similar patient, when the clinical presentation is unclear or more severe, perhaps the best "next step" may be diagnostic in nature such as thallium stress test, or even coronary angiography. The **next step** depends upon the **clinical state of the patient** (if unstable, the next step is therapeutic), the potential **severity** of the disease (the next step may be staging), or the **uncertainty of the diagnosis** (the next step is diagnostic).

Usually, the vague question, "What is your next step?" is the most difficult question, because the answer may be diagnostic, staging, or therapeutic.

WHAT IS THE LIKELY MECHANISM FOR THIS PROCESS?

This question goes further than making the diagnosis, but also requires the student to understand the underlying mechanism for the process. For example, a clinical scenario may describe an "18-year-old woman who presents with several months of severe epistaxis, heavy menses, petechiae, and a normal CBC except for a platelet count of $15,000/mm^3$." Answers that a student may consider to explain this condition include immune-mediated platelet destruction, drug-induced thrombocytopenia, bone marrow suppression, and platelet sequestration as a result of hypersplenism.

The student is advised to learn the mechanisms for each disease process, and not merely memorize a constellation of symptoms. In other words, rather than solely committing to memory the classic presentation of idiopathic thrombocytopenic purpura (ITP) (isolated thrombocytopenia without lymphadenopathy or offending drugs), the student should understand that ITP is an autoimmune process whereby the body produces IgG antibodies against the platelets. The platelets-antibody complexes are then taken from the circulation in the spleen. Because the disease process is specific for platelets, the other two cell lines (erythrocytes and leukocytes) are normal. Also, because the thrombocytopenia is caused by excessive platelet peripheral destruction, the bone marrow will show increased megakaryocytes (platelet precursors). Hence, treatment for ITP includes oral corticosteroid agents to decrease the immune process of antiplatelet IgG production, and, if refractory, then splenectomy.

WHAT ARE THE RISK FACTORS FOR THIS PROCESS?

Understanding the risk factors helps the practitioner to establish a diagnosis and to determine how to interpret tests. For example, understanding the risk factor analysis may help to manage a 45-year-old obese woman with sudden onset of dyspnea and pleuritic chest pain following an orthopedic surgery for a femur fracture. This patient has numerous risk factors for deep venous thrombosis and pulmonary embolism. The physician may want to pursue angiography

---

Clinical Pearl

➤ When the pretest probability of a disease is high based on risk factors, even with a negative initial test, more definitive testing may be indicated.

even if the ventilation/perfusion scan result is low probability. Thus, the number of risk factors helps to categorize the likelihood of a disease process.

WHAT ARE THE COMPLICATIONS TO THIS PROCESS?

A clinician must understand the complications of a disease so that one may monitor the patient. Sometimes the student has to make the diagnosis from clinical clues and then apply his/her knowledge of the sequelae of the pathological process. For example, the student should know that chronic hypertension may affect various end organs, such as the brain (encephalopathy or stroke), the eyes (vascular changes), the kidneys, and the heart. Understanding the types of consequences also helps the clinician to be aware of the dangers to a patient. The clinician is acutely aware of the need to monitor for the end-organ involvement and undertakes the appropriate intervention when involvement is present.

WHAT IS THE BEST THERAPY?

To answer this question, the clinician needs to reach the correct diagnosis, assess the severity of the condition, and weigh the situation to reach the appropriate intervention. For the student, knowing exact dosages is not as important as understanding the best medication, the route of delivery, mechanism of action, and possible complications. It is important for the student to be able to verbalize the diagnosis and the rationale for the therapy. A common error is for the student to "jump to a treatment," like a random guess, and therefore being given "right or wrong" feedback. In fact, the student's guess may be correct, but for the wrong reason; conversely, the answer may be a very reasonable one, with only one small error in thinking. Instead, the student should verbalize the steps so that feedback may be given at every reasoning point.

For example, if the question is, "What is the best therapy for a 25-year-old man who complains of a nontender penile ulcer?" the incorrect manner of response is for the student to blurt out "azithromycin." Rather, the student should reason it out in a way similar to this: "The most common cause of a nontender infectious ulcer of the penis is syphilis. Nontender adenopathy is usually associated. Therefore, the best treatment for this man with probable syphilis is intramuscular penicillin (but I would want to confirm the diagnosis). His partner also needs treatment."

Clinical Pearl

➤ Therapy should be logical based on the severity of disease. Antibiotic therapy should be tailored for specific organisms.

HOW WOULD YOU CONFIRM THE DIAGNOSIS?

In the scenario above, the man with a nontender penile ulcer is likely to have syphilis. Confirmation may be achieved by serology (rapid plasma reagent [RPR] or Venereal Disease Research Laboratory [VDRL] test); however, there is a significant possibility that patients with primary syphilis may not have developed antibody response yet, and have negative serology. Thus, confirmation of the diagnosis is attained with dark-field microscopy. Knowing the limitations of diagnostic tests and the manifestations of disease aids in this area.

Summary

1. There is no replacement for a careful history and physical examination.
2. There are four steps to the clinical approach to the patient: making the diagnosis, assessing severity, treating based on severity, and following response.
3. Assessment of pretest probability and knowledge of test characteristics are essential in the application of test results to the clinical situation.
4. There are seven questions that help to bridge the gap between the textbook and the clinical arena.

REFERENCES

Bordages G. Elaborated knowledge: a key to successful diagnostic thinking. *Acad Med.* 1994;69(11):883-885.

Bordages G. Why did I miss the diagnosis? Some cognitive explanations and educational implications. *Acad Med.* 1999;74(10):138-143.

Gross R. *Making Medical Decisions.* Philadelphia, PA: American College of Physicians; 1999.

Mark DB. Decision-making in clinical medicine. In: Fauci AS, Braunwald E, Kasper KL, et al., eds. *Harrison's Principles of Internal Medicine.* 17th ed. New York, NY: McGraw-Hill; 2008:16-23.

Clinical Cases

Case 1

A 56-year-old man comes to the emergency room complaining of chest discomfort. He describes the discomfort as a severe, retrosternal pressure sensation that had awakened him from sleep 3 hours earlier. He previously had been well but has a medical history of hypercholesterolemia and a 40-pack-per-year history of smoking. On examination, he appears uncomfortable and diaphoretic, with a heart rate of 116 bpm, blood pressure 166/102 mm Hg, respiratory rate 22 breaths per minute, and oxygen saturation of 96% on room air. Jugular venous pressure appears normal. Auscultation of the chest reveals clear lung fields, a regular rhythm with an S_4 gallop, and no murmurs or rubs. A chest radiograph shows clear lungs and a normal cardiac silhouette. The ECG is shown in Figure 1–1.

➤ What is the most likely diagnosis?

➤ What is the next step in therapy?

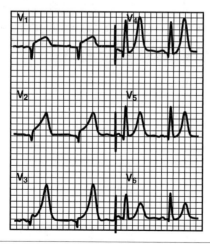

Figure 1–1. Electrocardiogram. *Reproduced, with permission, from Braunwald E, Fauci AS, Kasper DL, et al, eds.* Harrison's Principles of Internal Medicine. *16th ed. New York, NY: McGraw-Hill; 2005:1316.*

ANSWERS TO CASE 1:
Myocardial Infarction, Acute

Summary: This is a 56-year-old man with risk factors for coronary atherosclerosis (smoking and hypercholesterolemia) who has chest pain typical of cardiac ischemia, that is, retrosternal pressure sensation. Cardiac examination reveals an S_4 gallop, which may be seen with myocardial ischemia because of relative noncompliance of the ischemic heart, as well as hypertension, tachycardia, and diaphoresis, which all may represent sympathetic activation. The duration of the pain and the electrocardiographic (ECG) findings suggest an acute myocardial infarction (MI).

> **Most likely diagnosis:** Acute ST-segment elevation MI.

> **Next step in therapy:** Administer aspirin and a beta-blocker, and assess whether he is a candidate for rapid reperfusion of the myocardium, that is, treatment with thrombolytics or percutaneous coronary intervention.

ANALYSIS

Objectives

1. Know the diagnostic criteria for acute MI.
2. Know which patients should receive thrombolytics or undergo percutaneous coronary intervention, which may reduce mortality.
3. Be familiar with the complications of MI and their treatment options.
4. Understand post-MI risk stratification and secondary prevention strategies.

Considerations

The three most important issues for this patient are (1) the **suspicion of acute MI** based on the clinical and ECG findings, (2) deciding whether the patient has indications or contraindications for **thrombolytics or primary percutaneous coronary intervention**, and (3) **excluding other diagnoses** that might mimic acute MI but would not benefit or which might be worsened by anticoagulation or thrombolysis (eg, acute pericarditis, aortic dissection).

APPROACH TO
Suspected MI

DEFINITIONS

ACUTE CORONARY SYNDROME: Spectrum of acute cardiac ischemia ranging from **unstable angina** (ischemic pain at rest or at lower threshold of exertion or new onset of chest pain) to **acute MI** (death of cardiac tissue), usually precipitated by thrombus formation in a coronary artery with an atherosclerotic plaque.

ACUTE MYOCARDIAL INFARCTION: Death of myocardial tissue because of inadequate blood flow.

NON–ST-SEGMENT ELEVATION MYOCARDIAL INFARCTION (NSTEMI): MI, but without ST-segment elevation as defined below. May have other ECG changes, such as ST-segment depression or T-wave inversion. Previously referred to as non–Q wave or subendocardial MI.

PCI: Percutaneous coronary intervention (angioplasty and/or stenting.)

ST-SEGMENT ELEVATION MYOCARDIAL INFARCTION (STEMI): MI as defined as in acute myocardial infarction, with ST-segment elevation more than 0.1 mV in two or more contiguous leads. Previously referred to as Q-wave or transmural MI.

THROMBOLYTICS: Drugs such as tissue plasminogen activator (tPA), streptokinase, and reteplase (rPA), which act to lyse fibrin thrombi in order to restore patency of the coronary artery.

CLINICAL APPROACH

Pathophysiology

Acute coronary syndromes, which exist on a continuum ranging from **unstable angina** pectoris to **NSTEMI** to **STEMI**, usually are caused by **in situ thrombosis** at the site of a ruptured atherosclerotic plaque in a coronary artery. Occasionally, they are caused by embolic occlusion, coronary vasospasm, vasculitis, aortic root or coronary artery dissection, or cocaine use (which promotes both vasospasm and thrombosis). The resultant clinical syndrome is related to both the degree of atherosclerotic stenosis in the artery and to the duration and extent of sudden thrombotic occlusion of the artery. If the occlusion is incomplete or if the thrombus undergoes spontaneous lysis, unstable angina occurs. If the occlusion is complete and remains for more than 30 minutes, infarction occurs. In contrast, the mechanism of chronic stable angina usually is a flow-limiting stenosis caused by atherosclerotic plaque that causes ischemia during exercise without acute thrombosis (Table 1–1).

DIAGNOSTIC CRITERIA FOR ACUTE MI

History

Chest pain is the cardinal feature of MI, even though it is not universally present. It is of the same character as angina pectoris—described as heavy, squeezing, or crushing—and is localized to the retrosternal area or epigastrium, sometimes with radiation to the arm, lower jaw, or neck. **In contrast to stable angina, however, it persists for more than 30 minutes and is not relieved by rest.**

Table 1–1 CLINICAL MANIFESTATIONS OF CORONARY ARTERY DISEASE

VESSEL ARCHITECTURE	BLOOD FLOW	CLINICAL MANIFESTATION
Early plaque	Unobstructed	Asymptomatic
Critical coronary artery stenosis >70%	Blood flow limited during exertion	Stable angina
Unstable plaque rupture	Platelet thrombus begins to form and spasm limits blood flow at rest	Unstable angina
Unstable platelet thrombus on ruptured plaque	Transient or incomplete vessel occlusion (lysis occurs)	Non–ST-segment elevation (subendocardial) myocardial infarction
Platelet thrombus on ruptured plaque	Complete vessel occlusion (no lysis)	ST-segment elevation (transmural) myocardial infarction

The pain often is accompanied by sweating, nausea, vomiting, and/or the sense of impending doom. In a patient older than 70 years or who is diabetic, an acute MI may be painless or associated with only vague discomfort, but it may be heralded by the sudden onset of dyspnea, pulmonary edema, or ventricular arrhythmias.

Physical Findings

There are **no specific physical findings** in a patient with an acute MI. Many patients are anxious and diaphoretic. Cardiac auscultation may reveal an S_4 gallop, reflecting myocardial noncompliance because of ischemia; an S_3 gallop, representing severe systolic dysfunction; or a new apical systolic murmur of mitral regurgitation caused by ischemic papillary muscle dysfunction.

Electrocardiogram

The ECG often is critical in diagnosing acute MI and guiding therapy. A series of ECG changes reflect the evolution of the infarction (Figure 1–2).

1. The earliest changes are tall, positive, **hyperacute T waves** in the ischemic vascular territory.
2. This is followed by **elevation of the ST segments** (myocardial "injury pattern").
3. Over hours to days, **T-wave inversion** frequently develops.
4. Finally, diminished R-wave amplitude or **Q waves** occur, representing significant myocardial necrosis and replacement by scar tissue, and they are what one seeks to prevent in treating the acute MI (Figure 1–3).

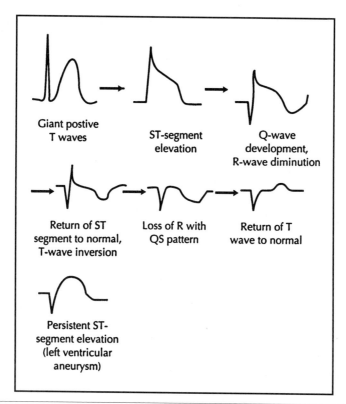

Figure 1–2. Temporal evolution of ECG changes in acute myocardial infarction. Note tall hyperacute T waves and loss of R-wave amplitude, followed by ST-segment elevation, T-wave inversion, and development of Q waves. Persistent ST-segment elevation suggests left ventricular aneurysm. *Reproduced from Alpert JS.* Cardiology for the Primary Care Physician. *2nd ed. Current Medicine/ Current Science; 1998:219-229 with kind permission from Current Medicine Group LLC.*

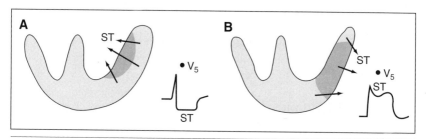

Figure 1–3. Subendocardial infarction produces an inward ST vector, resulting in ST-segment depression. Transmural infarction produces an outward ST vector, resulting in ST-segment elevation in the overlying leads. *Reproduced, with permission, from Braunwald E, Fauci AS, Kasper DL, et al, eds.* Harrison's Principles of Internal Medicine. *16th ed. New York, NY: McGraw-Hill; 2005:1316.*

Sometimes when acute ischemia is limited to the **subendocardium, ST-segment depression,** rather than ST-segment elevation, develops. **ST-segment elevation is typical of acute transmural ischemia,** that is, a greater degree of myocardial involvement than in NSTEMI.

From the ECG we can localize the ischemia related to a vascular territory supplied by one of the three major coronary arteries. **STEMI** is defined as ST-segment elevation more than 0.1 mV in two or more contiguous leads (ie, in the same vascular territory) and/or a new left bundle branch block (LBBB) (which obscures usual ST-segment analysis). As a general rule, **leads II, III, aVF** correspond to the **inferior** surface of the heart supplied by the **right coronary artery** (RCA), leads V_2 **to** V_4 correspond to the **anterior** surface supplied by the **left anterior descending coronary artery** (LAD), and **leads I, aVL, V_5 and V_6** correspond to the **lateral** surface, supplied by the **left circumflex coronary artery** (LCX).

Cardiac Enzymes

Certain proteins, referred to as cardiac enzymes, are released into blood from necrotic heart muscle after an acute MI. Creatine phosphokinase (CK) level rises within 4 to 8 hours and returns to normal by 48 to 72 hours. Creatine phosphokinase is found in skeletal muscle and other tissues, but the creatine kinase myocardial band (CK-MB) isoenzyme is not found in significant amounts outside of heart muscle, so elevation of this fraction is more specific for myocardial injury. Cardiac-specific troponin I (cTnI) and cardiac-specific troponin T (cTnT) are more specific to heart muscle and are the preferred markers of myocardial injury. These enzyme levels rise approximately 6 hours after infarct. Cardiac-specific troponin I levels may remain elevated for 7 to 10 days and cTnT levels for 10 to 14 days. They are very sensitive indicators of myocardial injury, and their levels may be elevated with even small amounts of myocardial necrosis. Generally, two sets of normal troponin levels 4 to 6 hours apart exclude MI.

The diagnosis of **acute MI** is made by finding **at least two of the following three features:** typical **chest pain persisting for more than 30 minutes,** typical **ECG findings,** and **elevated cardiac enzyme levels.** Because of the urgency in initiating treatment, diagnosis often rests upon the clinical history and the ECG findings, while determination of cardiac enzyme levels is pending. During the initial evaluation, one must consider and exclude other diagnoses that typically present with chest pain but would be worsened by the anticoagulation or thrombolysis usually used to treat acute MI. **Aortic dissection** often presents with **unequal pulses or blood pressures in the arms,** a **new murmur of aortic insufficiency,** or a **widened mediastinum** on chest X-ray film. Acute pericarditis often presents with chest pain and a pericardial friction rub, but the ECG findings show **diffuse ST-segment elevation** rather than those limited to a vascular territory.

TREATMENT OF ACUTE MI

Once an acute MI has been diagnosed based on history, ECG, or cardiac enzyme levels, several therapies are initiated. Because the process is caused by acute thrombosis, antiplatelet agents such as **aspirin** and anticoagulation with **heparin** are used. To limit infarct size, **beta-blockers** are used to decrease myocardial oxygen demand, and **nitrates** are given to increase coronary blood flow. All of these therapies appear to reduce mortality in patients with acute MI. In addition, morphine may be given to reduce pain and the consequent tachycardia, and patients are placed on supplemental oxygen (Figure 1–4).

Because prompt restoration of myocardial perfusion reduces mortality in STEMI, a decision should be made as to whether the patient can either receive thrombolytics or undergo primary percutaneous coronary intervention (PCI). **Individuals with ST-segment elevation MI benefit from thrombolytics, with a lower mortality, greater preservation of myocardial function, and fewer complications**; patients without ST-segment elevation do not receive the same mortality benefit. Because myocardium can be salvaged only before it is irreversibly injured ("time is muscle"), patients **benefit maximally** when the drug is given early, for example, **within 1 to 3 hours after the onset of chest pain**, and the relative benefits decline with time. Because systemic coagulopathy may develop, the **major risk of thrombolytics is bleeding**, which can be potentially disastrous, for example, intracranial hemorrhage. The risk of hemorrhage is relatively constant, so the risk begins to outweigh the benefit by 12 hours, at which time most infarctions are completed, that is, the at-risk myocardium is dead.

Thrombolytic therapy is indicated if all of the following criteria are met:

1. Clinical complaints are consistent with ischemic type chest pain.
2. ST-segment elevation more than 1 mm in at least two anatomically contiguous leads.
3. There are no contraindications to thrombolytic therapy.
4. Patient is younger than 75 years (greater risk of hemorrhage if >75).

Patients with STEMI should not receive thrombolytics if they have any of the absolute contraindications, such as recent major surgery or aortic dissection (Table 1–2).

Percutaneous coronary intervention is effective in restoring perfusion in patients with acute STEMI and has been shown in multiple trials to provide a greater survival benefit than thrombolysis and to have a lower risk for serious bleeding when performed by experienced operators in dedicated medical centers. If patients with an acute STEMI present within 2 to 3 hours of symptom onset and receive PCI ideally within 90 minutes, then PCI is the recommended reperfusion therapy. PCI also can be used in patients with a contraindication to thrombolytic therapy or who are hypotensive or in cardiogenic shock, for whom thrombolytics offer no survival benefit. PCI is accomplished by cardiac catheterization, in which a guidewire is inserted into the

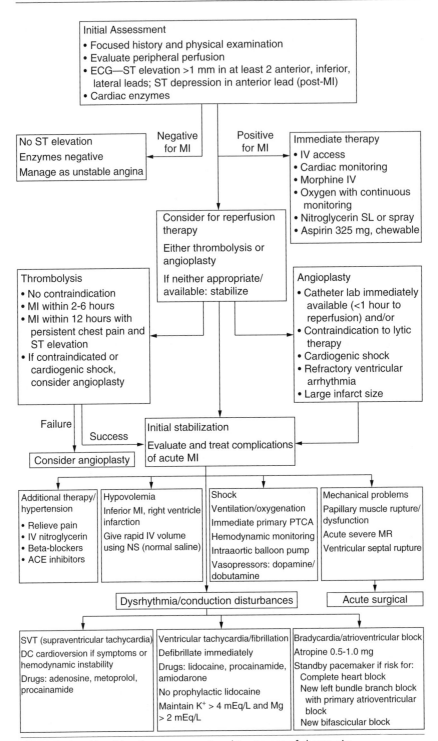

Figure 1–4. Algorithm for assessment and treatment of chest pain.

Table 1–2 CONTRAINDICATIONS TO THROMBOLYTIC THERAPY

Absolute contraindications
- Major surgery/trauma within past 2 weeks
- Aortic dissection
- Active internal bleeding (excluding menses)
- Pericarditis
- History of cerebral tumor/hemorrhage/arteriovenous malformation
- Prolonged, traumatic cardiopulmonary resuscitation
- Bleeding diathesis
- Allergy to agent/prior reaction
- Cerebrovascular accident known to be hemorrhage within past 12 months
- Pregnancy
- History of uncontrolled hypertension
- Recent hepatic/renal biopsy

Relative contraindications
- Blood pressure >180/110 mm Hg on >2 readings
- Bacterial endocarditis
- Diabetic retinopathy with recent bleed
- Severe renal/liver disease
- Chronic warfarin therapy
- Stroke/transient ischemic attack within past 12 months

occluded coronary artery and a small balloon threaded over the guidewire and inflated in an attempt to open the blockage and restore blood flow. Sometimes intraluminal expandable stents are deployed which may improve vessel patency. Use of primary PCI may be limited by the availability of the facilities and personnel required to perform the procedure in a timely fashion.

COMPLICATIONS OF ACUTE MI

Mortality in acute MI usually is a result of either myocardial pump failure and resultant cardiogenic shock or of ventricular arrhythmias.

Life-threatening **ventricular arrhythmias,** such as **ventricular tachycardia (VT)** and **ventricular fibrillation (VF),** are common, especially in the first 24 hours. Historically, the majority of deaths from acute MI occurred in the first hour and were caused by VT/VF. This has diminished in recent years with earlier and more aggressive treatment of ischemia and arrhythmias. Premature ventricular contractions (PVCs) are very common but generally they are not treated with antiarrhythmic agents unless they occur very frequently, are sustained, or induce hemodynamic compromise. Sustained VT (>30 seconds) and VF are life threatening because they prevent coordinated ventricular contraction and thus often cause pulselessness and cardiovascular collapse. They are treated with **direct current (DC) cardioversion**, followed by infusion of intravenous antiarrhythmics such as **amiodarone**. Electrolyte deficiency, such as hypokalemia or hypomagnesemia, which can potentiate ventricular arrhythmias, should be corrected. One benign ventricular arrhythmia that is generally not suppressed by antiarrhythmics is the **accelerated idioventricular rhythm**. This is a wide-complex escape rhythm between 60 and 110 bpm that frequently accompanies reperfusion of the myocardium but causes no hemodynamic compromise.

Supraventricular or atrial tachyarrhythmias are much less common after acute MI, but they can worsen ischemia and cause infarct extension as a consequence of the rate-related increase in myocardial oxygen demand. When they cause hemodynamic instability, they also are treated with immediate DC cardioversion. Other frequent rhythm disturbances are bradyarrhythmias. **Sinus bradycardia** is frequently seen in inferior MI because the right coronary artery supplies the sinoatrial node, but the condition generally requires no treatment unless it causes hypotension. If the rate is slow enough to cause cardiac output and blood pressure to fall, intravenous **atropine** usually is administered.

Bradyarrhythmias can be caused by atrioventricular (AV) conduction disturbances. **First-degree AV block** (PR-interval prolongation) and **Mobitz I second-degree AV block** (gradual prolongation of the PR interval before a nonconducted P wave) often are caused by AV nodal dysfunction, for example, nodal ischemia caused by inferior MI. Patients who are symptomatic can be treated with **atropine**.

AV conduction disturbances can be caused by dysfunction below the AV node, within the bundles of His, and typically produce a widened QRS complex. Examples include **Mobitz II second-degree AV block** (nonconducted P waves not preceded by PR prolongation) and **third-degree AV block** (complete AV dissociation with no P-wave conduction). Third-degree AV block also can be caused by AV nodal dysfunction. These arrhythmias are described more fully in Case 15. Conduction disturbances caused by involvement of the bundles of His include **LBBB** or **right bundle branch block (RBBB) with left anterior hemiblock**. All of these conduction disturbances have a worse prognosis than does AV nodal dysfunction because they are generally seen with anterior infarction in which a significant amount of myocardium is damaged. When symptomatic bradycardias such as third-degree AV block develop, they are best treated with external pacing or placement of a **temporary transvenous pacemaker**.

Cardiac Pump Failure and Cardiogenic Shock

Cardiogenic shock in acute MI usually is the most severe form of left ventricular (LV) pump failure. Ischemic reduction in ventricular diastolic compliance may lead to transient pulmonary congestion, associated with elevated left-sided filling pressures. Extensive myocardial necrosis and less contracting heart muscle may cause systolic failure and reduced cardiac output. Patients with hypotension frequently are evaluated by pulmonary artery (Swan-Ganz) catheterization to assess hemodynamic parameters. **Cardiogenic shock** is diagnosed when the patient has **hypotension** with systolic arterial pressure less than 80 mm Hg, **markedly reduced cardiac index** less than **1.8 L/min/m²**, and **elevated LV filling pressure** (measured indirectly with a pulmonary capillary wedge pressure >18 mm Hg). Clinically, such patients appear hypotensive, with cold extremities because of peripheral vasoconstriction, pulmonary edema, and elevated jugular venous pressure, reflecting high left- and right-sided filling pressures. Supportive treatment includes hemodynamic monitoring, adequate ventilation and oxygenation, and blood pressure support with vasopressors such as dobutamine and dopamine. These patients also may require mechanical assistance to augment blood pressure while providing afterload reduction, using intraaortic balloon counterpulsation. Cardiogenic shock may require urgent revascularization with primary percutaneous transluminal coronary angioplasty (PTCA) or coronary artery bypass surgery.

Hypotension may also be seen in patients with **right ventricular (RV) infarction**, which is a complication of right coronary artery occlusion and inferior infarction. In this case, LV function is not impaired, but LV filling is dramatically reduced because of the right-sided ventricular failure (the left heart can only pump out what it receives from the right heart). These patients can be recognized clinically as hypotensive, with markedly elevated jugular venous pressure but clear lung fields and no pulmonary edema seen radiographically (in contrast to the pulmonary edema seen in patients with hypotension to LV failure), and the diagnosis confirmed by observation of ST-segment elevation in a right-sided ECG. In this setting, RV function is impaired and highly dependent on adequate preload, so treatment requires support consisting of **volume replacement with saline** or colloid solution. Administration of diuretics or nitrates that might lower the preload can be disastrous in these patients by causing complete cardiovascular collapse.

A number of mechanical problems can complicate acute MI, usually within the first week. The most common is **papillary muscle dysfunction** caused by LV ischemia or infarction, leading to mitral regurgitation that may be hemodynamically significant. This is in contrast with **papillary muscle rupture**, which produces a flail mitral leaflet and acute mitral regurgitation with development of heart failure and cardiogenic shock. Development of acute heart failure and shock in association with a new holosystolic murmur also may signify **ventricular septal rupture**. Doppler echocardiography can be used to distinguish among these conditions. In all of them, stabilization of cardiogenic shock is accomplished using afterload reduction with intravenous nitroglycerin or nitroprusside and sometimes with aortic balloon counterpulsation until definitive, urgent, surgical repair can be accomplished.

The most catastrophic mechanical complication is **rupture of the ventricular free wall**. As blood fills the pericardium, cardiac tamponade develops rapidly, with sudden pulselessness, hypotension, and loss of consciousness. This complication nearly always is fatal.

Late complications that occur several weeks after an acute MI include development of a **ventricular aneurysm**, which should be suspected if ST-segment elevation persists weeks after the event, as well as **Dressler syndrome**, an immune phenomenon characterized by pericarditis, pleuritis, and fever. Dressler syndrome may remit and relapse, and it is treated with anti-inflammatory drugs, including nonsteroidal anti-inflammatory drugs (NSAIDs) and sometimes prednisone.

Post-MI Risk Stratification

The goal is to identify patients who are at high risk for subsequent cardiac events and who might benefit from revascularization. The initial evaluation involves noninvasive testing. **Submaximal exercise stress testing** is generally performed in stable patients before hospital discharge to detect residual ischemia and ventricular ectopy and to provide a guideline for exercise in the early recovery period. **Evaluation of LV systolic function**, usually with echocardiography, is routinely performed. High-risk patients include those with impaired systolic function, large areas of ischemic myocardium on stress testing or postinfarction angina, or ventricular ectopy who might benefit from coronary angiography to evaluate for revascularization. Percutaneous coronary intervention can be performed to reduce anginal symptoms, and **coronary artery bypass surgery** should be considered for patients with **multivessel atherosclerotic stenosis** and **impaired systolic function** because the surgery may reduce symptoms and prolong survival. Post-MI patients with **severe LV dysfunction** (LV ejection fraction <30%-35%) are at **increased risk for sudden cardiac death** from **ventricular arrhythmias** and may benefit from placement from an implantable cardioverter-defibrillator.

Secondary Prevention of Ischemic Heart Disease

Medical therapy to reduce modifiable risk factors is the cornerstone of post-MI care. In addition to symptom relief, the major goal of medical therapy is to prevent cardiac events: fatal or nonfatal MI. By far, the **most important risk factor is smoking cessation**. Quitting tobacco use can reduce the risk of fatal or nonfatal cardiac events by more than 50%, more than any other medical or surgical therapy available. A number of other therapies reduce the risk of recurrent cardiovascular events and prolong survival in patients with coronary artery disease. Antiplatelet agents such as **aspirin** and **clopidogrel** reduce the risk of thrombus formation, **beta-blockers** reduce myocardial oxygen demand and may help suppress ventricular arrhythmias, and cholesterol-lowering agents such as statins reduce the number of coronary events and prolong survival. Patients with established coronary artery disease (CAD) should have a low-density lipoprotein (LDL) cholesterol level less than 70 mg/dL. **Angiotensin-converting enzyme (ACE) inhibitors** are recommended for all patients after STEMI but are most important for patients with impaired systolic function (ejection fraction <40%), diabetes, or hypertension.

Comprehension Questions

1.1   A 36-year-old woman has severe burning chest pain that radiates to her neck. The pain occurs particularly after meals, especially when she lies down, and is not precipitated by exertion. She is admitted for observation. Serial ECG and troponin I levels are normal. Which of the following is the best next step?
   A. Stress thallium treadmill test
   B. Initiation of a proton pump inhibitor
   C. Coronary angiography
   D. Initiation of an antidepressant such as a selective serotonin reuptake inhibitor
   E. Referral to a psychiatrist

1.2   A 56-year-old man is admitted to the hospital for chest pain of 2-hour duration. His heart rate is 42 bpm, with sinus bradycardia on ECG, as well as ST-segment elevation in leads II, III, and aVF. Which of the following is the most likely diagnosis?
   A. He is likely in good physical condition with increased vagal tone.
   B. He likely has suffered an inferior wall MI.
   C. He likely has an LV aneurysm.
   D. The low heart rate is a reflection of a good cardiac ejection fraction.

1.3   A 59-year-old diabetic woman had suffered an acute anterior wall MI. Five days later, she gets into an argument with her husband and complains of chest pain. Her initial ECG shows no ischemic changes, but serum cardiac troponin I levels are drawn and return mildly elevated at this time. Which of the following is the best next step?
   A. Thrombolytic therapy.
   B. Percutaneous coronary intervention.
   C. Coronary artery bypass.
   D. Perform serial ECGs and obtain CK-MB.
   E. Prepare the patient for dialysis.

1.4   A 59-year-old male smoker complains of severe substernal squeezing
        chest pain of 30-minute duration. The paramedics have given sublin-
        gual nitroglycerin and oxygen by nasal cannula. His blood pressure is
        110/70 mm Hg and heart rate 90 bpm on arrival to the emergency room.
        The ECG is normal. Which of the following is the best next step?
        A. Echocardiography
        B. Thallium stress test
        C. Aspirin
        D. Coronary angiography
        E. Coronary artery bypass

ANSWERS

1.1   **B.** It is appropriate to evaluate chest pain to first rule out cardiac
        ischemia. One of the most common causes of "chest pain" particu-
        larly in a younger patient is esophageal spasm. This patient has clas-
        sic symptoms of reflux esophagitis and is best treated with a proton
        pump inhibitor. If the chest pain has the characteristics of angina
        pectoris (substernal location, precipitated by exertion, relieved by
        rest or nitroglycerin), it should be investigated with a stress test or
        coronary angiography.

1.2   **B.** Sinus bradycardia is often seen with inferior wall MI, because the
        right coronary artery supplies the inferior wall of the left ventricle
        and the sinoatrial node. The ischemic changes in leads II, III, and
        aVF are in the region of the inferior leads. Understanding which
        leads reflect which portion of the heart allows for an understanding
        of the aspect of the heart that is affected. Also understanding the
        area of the heart perfused by the various coronary arteries allows for
        correlation of associated symptoms or therapy.

1.3   **D.** Diabetic patients can have myocardial ischemia or infarction
        with atypical or absent symptoms. Clinical suspicion is required, and
        a liberal use of cardiac enzymes. Troponin levels often remain ele-
        vated for 7 to 10 days and should not be used to diagnose reinfarc-
        tion, especially if the levels are trending downward. New ECG
        findings or rapidly rising markers such as serum myoglobin or CK-MB
        can be used in this setting.

1.4   **C.** Aspirin is the first agent that should be used after oxygen and
        nitroglycerin. Aspirin use decreases mortality in the face of an acute
        coronary event. Because initial ECGs and cardiac enzymes may be
        normal in acute MI, serial studies are needed. Clinical assessment to
        exclude other causes of chest pain should be undertaken.

Clinical Pearls

➤ Acute coronary syndromes (unstable angina or acute myocardial infarction) occur when a thrombus forms at the site of rupture of an atherosclerotic plaque and acutely occludes a coronary artery.

➤ Acute myocardial infarction is diagnosed based on the presence of at least two of three criteria: typical symptoms, ECG findings, and cardiac enzymes. Initial ECG and enzyme levels may be normal, so serial studies are necessary.

➤ Early reperfusion with percutaneous coronary intervention or thrombolytics reduces mortality and preserves ventricular function in patients who have ST-segment elevation, have no contraindications, and receive treatment within the first 6 to 12 hours.

➤ The goal of secondary prevention after myocardial infarction is to prevent recurrent cardiac events and death. Smoking cessation, aspirin and clopidogrel, beta-blockers, and statins all reduce the rate of events and reduce mortality.

➤ After myocardial infarction, angioplasty can be performed to reduce ischemia and anginal symptoms. Bypass surgery may be indicated for patients with multivessel stenosis and impaired systolic function to reduce symptoms and prolong survival.

➤ The ECG can indicate the location of the ischemia or infarction: anterior (leads V_2 through V_4), lateral (leads I, aVL, V_5, and V_6), inferior (leads II, III, and aVF), and posterior (R waves in leads V_1 and V_2).

➤ An understanding of the portion of the heart affected by ischemia allows for identifying which coronary artery may be involved.

REFERENCES

Antman EM, Braunwald E. ST-segment elevation myocardial infarction. In: Kasper DL, Braunwald E, Fauci AS, et al., eds. *Harrison's Principles of Internal Medicine*. 17th ed. New York, NY: McGraw-Hill; 2008:1532-1544.

Antman EM, Hand M, Armstrong PW, et al. 2007 focused update of the ACC/AHA 2004 guidelines for the management of patients with ST-elevation myocardial infarction. *Circulation*. 117(2):296-329.

Antman EM, Selwyn AP, Braunwald E. Ischemic heart disease. In: Kasper DL, Braunwald E, Fauci AS, et al., eds. *Harrison's Principles of Internal Medicine*. 17th ed. New York, NY: McGraw-Hill; 2008:1514-1532.

Keeley EC, Boura JA, Grines CL. Primary angioplasty versus intravenous thrombolytic therapy for acute myocardial infarction: a quantitative review of 23 randomized trials. *Lancet*. 2003;361:13-20.

McClellan MB, Tunis SR. Medicare coverage of ICDs. *N Engl J Med*. 2005;352:222-224.

Tatum JL, Jesse RL, Kontos MC, et al. Comprehensive strategy for the evaluation and triage of the chest pain patient. *Ann Emerg Med*. 1997;29:116-125.

Case 2

A 72-year-old man presents to the office complaining of several weeks of worsening exertional dyspnea. Previously, he had been able to work in his garden and mow the lawn, but now he feels short of breath after walking 100 feet. He does not have chest pain when he walks, although in the past he has experienced episodes of retrosternal chest pressure with strenuous exertion. Once recently he had felt lightheaded, as if he were about to faint while climbing a flight of stairs, but the symptom passed after he sat down. He has been having some difficulty sleeping at night and has to prop himself up with two pillows. Occasionally, he wakes up at night feeling quite short of breath, which is relieved within minutes by sitting upright and dangling his legs over the bed. His feet have become swollen, especially by the end of the day. He denies any significant medical history, takes no medications, and prides himself on the fact that he has not seen a doctor in years. He does not smoke or drink alcohol.

On physical examination, he is afebrile, with a heart rate of 86 bpm, blood pressure 115/92 mm Hg, and respiratory rate 16 breaths per minute. Examination of the head and neck reveals pink mucosa without pallor, a normal thyroid gland, and distended neck veins. Bibasilar inspiratory crackles are heard on examination. On cardiac examination, his heart rhythm is regular with a normal S_1 and a second heart sound that splits during expiration, an S_4 at the apex, a nondisplaced apical impulse, and a late-peaking systolic murmur at the right upper sternal border that radiates to his carotids. The carotid upstrokes have diminished amplitude.

➤ What is the most likely diagnosis?

➤ What test would confirm the diagnosis?

ANSWERS TO CASE 2:
Congestive Heart Failure due to Critical Aortic Stenosis

Summary: A 72-year-old man complains of several weeks of worsening exertional dyspnea. He has experienced angina-like chest pressure with strenuous exertion and near-syncope while climbing a flight of stairs, and now he has symptoms of heart failure such as orthopnea and paroxysmal nocturnal dyspnea. Heart failure is also suggested by physical signs of volume overload (pedal edema, elevated jugular venous pressure, and crackles suggesting pulmonary edema). The cause of his heart failure may be aortic valvular stenosis, given the late systolic murmur radiating to his carotid, the paradoxical splitting of his second heart sound, and the diminished carotid upstrokes.

> **Most likely diagnosis:** Congestive heart failure (CHF), possibly as a result of aortic stenosis.

> **Diagnostic test:** Echocardiogram to assess the aortic valve area as well as the left ventricular systolic function.

ANALYSIS

Objectives

1. Know the causes of chronic heart failure (eg, ischemia, hypertension, valvular disease, alcohol abuse, cocaine, and thyrotoxicosis).
2. Recognize impaired systolic function versus diastolic dysfunction.
3. Be familiar with the treatment of acute and chronic heart failure.
4. Know the complications of treatment: hypokalemia and hyperkalemia, renal failure, digoxin toxicity.
5. Be familiar with the evaluation of aortic stenosis and the indications for valve replacement.

Considerations

This is an elderly patient with symptoms and signs of aortic stenosis. The valvular disorder has progressed from previous angina and presyncopal symptoms to heart failure, reflecting worsening severity of the stenosis and worsening prognosis for survival. This patient should undergo urgent evaluation of his aortic valve surface area and coronary artery status to assess the need for valve replacement.

APPROACH TO
Congestive Heart Failure

DEFINITIONS

ACUTE HEART FAILURE: Acute (hours, days) presentation of cardiac decompensation with pulmonary edema and low cardiac output, which may proceed to cardiogenic shock.

CHRONIC HEART FAILURE: Chronic (months, years) presence of cardiac dysfunction; symptoms may range from minimal to severe.

DIASTOLIC DYSFUNCTION: Increased diastolic filling pressures caused by impaired diastolic relaxation and decreased ventricular compliance.

SYSTOLIC DYSFUNCTION: Low cardiac output caused by impaired systolic function (low ejection fraction).

CARDIAC REMODELING: Changes to the heart due to increased cardiac loading (preload and afterload) which leads to cardiac dysfunction. Some medications can prevent or even reverse the remodeling.

CLINICAL APPROACH

Congestive heart failure (CHF) is a **clinical syndrome** that is produced when the heart is **unable to meet the metabolic needs of the body while maintaining normal ventricular filling pressures**. A series of **neurohumoral responses** develop, including activation of the renin-angiotensin-aldosterone axis and increased sympathetic activity, which initially may be compensatory but ultimately cause further cardiac decompensation. Symptoms may be a result of **forward failure** (low cardiac output or systolic dysfunction), including **fatigue, lethargy, and even hypotension**, or **backward failure** (increased filling pressures or diastolic dysfunction), including **dyspnea, peripheral edema, and ascites**. Some patients have isolated diastolic dysfunction with preserved left ventricular ejection fraction (LVEF>40%-50%), most often as a consequence of hypertension or simply of aging. Half of patients with CHF have impaired systolic dysfunction (LVEF <40%) with associated increased filling pressures. Some patients have isolated right-sided heart failure (with elevated jugular venous pressure, hepatic congestion, peripheral edema but no pulmonary edema), but more commonly patients have left ventricular failure (with low cardiac output and pulmonary edema) that progresses to biventricular failure.

Heart failure is a **chronic and progressive disease** that can be assessed by following the patient's exercise tolerance, such as the **New York Heart Association (NYHA) functional classification (Table 2–1)**. This functional

Table 2–1 NYHA FUNCTIONAL CLASSIFICATION

Class I: No limitation during ordinary physical activity.
Class II: Slight limitation of physical activity. Develops fatigue or dyspnea with moderate
  exertion.
Class III: Marked limitation of physical activity. Even light activity produces symptoms.
Class IV: Symptoms at rest. Any activity causes worsening.

classification carries prognostic significance. Individuals in class III who have low oxygen consumption during exercise have an annual mortality rate of 20%; in class IV, the rate is 60% annually. Patients with a low ejection fraction (LVEF <20%) also have very high mortality risks. Death associated with CHF may occur from the underlying disease process, cardiogenic shock, or sudden death as a result of ventricular arrhythmias.

Although heart failure has many causes (Table 2–2), identification of the underlying treatable or reversible causes of disease is essential. For example, heart failure related to tachycardia, alcohol consumption, or viral myocarditis may be reversible with removal of the inciting factor. In patients with underlying multivessel atherosclerotic coronary disease and a low ejection fraction, revascularization with coronary artery bypass grafting improves cardiac function and prolongs survival. For patients with heart failure, appropriate investigation is guided by the history but may include echocardiography to assess ejection

Table 2–2 SELECTED CAUSES OF CONGESTIVE HEART FAILURE

Myocardial Injury
• Adriamycin
• Alcohol use
• Cocaine
• Ischemic cardiomyopathy (atherosclerotic coronary artery disease)
• Rheumatic fever
• Viral myocarditis
Chronic Pressure Overload
• Aortic stenosis
• Hypertension
Chronic Volume Overload
• Mitral regurgitation
Infiltrative Diseases
• Amyloidosis
• Hemochromatosis
Chronic Tachyarrhythmia or Bradyarrhythmia

fraction and valvular function, cardiac stress testing, or coronary angiography as indicated, and, in some cases, endomyocardial biopsy.

The three major treatment goals for patients with chronic heart failure are relief of symptoms, preventing disease progression, and a reduction in mortality risk. The heart failure symptoms, which are mainly caused by low cardiac output and fluid overload, usually are relieved with dietary sodium restriction and loop diuretics. Because heart failure has such a substantial mortality, however, measures in an attempt to halt or reverse disease progression are necessary. Reversible causes should be aggressively sought and treated. Use of **angiotensin-converting enzyme (ACE) inhibitors or angiotensin receptor blockers (ARBs) and some beta-blockers, such as carvedilol, metoprolol, or bisoprolol, have been shown to reduce mortality in patients with impaired systolic function and moderate to severe symptoms.** In patients who cannot tolerate ACE inhibition (or in black patients in whom ACE inhibitors appear to confer less benefit), the use of hydralazine with nitrates has been shown to decrease mortality. Digoxin can be added to these regimens for additional symptom relief, but it provides no survival benefit.

The mechanism of the various agents are as follows:

Beta-blockers: Prevent and reverse adrenergically mediated intrinsic myocardial dysfunction and remodeling.

ACE inhibitors: Reduces preload and afterload, thereby reducing right atrial, pulmonary arterial, and pulmonary capillary wedge pressures along with systemic vascular resistance, and prevents remodeling. These **agents are the initial drugs of choice in treating CHF since there is survival advantage with their use.**

Nitrates and nitrites: (not as commonly used) Reduce preload and clear pulmonary congestion.

Diuretics: Used to decrease preload, used especially acutely.

Digoxin: Acts to improve the cardiac contractility somewhat.

Aortic Stenosis

The history and physical findings presented in the scenario suggest that this patient's heart failure may be a result of aortic stenosis. This is the **most common valvular abnormality in adults.** The large majority of cases occur in men. The causes of the valvular stenosis vary depending on the typical age of presentation: stenosis in patients **younger than 30 years** usually is caused by a **congenital bicuspid valve;** in patients 30 to 70 years old, it usually is caused by congenital stenosis or acquired rheumatic heart disease; and in patients **older than 70 years, it usually is caused by degenerative calcific stenosis.**

Typical physical findings include a **narrow pulse pressure,** a **harsh late-peaking systolic murmur** heard best at the right second intercostal space with radiation to the carotid arteries and a delayed slow-rising carotid upstroke (pulsus parvus et tardus). The electrocardiogram (ECG) often shows left ventricular hypertrophy. Doppler echocardiography reveals a thickened abnormal valve and can define severity as assessed by the aortic valve area and by estimating the transvalvular pressure gradient. As the valve orifice narrows, the pressure gradient increases in an attempt to maintain cardiac output. Severe aortic stenosis often has valve areas less than 1 cm^2 (normal 3-4 cm^2) and mean pressure gradients more than 40 mm Hg.

Symptoms of aortic stenosis develop as a consequence of the resulting left ventricular hypertrophy as well as the diminished cardiac output caused by the flow-limiting valvular stenosis. The first symptoms typically are **angina pectoris**, that is, retrosternal chest pain precipitated by exercise and relieved by rest. As the stenosis worsens and cardiac output falls, patients may experience **syncopal episodes**, typically precipitated by exertion. Finally, because of the low cardiac output and high diastolic filling pressures, patients develop clinically apparent **heart failure** as described earlier. The prognosis for patients worsens as symptoms develop, with mean survival with angina, syncope, or heart failure of 5 years, 3 years, and 2 years, respectively.

Patients with severe stenosis who are symptomatic should be considered for aortic valve replacement. Preoperative cardiac catheterization is routinely performed to provide definitive assessment of aortic valve area and the pressure gradient, as well as to assess the coronary arteries for significant stenosis. In patients who are not good candidates for valve replacement, the stenotic valve can be enlarged using balloon valvuloplasty, but this will provide only temporary relief of symptoms.

Comprehension Questions

2.1   A 55-year-old man is noted to have moderately severe congestive heart failure with impaired systolic function. Which of the following drugs would most likely lower his risk of mortality?

A. Angiotensin-converting enzyme inhibitors
B. Loop diuretics
C. Digoxin
D. Aspirin

2.2   In the United States, which of the following is most likely to have caused the congestive heart failure in the patient described in Question 2.1?

A. Diabetes
B. Atherosclerosis
C. Alcohol
D. Rheumatic heart disease

2.3   A 35-year-old woman is noted to have chest pain with exertion, and has been passing out recently. On examination she is noted to have a harsh systolic murmur. Which of the following is the best therapy for her condition?

    A. Coronary artery bypass
    B. Angioplasty
    C. Valve replacement
    D. Carotid endarterectomy

2.4   A 55-year-old man is noted to have congestive heart failure and states that he is comfortable at rest but becomes dyspneic even with walking to bathroom. On echocardiography, he is noted to have an ejection fraction of 47%. Which of the following is the more accurate description of this patient's condition?

    A. Diastolic dysfunction
    B. Systolic dysfunction
    C. Dilated cardiomyopathy
    D. Pericardial disease

ANSWERS

2.1   **A.** Angiotensin-converting enzyme inhibitor and beta-blockers decrease the risk of mortality when used to treat CHF with impaired systolic function. For this reason, these agents are the initial choice to treat CHF. They both prevent and can even, in some circumstances, reverse the cardiac remodeling.

2.2   **B.** In the United States, the most common cause of CHF associated with impaired systolic function is ischemic cardiomyopathy due to coronary atherosclerosis.

2.3   **C.** The symptoms of aortic stenosis classically progress through angina, syncope, and, finally, congestive heart failure, which has the worse prognosis for survival. This patient's systolic murmur is consistent with aortic stenosis. An evaluation should include echocardiography to confirm the diagnosis, and then aortic valve replacement.

2.4   **A.** When the ejection fraction exceeds 40%, there is likely diastolic dysfunction, with stiff ventricles. The stiff thickened ventricles do not accept blood very readily. This patient has symptoms with mild exertion which are indicative of functional class III. The worst class is level IV, manifested as symptoms at rest or with minimal exertion. ACE inhibitors are important agents in patients with diastolic dysfunction.

Clinical Pearls

➤ Congestive heart failure is a clinical syndrome that is always caused by some underlying heart disease, most commonly ischemic cardiomyopathy as a result of atherosclerotic coronary disease or hypertension.

➤ Heart failure can be caused by impaired systolic function (ejection fraction <40%) or impaired diastolic function (with preserved systolic ejection fraction).

➤ Chronic heart failure is a progressive disease with a high mortality. A patient's functional class, that is, his or her exercise tolerance, is the best predictor of mortality and often guides therapy.

➤ The primary goals of therapy are to relieve congestive symptoms with salt restriction, diuretics, digoxin, and vasodilators and to prolong survival with angiotensin-converting enzyme inhibitors or certain beta-blockers.

➤ Angiotensin-converting enzyme inhibitors together with beta blockers are the agents of choice for CHF.

➤ Aortic stenosis produces progressive symptoms such as angina, exertional syncope, and heart failure, with increasingly higher risk of mortality. Valve replacement should be considered for patients with symptoms and severe aortic stenosis, for example, an aortic valve area less than 1 cm^2.

REFERENCES

Asif M, Regan TJ. Congestive cardiomyopathy. In: Alpert JS, ed. *Cardiology for the Primary Care Physician*. 2nd ed. Stamford, CT: Appleton and Lange; 1998:219-229.

Carabello, BA. Clinical practice: aortic stenosis. *N Engl J Med*. 2002;346:677-682.

Jessup M, Brozena S. Heart failure. *N Engl J Med*. 2003;348:2007-2018.

Lejemtel TH, Sonnenblick EH, Frishman WH. Diagnosis and management of heart failure. In: Fuster V, Alexander RX, O'Rourke RA, eds. *Hurst's the Heart*. 10th ed. New York, NY: McGraw-Hill; 2001:6.

Mann DL. Heart failure and cor pulmonale. In: Fauci AS, Braunwald E, Kasper DL, et al., eds. *Harrison's Principles of Internal Medicine*. 17th ed. New York, NY: McGraw-Hill; 2008:1443-1457.

Case 3

A 26-year-old woman presents to the emergency room complaining of sudden onset of palpitations and severe shortness of breath and coughing. She reports that she has experienced several episodes of palpitations in the past, often lasting a day or two, but never with dyspnea like this. She has a history of rheumatic fever at the age of 14 years. She is now 20 weeks pregnant with her first child and takes prenatal vitamins. She denies use of any other medications, tobacco, alcohol, or illicit drugs.

On examination, her heart rate is between 110 and 130 bpm and is irregularly irregular, with blood pressure 92/65 mm Hg, respiratory rate 24 breaths per minute, and oxygen saturation of 94% on room air. She appears uncomfortable, with labored respirations. She is coughing, producing scant amounts of frothy sputum with a pinkish tint. She has ruddy cheeks and a normal jugular venous pressure. She has bilateral inspiratory crackles in the lower lung fields. On cardiac examination, her heart rhythm is irregularly irregular with a loud S_1 and low-pitched diastolic murmur at the apex. Her apical impulse is nondisplaced. Her uterine fundus is palpable at the umbilicus, and she has no peripheral edema. An electrocardiogram (ECG) is obtained (Figure 3–1).

➤ What is the most likely diagnosis?

➤ What is your next step?

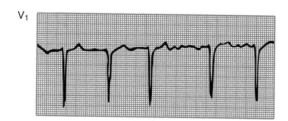

V_1

Figure 3–1. Electrocardiogram. *Reproduced, with permission, from Braunwald E, Fauci AS, Kasper DL, et al, eds.* Harrison's Principles of Internal Medicine. *16th ed. New York, NY: McGraw-Hill; 2005:1345.*

ANSWERS TO CASE 3:
Atrial Fibrillation, Mitral Stenosis

Summary: This 26-year-old woman, with a history of rheumatic fever during adolescence, is now in the second trimester of pregnancy and presents with acute onset of palpitations. She is found to have atrial fibrillation (AF) with a rapid ventricular response. She has a diastolic rumble and "ruddy cheeks," both features of mitral stenosis, which is the likely cause of her atrial fibrillation as a result of left atrial enlargement. Because of the increased blood volume associated with pregnancy and the onset of tachycardia and loss of atrial contraction, the atrial fibrillation has caused her to develop pulmonary edema.

➤ **Most likely diagnosis:** Atrial fibrillation caused by rheumatic heart disease.

➤ **Next step:** Cardiac rate control with intravenous beta-blockers.

ANALYSIS

Objectives

1. Know the causes of atrial fibrillation.
2. Understand the management of acute atrial fibrillation with rapid ventricular response.
3. Understand the rationale for anticoagulation in chronic atrial fibrillation.
4. Know the typical cardiac lesions of rheumatic heart disease and the physical findings in mitral stenosis.
5. Understand the physiologic basis of Wolff-Parkinson-White syndrome and the special considerations in atrial fibrillation.

APPROACH TO
Atrial Fibrillation

DEFINITIONS

ATRIAL FIBRILLATION: Abnormal irregular heart rhythm with chaotic generation of electrical signals in the atria of the heart.

DC CARDIOVERSION: Converting the rhythm of the heart to normal by applying direct-current electrical shock.

CLINICAL APPROACH

Atrial fibrillation (AF) is the most common arrhythmia for which patients seek treatment; it occurs in acute, paroxysmal, and chronic forms. During AF, disordered atrial depolarization, often at rates exceeding 300 to 400 bpm, produces an irregular ventricular response, depending on the number of impulses that are conducted through the atrioventricular (AV) node. The ECG is characterized by **absence of discrete P waves** and an **irregularly irregular ventricular response**. The incidence of AF increases with age, affecting 5% to 10% of patients older than 75 years. Although many patients can maintain a normal activity level and remain essentially asymptomatic with chronic AF, there are several causes of morbidity from this arrhythmia: it may trigger a rapid ventricular rate leading to myocardial ischemia or exacerbation of heart failure in patients with heart disease, and **thrombus formation** in the noncontractile atria can lead to systemic embolization (AF is a common cause of stroke).

Anything that causes atrial dilation or excessive sympathetic tone can lead to AF, but the **two most common causes** of AF are **hypertension and coronary atherosclerosis**. The **causes of AF** can be remembered with the **mnemonic "I SMART CHAP"** (Table 3–1).

Acute AF with rapid ventricular response must be addressed quickly. The four major goals are (1) stabilization, (2) rate control, (3) conversion to sinus rhythm, and (4) anticoagulation. If a patient is **hemodynamically unstable** (hypotensive, angina pectoris, pulmonary edema), **urgent direct current (DC) cardioversion** is indicated. If the patient is hemodynamically stable, **ventricular rate control** can generally be achieved with **intravenous beta-blockers, calcium channel blockers, or digoxin**, which slow conduction through the AV node. Once the ventricular rate has been controlled, consideration can be given to reversing the underlying causes (eg, thyrotoxicosis,

Table 3–1 CAUSES OF ATRIAL FIBRILLATION

Inflammatory disease (pericarditis, myocarditis)
Surgery (postbypass surgery, postvalvular surgery)
Medications (theophylline, caffeine, digitalis)
Atherosclerotic coronary artery disease
Rheumatic heart disease (especially with mitral stenosis)
Thyrotoxicosis
Congenital heart disease (atrial septal defect, Ebstein anomaly)
Hypertensive heart disease
Alcohol consumption (holiday heart syndrome, alcoholic cardiomyopathy)
Pulmonary disease, especially pulmonary embolus

use of adrenergic stimulants, or worsening heart failure) so that patients can undergo **cardioversion** to sinus rhythm. This may occur spontaneously or after correction of underlying abnormalities, or it may require pharmacologic or electrical cardioversion. If the duration of **AF exceeds 48 hours, the risk of intraatrial thrombus formation increases.**

Cardioverting the patient back to sinus rhythm, the return of coordinated atrial contraction in the presence of an atrial thrombus, may result in clot embolization, leading to a cerebral infarction or other distant ischemic event. Therefore, after 48 hours of AF, patients should receive 3 to 4 weeks of warfarin therapy prior to and after cardioversion to reduce the risk of thromboembolic phenomena. Alternatively, low-risk patients can undergo transesophageal echocardiography to exclude the presence of an atrial appendage thrombus prior to cardioversion. Postcardioversion anticoagulation is still required for 4 weeks, because even though the rhythm returns to sinus, the atria do not contract normally for some time. Pharmacologic cardioverting agents, though not as effective, include procainamide, sotalol, and amiodarone.

Many patients with AF cannot be cardioverted and be expected to remain in sinus rhythm. **Two important prognostic factors** are **left atrial dilation** (atrial diameter >4.5 cm predicts failure of cardioversion) and **duration of AF**. The longer the patient is in fibrillation, the more likely the patient is to stay there ("atrial fibrillation begets atrial fibrillation") as a consequence of electrical remodeling of the heart. In patients with chronic AF, the management goals are rate control, using drugs to reduce AV nodal conduction as described earlier, and anticoagulation. Patients with chronic AF who are not anticoagulated have a 5% per year incidence of clinically evident embolization such as stroke. For chronic AF caused by valvular disease such as mitral stenosis, the annual risk of stroke is substantially higher. **Warfarin anticoagulation reduces the risk of stroke in patients with chronic AF by two-thirds.** Warfarin does not produce a predictable dose-related response; therefore, the level of anticoagulation needs to be monitored by regular laboratory testing using the international normalized ratio (INR). In AF not caused by valvular disease, the goal INR is 2 to 3. AF that develops in patients younger than 60 years without evidence of structural heart disease, hypertension, or other factors for stroke is termed **lone AF**, and the **risk of stroke is very low**, so anticoagulation with warfarin is not used. Instead, low-dose aspirin may be used.

The major complication of warfarin therapy is bleeding as a consequence of excessive anticoagulation. The risk of bleeding increases as the INR increases. If the INR is markedly elevated (eg, INR >6) but there is no apparent bleeding, the values will return to normal over several days if the warfarin is held. For higher levels of INR but without bleeding, vitamin K can be administered. If clinically significant bleeding is present, warfarin toxicity can be rapidly reversed with administration of vitamin K and fresh-frozen plasma to replace clotting factors and provide intravascular volume replacement.

RHEUMATIC HEART DISEASE

In the case presented in the scenario, the cause of this patient's AF appears to be mitral stenosis. Because she has a history of acute rheumatic fever, her mitral stenosis almost certainly is a result of rheumatic heart disease. **Rheumatic heart disease** is a late sequela of acute rheumatic fever, arising many years after the original attack. Valvular thickening, fibrosis, and calcifications lead to valvular stenosis. The **mitral valve is most frequently involved**. The aortic valve may also develop stenosis, but usually in combination with the mitral valve. The right side of the heart is rarely involved.

Almost all cases of **mitral stenosis** in adults are secondary to **rheumatic heart disease**, usually involving women. The physical signs of mitral stenosis are a **loud S₁** and an **opening snap following S₂**. The S_2-OS (mitral valve opening snap) interval narrows as the severity of the stenosis increases. There is a **low-pitched diastolic rumble** after the opening snap, heard best at the apex with the bell of the stethoscope. Because of the stenotic valve, pressure in the left atrium is increased, leading to left atrial dilation and, ultimately, to pulmonary hypertension. Pulmonary hypertension can cause hemoptysis and signs of right-sided heart failure such as peripheral edema. When AF develops, the rapid ventricular response produces pulmonary congestion as a consequence of shortened diastolic filling time. Rate control with intravenous digoxin, beta-blockers, or calcium channel blockers is essential to relief of pulmonary symptoms.

WOLFF-PARKINSON-WHITE SYNDROME

Another cause of AF is the **Wolff-Parkinson-White (WPW) syndrome**. In patients with this condition, AF may be life-threatening. In addition to the AV node, patients with WPW have an **accessory pathway** that provides an alternate route for electrical communication between the atria and ventricles, leading to **preexcitation**, that is, early ventricular depolarization that begins prior to normal AV nodal conduction. A portion of ventricular activation occurs over the accessory pathway, with the remaining occurring normally through the His-Purkinje system. This preexcitation is recognized on the ECG as a **delta wave**, or early up-slurring of the R wave, which both **widens the QRS complex** and **shortens the PR interval**, which represents the normal AV nodal conduction time (Figure 3–2). Some patients with the ECG abnormalities of WPW syndrome are asymptomatic; others have recurrent tachyarrhythmias. Most of the tachycardia is caused by paroxysmal supraventricular tachycardia; one third of patients will have AF. AF with conduction to the ventricles over an accessory pathway is a special case for two reasons. First, when conducted through the accessory pathway, the **widened QRS** may look like ventricular tachycardia, except that it will have the **irregular RR**

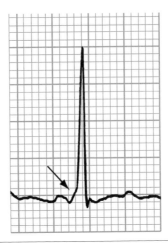

Figure 3–2.   Electrocardiogram revealing the delta wave of Wolff-Parkinson-White syndrome. *Reproduced, with permission, from Stead LG, Stead SM, Kaufman MS. First Aid for the Medicine Clerkship. 2nd ed. New York, NY: McGraw-Hill; 2006:44.*

interval of AF. Second, because the AV conduction is occurring through the accessory pathway rather than through the AV node, the ventricular rate may be very rapid, and the usual AV nodal–blocking drugs given for ventricular rate control will not affect the accessory pathway. In fact, **digoxin, verapamil**, and other AV nodal–blocking agents can, **paradoxically, increase the ventricular rate** and **should be avoided in WPW patients with AF**. If hemodynamically unstable, **DC cardioversion** should be performed. If hemodynamically stable, the agent of choice is **procainamide or ibutilide**, to slow conduction and convert the rhythm to sinus.

Comprehension Questions

3.1   A 28-year-old woman has been told she has rheumatic heart disease, specifically mitral stenosis. Which of the following murmurs is most likely present?

A. Diastolic rumble at apex of the heart
B. Early diastolic decrescendo at right upper sternal border
C. Holosystolic murmur at apex
D. Late-peaking systolic murmur at right upper sternal border

3.2   A 48-year-old woman is noted to have atrial fibrillation with a ventricular heart rate of 140 bpm. She is slightly dizzy with a systolic blood pressure of 75/48 mm Hg. Which of the following is the most appropriate next step?

A. Intravenous digoxin.
B. DC cardioversion.
C. Initiate vagal maneuvers.
D. Intravenous diltiazem (Cardizem).

3.3   A third-year medical student has been reading about the dangers of excessive anticoagulation and bleeding potential. He reviews the charts of several patients with atrial fibrillation currently taking Coumadin. Which of the following patients is best suited to have anticoagulation discontinued?

A. A 45-year-old man who has normal echocardiographic findings and no history of heart disease or hypertension, but a family history of hyperlipidemia
B. A 62-year-old man with mild chronic hypertension and dilated left atrium, but normal ejection fraction
C. A 75-year-old woman who is in good health except for a prior stroke, from which she has recovered nearly all function
D. A 52-year-old man with orthopnea and paroxysmal nocturnal dyspnea

3.4   A 59-year-old woman has been placed on warfarin (Coumadin) after being found to have had chronic atrial fibrillation. She is noted to have an INR of 5.8, is asymptomatic, and has no overt bleeding. Which of the following is the best management for this patient?

A. Transfuse with erythrocytes.
B. Give vitamin K.
C. Give fresh frozen plasma.
D. Hold warfarin.

3.5   A 45-year-old woman is noted to have dizziness, pounding of the chest, and fatigue of 3 hours duration. On examination, she is noted to have a blood pressure (BP) of 110/70 mm Hg and heart rate of 180 bpm. She is noted on ECG to have atrial fibrillation with delta waves. The emergency room physician counsels the patient regarding cardioversion, but the patient declines. Which of the following is the best therapy for her condition?

A. Digoxin
B. Angiotensin-converting enzyme (ACE) inhibitor
C. Calcium channel blocker
D. Procainamide

ANSWERS

3.1   **A.** A diastolic rumble at the cardiac apex suggests mitral stenosis. The early diastolic decrescendo murmur is typical of aortic regurgitation, holosystolic murmur at the apex that of mitral regurgitation, and late-peaking systolic murmur at the upper sternal border that of aortic stenosis.

3.2   **B.** This individual has significant symptoms and hypotension caused by the atrial fibrillation and rapid ventricular rate; consequently, DC cardioversion is the treatment of choice.

3.3   **A.** Conditions associated with a high risk for embolic stroke include a dilated left atrium, congestive heart failure, prior stroke, and the presence of a thrombus by echocardiogram. The man in answer A has "lone atrial fibrillation" and has a low risk for stroke and thus would not benefit from anticoagulation.

3.4   **D.** The target INR with warfarin is 2 to 3; thus, 5.8 is markedly elevated. However, because she has no overt bleeding and is asymptomatic, holding the warfarin until the INR reaches the acceptable range is a reasonable approach.

3.5   **D.** This patient has atrial fibrillation but with WPW as indicated by the delta wave. In this setting, the typical agents used to treat atrial fibrillation that slow the AV node are contraindicated since the WPW would worsen. DC cardioversion is an option; however in a hemodynamically stable patient, procainamide may be used since it will slow propagation through the accessory pathway. Because this patient declines cardioversion, procainamide is the best choice. Procainamide may cause hypotension, widen the QRS complex, and sometimes cause greater propagation through the AV node.

Clinical Pearls

➤ The two most common causes of atrial fibrillation are hypertension and atherosclerotic heart disease. The other causes can be remembered with the mnemonic "I SMART CHAP."

➤ Acute atrial fibrillation is treated with direct current cardioversion if the patient is unstable. If the patient is stable, initial management is ventricular rate control with an atrioventricular nodal-blocking agent, such as digoxin, beta-blockers, diltiazem, or verapamil.

➤ Patients with chronic atrial fibrillation generally require long-term anticoagulation to prevent embolic strokes. An exception is "lone atrial fibrillation," in which the risk of stroke is low.

➤ Wolff-Parkinson-White syndrome is a ventricular preexcitation syndrome defined as symptomatic tachycardia, with a delta wave, short PR interval (<0.12 seconds), and prolonged QRS interval (>0.12 seconds).

➤ Atrial fibrillation in Wolff-Parkinson-White syndrome is treated with direct current cardioversion or with procainamide or ibutilide. AV nodal–blocking agents can, paradoxically, increase the ventricular rate.

REFERENCES

Feldman T. Rheumatic mitral stenosis. On the rise again. *Postgrad Med.* 1993;93:93-104.

Marchlinski F. The tachyarrhythmias. In: Kasper DL, Braunwald E, Fauci AS, et al, eds. *Harrison's Principles of Internal Medicine.* 17th ed. New York, NY: McGraw-Hill; 2008:1425-1443.

O'Gara P, Braunwald E. Valvular heart disease. In: Kasper DL, Braunwald E, Fauci AS, et al, eds. *Harrison's Principles of Internal Medicine.* 17th ed. New York, NY: McGraw-Hill; 2008:1465-1480.

Snow V, Weiss KB, LeFevre M, et al. Management of newly detected atrial fibrillation: a clinical practice guideline from the American Academy of Family Physicians and the American College of Physicians. *Ann Intern Med.* 2003;139:1009-1017.

Van Gelder IC, Hagens VE, Bosker, HA, et al. A comparison of rate control and rhythm control in patients with recurrent persistent atrial fibrillation. *N Engl J Med.* 2002;347:1834-1840.

Case 4

A 37-year-old executive returns to your office for follow-up of recurrent upper abdominal pain. He initially presented 6 weeks ago, complaining of an increase in frequency and severity of burning epigastric pain, which he has experienced occasionally for more than 2 years. Now the pain occurs three or four times per week, usually when he has an empty stomach, and it often awakens him at night. The pain usually is relieved within minutes by food or over-the-counter antacids but then recurs within 2 to 3 hours. He admitted that stress at work had recently increased and that because of long working hours, he was drinking more caffeine and eating a lot of take-out foods. His medical history and review of systems were otherwise unremarkable, and, other than the antacids, he takes no medications. His physical examination was normal, including stool guaiac that was negative for occult blood. You advised a change in diet and started him on an H_2 blocker. His symptoms resolved completely with the diet changes and daily use of the medication. Results of laboratory tests performed at his first visit show no anemia, but his serum *Helicobacter pylori* antibody test was positive.

➤ What is your diagnosis?

➤ What is your next step?

ANSWERS TO CASE 4:
Peptic Ulcer Disease

Summary: A 37-year-old man presents with complaints of chronic and recurrent upper abdominal pain with characteristics suggestive of duodenal ulcer: the pain is burning, occurs when the stomach is empty, and is relieved within minutes by food or antacids. He does not have evidence of gastrointestinal bleeding or anemia. He does not take nonsteroidal anti-inflammatory drugs, which might cause ulcer formation, but he does have serologic evidence of *H pylori* infection.

> **Most likely diagnosis:** Peptic ulcer disease (PUD)

> **Next step:** Antibiotic therapy for *H pylori* infection

ANALYSIS

Objectives

1. Know how to differentiate common causes of abdominal pain by historical clues.
2. Recognize clinical features of duodenal ulcer, gastric ulcer, and features that increase concern for gastric cancer.
3. Understand the role of *H pylori* infection and use of nonsteroidal anti-inflammatory drugs (NSAIDs) in the etiology of PUD.
4. Understand the use and interpretation of tests for *H. pylori*.

Considerations

In this patient, the symptoms are suggestive of duodenal ulcer. He does not have "alarm symptoms," such as weight loss, bleeding, or anemia, and his young age and chronicity of symptoms make gastric malignancy an unlikely cause for his symptoms. *Helicobacter pylori* commonly is associated with PUD and requires treatment for cure of the ulcer and prevention of recurrence. This patient's symptoms are also consistent with nonulcer dyspepsia.

APPROACH TO
Peptic Ulcer Disease

DEFINITIONS

DYSPEPSIA: Pain or discomfort centered in the upper abdomen (mainly in or around the midline), which can be associated with fullness, early satiety, bloating, or nausea. Dyspepsia can be intermittent or continuous, and it may or may not be related to meals.

FUNCTIONAL (NONULCER) DYSPEPSIA: Symptoms as described for dyspepsia, persisting for at least 12 weeks but without evidence of ulcer on endoscopy.

HELICOBACTER PYLORI: A gram-negative microaerophilic bacillus that resides within the mucus layer of the gastric mucosa and causes persistent gastric infection and chronic inflammation. It produces a urease enzyme that splits urea, raising local pH and allowing it to survive in the acidic environment.

PEPTIC ULCER DISEASE (PUD): Presence of gastric or duodenal ulcers as demonstrated by endoscopy or by upper gastrointestinal barium study.

CLINICAL APPROACH

Upper abdominal pain is one of the most common complaints encountered in primary care practice. Many patients have benign functional disorders (ie, no specific pathology can be identified after diagnostic testing), but others have potentially more serious conditions such as PUD or gastric cancer. Historical clues, knowledge of the epidemiology of diseases, and some simple laboratory assessments can help to separate benign from serious causes of pain. However, endoscopy is often necessary to confirm the diagnosis.

Dyspepsia refers to upper abdominal pain or discomfort that can be caused by PUD, but it also can be produced by a number of other gastrointestinal disorders. **Gastroesophageal reflux** typically produces "heartburn," or burning epigastric or mid chest pain, usually occurring after meals and worsening with recumbency. **Biliary colic** caused by gallstones typically has acute onset of severe pain located in the right upper quadrant or epigastrium, usually is precipitated by meals, especially fatty foods, lasts 30 to 60 minutes with spontaneous resolution, and is more common in women. **Irritable bowel syndrome** is a diagnosis of exclusion but is suggested by chronic dysmotility symptoms, (bloating, cramping) often relieved with defecation, without weight loss or bleeding. If these causes are excluded by history or other investigations, it is still difficult to clinically distinguish by symptoms the patients with PUD and those without ulcers, termed *nonulcer dyspepsia*.

The classic symptoms of **duodenal ulcers** are caused by the presence of acid without food or other buffers. Symptoms are typically produced after the stomach is emptied but food-stimulated acid production still persists, typically 2 to 5 hours after a meal. They may awaken patients at night, when circadian rhythms increase acid production. The pain is typically relieved within minutes by neutralization of acid by food or antacids (eg, calcium carbonate, aluminum-magnesium hydroxide). **Gastric ulcers**, by contrast, are more variable in their presentation. Food may actually worsen symptoms in patients with gastric ulcer, or pain might not be relieved by antacids. In fact, many patients with PUD have no symptoms at all. **Gastric cancers** may present with dysphagia if they are located in the cardiac region of the stomach, with persistent vomiting if they block the pyloric channel, or with early satiety by their mass effect or infiltration of the stomach wall. They may present with pain symptoms as a result of ulcer formation.

Because the incidence of gastric cancer increases with age, patients **older than 45 years** who present with **new-onset dyspepsia** should generally undergo endoscopy. In addition, patients with **alarm symptoms** (eg, weight loss, recurrent vomiting, dysphagia, evidence of bleeding, or anemia) should be referred for prompt endoscopy. Finally, endoscopy should be recommended for patients whose symptoms have **failed to respond** to empiric therapy. When endoscopy is undertaken, besides visualization of the ulcer, biopsy samples can be taken to exclude the possibility of malignancy as the cause of a gastric ulcer, and biopsy specimens can be obtained for urease testing or microscopic examination to prove current H pylori infection.

In **younger patients with no alarm features**, an acceptable strategy is to perform a noninvasive **H pylori antibody test** to determine if the patient is infected. Helicobacter pylori is more common in older patients, in lower socioeconomic groups, in institutionalized patients, and in developing countries. It has been established as the causative agent in the majority of duodenal and gastric ulcers, and it is associated with the development of gastric carcinoma and gastric mucosa–associated lymphoid tissue (MALT) lymphoma. The two most common tests are the **urea breath test**, which provides evidence of current active infection, and **H pylori antibody** tests, which provide evidence of prior infection but will remain positive for life, even after successful treatment. Because chronic infection with H pylori is found in 90% to 95% of duodenal ulcers and in 80% of patients with gastric ulcers not related to NSAID use, a suggested strategy is to test for infection and, if present, to treat it with an antibiotic regimen such as clarithromycin and amoxicillin, as well as acid suppression with a proton pump inhibitor. The reason for treating infection with antibiotics is that eradication of the infection will largely prevent recurrence. Whether treatment of H pylori infection reduces or eliminates dyspeptic symptoms in the absence of ulcers (nonulcer dyspepsia) is uncertain. Similarly, whether treatment of asymptomatic patients found to be H pylori positive is beneficial is unclear. In H. pylori–positive patients with dyspepsia, antibiotic treatment may be considered, but a follow-up visit is recommended within 4 to 8 weeks. If symptoms persist or alarm features develop, then prompt upper endoscopy is indicated.

In addition to H. pylori, the other major cause of duodenal and gastric ulcers is the use of **NSAIDs**. They promote ulcer formation by inhibiting gastroduodenal prostaglandin synthesis, resulting in reduced secretion of mucus and bicarbonate and decreased mucosal blood flow. In other words, they impair local defenses against acid damage. The risk of ulcer formation caused by NSAID use is dose dependent and can occur within days after treatment is initiated. If ulceration occurs, the NSAID should be discontinued if possible, and acid-suppression therapy with an H_2-receptor antagonist or proton pump inhibitor should be initiated.

A rare cause of ulcer is the **Zollinger-Ellison syndrome**, a condition in which a gastrin-producing tumor (usually pancreatic) causes acid hypersecretion, peptic ulceration, and often diarrhea. This condition should be suspected if ulcer disease occurs and the patient is *H pylori* negative and does not use NSAIDs. To diagnose this condition, one should measure serum gastrin levels, which are markedly elevated (>1000 pg/mL), and then try to localize the tumor with an imaging study.

Hemorrhage is the most common severe complication of PUD and can present with hematemesis or melena. **Free perforation** into the abdominal cavity may occur in association with hemorrhage, with sudden onset of pain and development of peritonitis. If the perforation occurs adjacent to the pancreas, it may induce pancreatitis. Some patients with chronic ulcers later develop **gastric outlet obstruction**, with persistent vomiting and weight loss but no abdominal distention. Perforation and obstruction are indications for surgical intervention.

Comprehension Questions

4.1   A 42-year-old overweight but otherwise healthy woman presents with sudden onset of right upper abdominal colicky pain 45 minutes after a meal of fried chicken. The pain is associated with nausea and vomiting, and any attempt to eat since has caused increased pain. Which of the following is the most likely cause?

A. Gastric ulcer
B. Cholelithiasis
C. Duodenal ulcer
D. Acute hepatitis

4.2   Which of the following is the most accurate statement regarding *H pylori* infection?

A. It is more common in developed than underdeveloped countries.
B. It is associated with the development of colon cancer.
C. It is believed to be the cause of nonulcer dyspepsia.
D. The route of transmission is believed to be sexually transmitted.
E. It is believed to be a common cause of both duodenal and gastric ulcers.

4.3   A 45-year-old man was brought to the emergency room after vomiting bright red blood. He has a blood pressure of 88/46 mm Hg and heart rate of 120 bpm. Which of the following is the best next step?

A. Intravenous fluid resuscitation and preparation for a transfusion
B. Administration of a proton pump inhibitor
C. Guaiac test of the stool
D. Treatment for *H. pylori*

4.4   Which one of the following patients should be promptly referred for
       endoscopy?
       A. A 65-year-old man with new onset of epigastric pain and weight loss
       B. A 32-year-old patient whose symptoms are not relieved with ranitidine
       C. A 29-year-old *H. pylori*-positive patient with dyspeptic symptoms
       D. A 49-year-old woman with intermittent right upper quadrant pain
          following meals

ANSWERS

4.1   **B.** Right upper abdominal pain of acute onset that occurs after inges-
       tion of a fatty meal and is associated with nausea and vomiting is
       most suggestive of biliary colic as a result of gallstones. Duodenal
       ulcer pain is likely to be diminished with food, and gastric ulcer pain
       is not likely to have acute severe onset. Acute hepatitis is more likely
       to produce dull ache and tenderness.

4.2   **E.** Although *H pylori* is clearly linked to gastric and duodenal ulcers
       and probably to gastric carcinoma and lymphoma, whether it is more
       common in patients with nonulcer dyspepsia and whether treatment
       in those patients reduces symptoms are unclear. It is more common
       in underdeveloped or developing countries.

4.3   **A.** This patient is hemodynamically unstable with hypotension and
       tachycardia as a consequence of the acute blood loss. Volume resusci-
       tation, immediately with crystalloid or colloid solution, followed by
       blood transfusion, if necessary, is the initial step to prevent irreversible
       shock and death. Later, after stabilization, acid suppression and *H pylori*
       treatment might be useful to heal an ulcer, if one is present.

4.4   **A.** Patient in answer A has "red flag" symptoms: he is older than 45 years
       and has new onset symptoms. Patient in answer B may benefit from
       the reassurance of a negative endoscopic examination. Patient in
       answer C, however, may benefit from treatment of her *H pylori* first.
       Some studies indicate this approach may be cost-saving overall. This
       patient could be sent for an endoscopic examination if she does not
       improve following the therapy.

Clinical Pearls

➤ The most common causes of duodenal and gastric ulcers are *Helicobacter pylori* infection and use of nonsteroidal anti-inflammatory drugs.

➤ *Helicobacter pylori* is associated with duodenal and gastric ulcers, chronic active gastritis, gastric adenocarcinoma, and gastric mucosa–associated lymphoid tissue lymphoma. It is not definitively associated with nonulcer dyspepsia.

➤ Treatment of peptic ulcers requires acid suppression with an H_2 blocker or proton-pump inhibitor to heal the ulcer, as well as antibiotic therapy of *Helicobacter pylori* infection, if present, to prevent recurrence.

➤ Patients with dyspepsia who have "red flag" symptoms (new dyspepsia after age 45 years, weight loss, dysphagia, evidence of bleeding or anemia) should be referred for an early endoscopic examination.

➤ Other patients (patients with dyspepsia who does not have "red flag" symptoms) may be tested for *Helicobacter pylori* and treated first. Antibody tests show evidence of infection but remain positive for life, even after successful treatment. Urea breath tests are evidence of current infection.

➤ Common treatment regimens for *Helicobacter pylori* infection include a 14-day course of a proton-pump inhibitor in high doses (e.g., lansoprazole 30 mg twice daily or omeprazole 20 mg twice daily) along with antibiotic therapy, usually clarithromycin and amoxicillin.

REFERENCES

Bytzer P, Talley NJ. Dyspepsia. *Ann Intern Med*. 2001;134:815.

Del Valle J. Peptic ulcer disease and related disorders. In: Kasper DL, Braunwald E, Fauci AS, et al, eds. *Harrison's Principles of Internal Medicine*. 17th ed. New York, NY: McGraw-Hill; 2008:1855-1872.

Suerbaum S, Michetti P. Medical progress: *Helicobacter pylori* infection. *N Engl J Med*. 2002;347:1175-1186.

Vakil N, Connor J. *Helicobacter pylori* eradication: equivalence trials and the optimal duration of therapy. *Am J Gastroenterol*. 2005;100:702.

Case 5

A 65-year-old white woman is brought to the emergency room by her family for increasing confusion and lethargy over the past week. She was recently diagnosed with small cell cancer of the lung. She has not been febrile or had any other recent illnesses. She is not taking any medications. Her blood pressure is 136/82 mm Hg, heart rate 84 bpm, and respiratory rate 14 breaths per minute and unlabored. She is afebrile. On examination, she is an elderly appearing woman who is difficult to arouse and reacts only to painful stimuli. She is able to move her extremities without apparent motor deficits, and her deep tendon reflexes are decreased symmetrically. The remainder of her examination is normal, with a normal jugular venous pressure and no extremity edema. You order some laboratory tests, which reveal the serum sodium level is 108 mmol/L, potassium 3.8 mmol/L, bicarbonate 24 mEq/L, blood urea nitrogen 5 mg/dL, and creatinine 0.5 mg/dL. Serum osmolality is 220 mOsm/kg, and urine osmolality is 400 mOsm/kg. A computed tomographic (CT) scan of the brain shows no masses or hydrocephalus.

➤ What is the most likely diagnosis?

➤ What is your next step in therapy?

➤ What are the complications of therapy?

ANSWERS TO CASE 5:

Hyponatremia, Syndrome of Inappropriate Secretion of Antidiuretic Hormone

Summary: A 65-year-old white woman with small cell lung cancer has increasing confusion and lethargy over the past week. She is afebrile and normotensive, and she has no edema or jugular venous distention. She is lethargic but is able to move her extremities without apparent motor deficits, and her deep tendon reflexes are decreased symmetrically. Her serum sodium level is 108 mmol/L, potassium 3.8 mmol/L, bicarbonate 24 mEq/L, blood urea nitrogen (BUN) 5 mg/dL, and creatinine 0.5 mg/dL; serum osmolality is 220 mOsm/kg, and urine osmolality is 400 mOsm/kg. A CT scan of the brain shows no masses or hydrocephalus.

➤ **Most likely diagnosis:** Coma/lethargy secondary to severe hyponatremia, which is most likely caused by a tumor-related syndrome of inappropriate secretion of antidiuretic hormone (SIADH).

➤ **Next therapeutic step:** Treat the hyponatremia with hypertonic saline.

➤ **Most serious complication of this therapy:** Osmotic cerebral demyelination, also referred to as central pontine myelinolysis.

ANALYSIS

Objectives

1. Learn the causes of hyponatremia.
2. Understand the use of laboratory testing in the diagnosis of hyponatremia.
3. Know how to treat hyponatremia, and some of the potential complications of therapy.

Considerations

This elderly woman with small cell lung cancer presents in a stuporous state with hypotonic hyponatremia. She appears euvolemic, as she does not have findings suggestive of either volume overload (jugular venous distention or peripheral edema) or volume depletion. She has no focal neurologic deficits or apparent masses on CT scan of the brain suggesting cerebral metastases. The most likely cause for her mental status alteration is the hyponatremia. The patient does not take medications; thus, with the situation of hypotonic hyponatremia in a euvolemic state and with inappropriately concentrated urine, the most likely etiology is inappropriate antidiuretic hormone produced by the lung cancer. Therapy is guided by the severity of the hyponatremia and the symptoms. Because this individual is stuporous and the sodium level is severely decreased, hypertonic saline is required with fairly rapid partial correction. This therapy is not benign and requires monitoring in intensive care unit (ICU). Also, the target is not correction of the sodium level to normal but rather to a level of safety, such as 120 to 125 mmol/L.

APPROACH TO
Hyponatremia

DEFINITIONS

ANTIDIURETIC HORMONE (ADH): Also referred to as arginine vasopressin (AVP), ADH is the posterior pituitary hormone that controls excretion of free water and thus, indirectly, sodium concentration and serum tonicity.

OSMOLALITY: Concentration of osmotically active particles, which draw water into a compartment; normal range is 280 to 300 mOsm/kg.

SYNDROME OF INAPPROPRIATE SECRETION OF ANTIDIURETIC HORMONE (SIADH): Nonphysiologic elevation of ADH levels as a consequence of ectopic production, as in malignancy, or stimulation of excess pituitary production by various pulmonary or central nervous system (CNS) diseases.

CLINICAL APPROACH

Hyponatremia is defined as a serum sodium level <135 mmol/L and is, by far, the **most common electrolyte disturbance among hospitalized patients**. Patients are often asymptomatic, especially if the hyponatremia develops slowly. Depending on the rapidity with which the hyponatremia develops, most patients do not have symptoms until the serum sodium level is in the low 120 mmol/L range. The clinical manifestations are related to osmotic water shifts leading to cerebral edema; thus, the symptoms are mainly neurological: lethargy, confusion, seizures, or coma.

Serum sodium concentrations are important because they almost always reflect tonicity, the effect of extracellular fluid on cells that will cause the cells (eg, brain cells) to swell (hypotonicity) or to shrink (hypertonicity). For purposes of this discussion, we use serum osmolality as a valid indicator of tonicity, which is almost always true, so we use the terms interchangeably. Whereas hypernatremia always reflects hyperosmolality, hyponatremia may occur in the setting of hyperosmolality, normal osmolality, or hypoosmolality (Table 5–1).

Hyponatremia associated with a hypoosmolar state is more common and more dangerous. Some hyponatremic conditions are associated with hyperosmolarity or with normal osmolarity. **Hyperosmolar hyponatremia** is most often caused by an increase in the serum level of an osmotically active

Table 5–1 CAUSES OF HYPONATREMIA

Pseudohyponatremia

Normal plasma osmolarity
- -Hyperlipidemia
- Hyperproteinemia
- Posttransurethral resection of prostate/bladder tumor

Increased plasma osmolarity
- Hyperglycemia
- Mannitol

Hypoosmolar hyponatremia

Primary Na⁺ loss (secondary water gain)
- Integumentary loss: sweating, burns
- Gastrointestinal loss: vomiting, tube drainage, fistula, obstruction, diarrhea
- Renal loss: diuretics, osmotic diuresis, hypoaldosteronism, salt-wasting nephropathy, postobstructive diuresis, nonoliguric acute tubular necrosis

Primary water gain (secondary Na⁺ loss)
- Primary polydipsia
- Decreased solute intake (eg, beer potomania)
- AVP release as a result of pain, nausea, drugs, etc
- Syndrome of inappropriate AVP secretion
- Glucocorticoid deficiency
- Hypothyroidism
- Chronic renal insufficiency

Primary Na⁺ gain (exceeded by secondary water gain)
- Heart failure
- Hepatic cirrhosis
- Nephrotic syndrome

Reproduced, with permission, from Braunwald E, Fauci AS, Kasper KL, et al, eds. Harrison's Principles of Internal Medicine. *17th ed. New York, NY: McGraw-Hill; 2008:277.*

molecule that is confined to the extracellular space and that cannot readily cross cell membranes, such as glucose or mannitol. These solutes draw water out from the intracellular space, leading to relative hyponatremia. Hyperglycemia occurs in the setting of insulin-deficient states, such as uncontrolled diabetes mellitus. For glucose, each 100 mg/dL increase in serum glucose leads to an approximately 1.6 mmol/L decrease in the serum sodium level. Transurethral resection of the prostate is a common cause of hyponatremia because of the large volume of mannitol-containing bladder irrigation fluid used intraoperatively. For either of these states, correction of the glucose level (or excretion of the mannitol) corrects the hyponatremia.

Pseudohyponatremia refers to an artifact of measurement in states where the serum sodium level and, thus, the tonicity are, in fact, normal. In the past this occurred when high serum proteins levels (as in a paraproteinemia such as multiple myeloma) or very high lipid levels interfered with measurement of the serum sodium level. With current laboratory technology, the sodium level is directly measured, so pseudohyponatremia is not common. One can suspect pseudohyponatremia if the measured and calculated serum osmolarities are different.

Hypotonic hyponatremia *always* occurs because there is water gain, that is, restriction or impairment of free water excretion. If one considers that the normal kidney capacity to excrete free water is approximately 18 to 20 L/d, it becomes apparent that it is very difficult to overwhelm this capacity solely through excessive water intake. Therefore, when hyponatremia develops, the kidney is usually holding on to free water, either pathologically, as in SIADH, or physiologically, as an attempt to maintain effective circulating volume when patients are significantly volume depleted. Hyponatremia can also occur in cases of sodium loss, for example, as a consequence of diuretic use, or because of aldosterone deficiency. However, in those cases, there is then a secondary gain of free water.

To determine the cause of the hypotonic hyponatremia, the physician must clinically assess the volume status of the patient by history and physical examination. A history of vomiting, diarrhea, or other losses, such as profuse sweating, suggests hypovolemia, as do flat neck veins, dry oral mucous membranes, and diminished urine output. In cases of significant hypovolemia, there is a physiologic increase in ADH in an attempt to retain free water to maintain circulating volume, even at the expense of hypotonicity. In these cases, the excess ADH is not "inappropriate" as in SIADH, but extremely appropriate. At this point, one can check the urinary sodium levels. In hypovolemia, the kidney should be avidly retaining sodium, so the urine sodium level should be less than 20 mmol/L. If the patient is hypovolemic, yet the urine sodium level is more than 20 mmol/L, then kidneys do not have the ability to retain sodium normally. Either kidney function is impaired by the use of diuretics, or the kidney is lacking necessary hormonal stimulation, as in adrenal insufficiency, or there is a primary renal problem, such as tubular damage from acute tubular necrosis. When patients are **hypovolemic,** treatment of the hyponatremia requires **correction of the volume status, usually replacement with isotonic (0.9%) or "normal" saline.**

Hypervolemia is usually apparent as edema or elevated jugular venous pressure. It commonly occurs as a result **of congestive heart failure, cirrhosis of the liver, or the nephrotic syndrome**. In these edematous disorders, there is usually a total body excess of both sodium and water, yet arterial baroreceptors perceive hypoperfusion or a decrease in intravascular volume, which leads to an increase in the level of ADH and, therefore, retention of free water by the kidneys. Renal failure itself can lead to hypotonic hyponatremia because of an inability to excrete dilute urine. In any of these cases, the usual initial treatment of hyponatremia is administration of diuretics to reduce excess salt and water. Thus, hypovolemic or hypervolemic hyponatremia is often apparent clinically and often does not present a diagnostic challenge. Euvolemic hyponatremia, however, is a frequent problem that is not so easily diagnosed. Once the clinician has diagnosed the patient with euvolemic hypotonic hyponatremia, the next step is to measure the urine osmolarity. This measurement is taken to determine whether the kidney is actually capable of excreting the free water normally (osmolality should be maximally dilute, <100 mOsm/kg in the face of hyposmolality or excess free water) or whether the free water excretion is impaired (urine not maximally concentrated, >150-200 mOsm/kg). If the urine is maximally dilute, it is handling free water normally but its capacity for excretion has been overwhelmed, as in central polydipsia. More commonly, free water excretion is impaired and the urine is not maximally dilute as it should be. Two important diagnoses must be considered at this point: **hypothyroidism** and **adrenal insufficiency. Thyroid hormone and cortisol both are permissive for free water excretion, so their deficiency causes water retention.** Isolated cortisol deficiency can mimic SIADH. In contrast, patients with Addison disease also lack aldosterone, so they have impaired ability to retain sodium. Patients with adrenal insufficiency are usually hypovolemic and often present in shock.

Euvolemic hyponatremia is most commonly caused by **SIADH.** Nonphysiologic nonosmotically mediated (therefore "inappropriate") secretion can occur in the setting of pulmonary disease, CNS disease, pain, in the postoperative period, or as part of a paraneoplastic syndrome. Because of retention of free water, patients actually have mild (although clinically inapparent) volume expansion. Additionally, if they have a normal dietary sodium intake, the kidneys do not retain sodium avidly. Therefore, modest natriuresis occurs so that the urine sodium level is elevated to more than 20 mmol/L. **SIADH is a diagnosis of exclusion:** the patient must be hypoosmolar but euvolemic, with urine that is not maximally dilute (osmolality >150-200 mOsm/L), urine sodium more than 20 mmol/L, and normal adrenal and thyroid function. Some laboratory clues to SIADH are low BUN and low uric acid levels. Unless the patient has severe neurologic symptoms, the treatment of SIADH is water restriction.

Patients with **severe neurologic symptoms**, such as seizures or coma, require **rapid** partial correction of the sodium level. The treatment of choice is hypertonic (eg, 3%) saline. When there is concern that the saline infusion might cause volume overload, the infusion can be administered with a loop diuretic such as furosemide. The diuretic will cause the excretion of hypotonic urine that is essentially "half-normal saline," so a greater portion of sodium than water will be retained, helping to correct the serum sodium level.

When hyponatremia occurs for any reason, especially when it occurs slowly, the brain adapts to prevent cerebral edema. Solutes leave the intracellular compartment of the brain over hours to days, so patients may have few neurologic symptoms despite very low serum sodium levels. If the serum sodium level is corrected rapidly, the brain does not have time to readjust, and it may shrink rapidly as it loses fluid to the extracellular space. It is believed that this rapid shrinkage may trigger demyelination of the cerebellar and pontine neurons. This **osmotic cerebral demyelination**, or **central pontine**

myelinolysis, may cause **quadriplegia, pseudobulbar palsies, a "locked-in" syndrome, coma, or death**. Demyelination can occur even when fluid restriction is the treatment used to correct the serum sodium level. Therefore, several expert authors have published formulas and guidelines for the slow and judicious correction of hyponatremia, but the general rule is not to correct the serum sodium concentration faster than 0.5 to 1 mEq/h.

Comprehension Questions

5.1   A 24-year-old man develops seizures following an emergent splenectomy after a car accident. His serum sodium level is initially 116 mEq/L and is corrected to 120 mEq/L over the next 3 hours with hypertonic saline. Which of the following factors most likely led to his hyponatremia?

   A. Elevation of serum vasopressin
   B. Administration of hypertonic solutions
   C. Volume depletion
   D. Seizure-induced hyponatremia

5.2   A 56-year-old man presents to the doctor for the first time complaining of fatigue and weight loss. He has never had any health problems, but he has smoked a pack of cigarettes per day for about 35 years. He is a day laborer and is currently homeless and living in a shelter. His physical examination is notable for a low to normal blood pressure, skin hyperpigmentation, and digital clubbing. He appears euvolemic. You tell him you are not sure of the problem as yet, but you will draw some blood tests and schedule him for follow-up in 1 week. The laboratory calls that night and informs you that the patient's sodium level is 126 mEq/L, potassium level is 6.7 mEq/L, creatine level is normal, and bicarbonate and chloride levels are low. Which of the following is the likely cause of his hyponatremia given his presentation?

   A. SIADH
   B. Hypothyroidism
   C. Gastrointestinal losses
   D. Adrenal insufficiency
   E. Renal insufficiency

5.3   An 83-year-old woman comes to your office complaining of a
       headache and mild confusion. Her medical history is remarkable only
       for hypertension, which is well controlled with hydrochlorothiazide.
       Her examination and laboratory tests show no signs of infection, but her
       serum sodium level is 119 mEq/L, and plasma osmolarity is 245 mOsm/kg.
       She appears to be clinically hypovolemic. Which of the following is
       the best initial therapy?
       A. Fluid restriction
       B. Infusion of 0.9% saline
       C. Infusion of 3% saline
       D. Infusion of 3% saline with furosemide

5.4   A 58-year-old man has undergone a lengthy colon cancer surgery. On
       the first postoperative day, he is noted to have significant hypona-
       tremia with a sodium level of 128 mEq/L. You suspect that the hypona-
       tremia is due to the intravenous infusion of hypotonic solution. Which
       of the following laboratory findings supports your diagnosis?
       A. Urine sodium >20mmol/L
       B. Urine osmolality >200 mOsm/L
       C. Serum osmolarity <280 mOsm/kg
       D. Serum potassium >5.0 mEq/L

ANSWERS

5.1   **A.** In the postoperative state or in situations where the patient is in
       pain, the serum vasopressin level may rise, leading to inappropriate
       retention of free water, which leads to dilution of the serum.
       Concomitant administration of hypotonic fluids may exacerbate the
       situation.

5.2   **D.** Hyponatremia in the setting of hyperkalemia and acidosis is sus-
       picious for adrenal insufficiency. This patient's examination is also
       suggestive of the diagnosis, given his complaints of fatigue, weight
       loss, low blood pressure, and hyperpigmentation. The diagnosis is
       made by a 24-hour urine cortisol test or by measuring the response to
       adrenocorticotropic hormone (ACTH) stimulation. The underlying
       cause of the adrenal gland destruction in this patient probably is
       either tuberculosis or malignancy.

5.3   **B.** Because the patient is hypovolemic, probably as a result of the use
       of diuretics, volume replacement with isotonic saline is the best ini-
       tial therapy. Hyponatremia caused by thiazide diuretics can occur by
       several mechanisms, including volume depletion. It is most common
       in elderly women.

5.4   **C.** In a patient with hyponatremia due to the infusion of excessive hypotonic solution, the serum osmolality should be low. The kidneys in responding normally should attempt to retain sodium and excrete water; hence, the urine sodium concentration should be low, and the urine osmolality should be low. When the infusion of hypotonic solution is used, the serum potassium level will also be low. This is in contrast to a situation of mineralocorticoid deficiency in which the sodium level will be decreased and potassium level may be elevated. Similarly, hyperaldosteronism can lead to hypertension and hypokalemia (Conn syndrome).

Clinical Pearls

➤ Hyponatremia almost always occurs by impairment of free water excretion.

➤ Syndrome of inappropriate secretion of antidiuretic hormone is a diagnosis of exclusion. Criteria include euvolemic patient, serum hypoosmolarity, urine that is not maximally dilute (osmolality >150-200 mmol/L), urine sodium more than 20 mmol/L, and normal adrenal and thyroid function.

➤ Hypovolemic patients with hyponatremia should be treated with volume replacement, typically with isotonic (0.9%) saline.

➤ Euvolemic patients with asymptomatic hyponatremia can be treated with fluid restriction. Patients with severe symptoms, such as coma or seizures, should be treated with hypertonic (3%) saline.

➤ The rate of sodium correction generally should not exceed 0.5 to 1 mEq/h, otherwise central pontine myelinolysis (osmotic demyelination) can occur.

REFERENCES

Androgue H, Madias N. Hyponatremia. *N Engl J Med.* 2000;342:1581-1589.

Lin M, Liu SJ, Lim IT. Disorders of water imbalance. *Emerg Med Clin North Am.* 2005;23:749-770.

Robertson G. Disorders of the neurohypophysis. In: Kasper DL, Braunwald E, Fauci AS, et al, eds. *Harrison's Principles of Internal Medicine.*17th ed. New York, NY: McGraw-Hill; 2008:2217-2224.

Singer G, Brenner B. Fluid and electrolyte disturbances. In: Kasper DL, Braunwald E, Fauci AS, et al, eds. *Harrison's Principles of Internal Medicine.* 17th ed. New York, NY: McGraw-Hill; 2008:274-285.

Case 6

A 42-year-old man is brought to the emergency room by ambulance after a sudden onset of severe retrosternal chest pain that began an hour ago while he was at home mowing the lawn. He describes the pain as sharp, constant, and unrelated to movement. It was not relieved by three doses of sublingual nitroglycerin administered by the paramedics while en route to the hospital. He has never had symptoms like this before. His only medical history is hypertension, for which he takes enalapril. There is no cardiac disease in his family. He does not smoke, drink alcohol, or use illicit drugs. He is a basketball coach at a local high school, and is usually physically very active.

On physical examination, he is a tall man with long arms and legs who appears uncomfortable and diaphoretic; he is lying on the stretcher with his eyes closed. He is afebrile, with a heart rate of 118 bpm, and blood pressure of 156/100 mm Hg in the right arm and 188/94 mm Hg in the left arm. His head and neck examination is unremarkable. His chest is clear to auscultation bilaterally, and incidental note is made of pectus excavatum. His heart rate is tachycardic and regular, with a soft, early diastolic murmur at the right sternal border. His abdominal examination is benign, and neurologic examination is nonfocal. His chest X-ray shows a widened mediastinum.

➤ What is the most likely diagnosis?

➤ What is your next step?

ANSWERS TO CASE 6:

Aortic Dissection, Marfan Syndrome

Summary: A 42-year-old man is brought in to the emergency room with severe chest pain, which was unrelieved by nitroglycerin. His blood pressure is elevated but asymmetric in his arms, and he has a new murmur of aortic insufficiency. The chest X-ray shows a widened mediastinum. All of these features strongly suggest aortic dissection as the cause of his pain. He is tall with pectus excavatum and other features of Marfan syndrome, which may be the underlying cause of his dissection.

➤ **Most likely diagnosis:** Aortic dissection.

➤ **Next step:** Administer an intravenous beta-blocker and perform a noninvasive imaging procedure, such as transesophageal echocardiography (TEE), CT (computed tomography) angiography, or magnetic resonance imaging (MRI).

ANALYSIS

Objectives

1. Learn the clinical and radiographic features of aortic dissection as well as complications of dissection.
2. Know the risk factors for aortic dissection.
3. Understand the management of dissection and the indications for surgical versus medical treatment.
4. Learn about other aortic diseases, such as abdominal aortic aneurysm (AAA), the role of surveillance, and indications for surgical repair.

Considerations

Most patients with chest pain seek medical attention because they are concerned about a myocardial infarction (MI). Differentiating other conditions of chest pain is important because some underlying conditions, such as aortic dissection, could be worsened by the treatment of MI, for example, by anticoagulation with heparin or use of thrombolytics. In hypertensive patients with dissection, urgent blood pressure lowering is indicated to limit propagation of the dissection.

APPROACH TO
Aortic Aneurysm and Dissection

DEFINITIONS

ABDOMINAL AORTIC ANEURYSM (AAA): Defined as a pathologic dilation to more than 1.5 times the normal diameter of the aorta. Aneurysms can occur anywhere in the thoracic or abdominal aorta, but the large majority occur in the abdomen, below the renal arteries.

AORTIC DISSECTION (DISSECTING HEMATOMA): Tear or ulceration of the aortic intima that allows pulsatile aortic flow to dissect longitudinally along elastic planes of the media, creating a false lumen or channel for blood flow. Sometimes referred to as a "dissecting aneurysm," although the term is misleading because the dissection typically produces the aneurysmal dilation rather than the reverse.

CLINICAL APPROACH

The aorta is the largest conductance vessel in the body. It receives most of the shear forces generated by the heart with every heartbeat throughout the lifetime of an individual. The wall of the aorta is composed of three layers: the intima, the media, and the adventitia. These specialized layers allow the aortic wall to distend under the great pressure created by every heartbeat. Some of this kinetic energy is stored as potential energy, thus allowing forward flow to be maintained during the cardiac cycle. One must consider the great tensile stress that the walls of this vessel faces when considering the pathologic processes that affect it.

Cystic degeneration of the elastic media predisposes patients to aortic dissection. This occurs in various connective tissue disorders that cause cystic medial degeneration, such as Marfan and Ehlers-Danlos syndrome. Other factors predisposing to aortic dissection are hypertension, aortic valvular abnormalities such as aortic stenosis and congenital bicuspid aortic valve, coarctation of the aorta, pregnancy, and atherosclerotic disease. Aortic dissection may occur iatrogenically after cardiac surgery or catheterization.

A dissection occurs when there is a sudden intimal tear or rupture followed by the formation of a dissecting hematoma within the aortic media, separating the intima from the adventitia and propagating distally. The presence of hypertension and associated shear forces are the most important factors causing propagation of the dissection. Aortic dissection can produce several devastating or fatal complications. It can produce an intraluminal intimal flap, which can occlude branch arteries and cause organ ischemia or infarction. The hematoma may rupture into the pericardial sac, causing cardiac tamponade, or into the pleural space, causing exsanguination. It can produce severe acute aortic regurgitation leading to fulminant heart failure.

The clinical features of aortic dissection typically include a **sudden onset of ripping or tearing pain in the chest, which often radiates to the back** and may radiate to the neck or extremities as the dissection extends (Table 6–1). Differentiating the pain of dissection from the pain of myocardial ischemia or infarction is essential because **the use of anticoagulation or thrombolytics in a patient with a dissection may be devastating**. In contrast to anginal pain, which often builds over minutes, the pain of dissection is **often maximal at onset**. In addition, myocardial ischemia pain usually is relieved with nitrates, whereas the pain of dissection is not. Also, because most dissections begin very close to the aortic valve, a dissection may produce the **early diastolic murmur of aortic insufficiency**; if it occludes branch arteries, it can produce dramatically different pulses and blood pressures in the extremities. Most patients with dissection are hypertensive; if hypotension is present, one must suspect aortic rupture, cardiac tamponade, or dissection of the subclavian artery supplying the arm where the blood pressure is being measured. Often a widened superior mediastinum is noted on plain chest film because of dissection of the ascending aorta.

When aortic dissection is suspected, confirming the diagnosis with an imaging study is essential. Conventional aortography was the traditional diagnostic "gold standard," but in recent years, very sensitive noninvasive studies, such as TEE, dynamic CT scanning, and MRI, have gained widespread use. Because of the emergent nature of the condition, the best initial study is the one that can be obtained and interpreted quickly in the given hospital setting.

Several classification schemes describe the different types of aortic dissections. Figure 6–1 shows the Stanford classification. Type A dissection always involves the ascending aorta but can involve any other part. Type B dissection does not involve the ascending aorta but can involve any other part.

Table 6–1 CLINICAL MANIFESTATION OF AORTIC DISSECTION

Horner syndrome	Compression of the superior cervical ganglion
Superior vena cava syndrome	Compression of the superior vena cava
Hemopericardium, pericardial tamponade	Thoracic dissection with retrograde flow into the pericardium
Aortic regurgitation	Thoracic dissection involving the aortic root
Bowel ischemia, hematuria	Dissection involving the mesenteric arteries or renal arteries
Hypertension, different blood pressures in arms	Thoracic dissection involving brachiocephalic artery
Hemiplegia	Carotid artery involvement

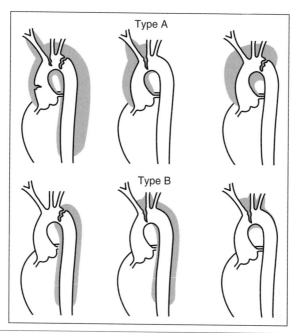

Figure 6–1. Classification of aortic aneurysms. *Reproduced, with permission, from Doroghazi RM, Slater EE. Aortic dissection. In: Braunwald E, Fauci AS, Kasper DL, et al, eds.* Harrison's Principles of Internal Medicine. *17th ed. New York, NY: McGraw-Hill; 2008:1566.*

Two-thirds of aortic dissections originate in the ascending aorta a few centimeters above the aortic valve. The classification system is important because it guides therapy. Virtually all **type A (proximal or ascending) dissections require urgent surgical therapy** with replacement of the involved aorta and sometimes the aortic valve. Without surgery, the mortality rate for type A dissections is 90%. Type B dissections do not involve the ascending aorta and typically originate in the aortic arch distal to the left subclavian artery. Type B dissections usually are first managed medically, and surgery usually is performed only for complications such as rupture or ischemia of a branch artery of the aorta. The aim of medical therapy is to prevent propagation of the dissection by reducing mean arterial pressure and the rate of rise (dP/dT) of arterial pressure, which correlates with arterial shear forces. Intravenous vasodilators, such as sodium nitroprusside to lower blood pressure, can be administered, along with intravenous beta-blockers, such as metoprolol, to reduce shear forces. Alternatively, one can administer intravenous labetalol, which accomplishes both tasks.

In marked contrast to the dramatic presentation of dissection of the thoracic aorta, patients with **AAAs typically are asymptomatic**; their **AAAs** often are detected by physical examination, with detection of a midline pulsatile mass, or are noted incidentally on ultrasound or other imaging procedure. The AAA usually is defined as a dilation of the aorta with a diameter more than 3 cm. It is found in 1.5% to 3% of older adults but in 5% to 10% of higher risk patients, such as those with known atherosclerotic disease. It is a degenerative condition typically found in older men (>50 years), most commonly in smokers, who often have atherosclerotic disease elsewhere, such as coronary artery disease or peripheral vascular disease.

The feared complication of AAA is spontaneous rupture. If the AAA ruptures anteriorly into the peritoneal cavity, the patient usually exsanguinates and dies within minutes. If the AAA ruptures posteriorly and the bleeding is confined to the retroperitoneum, the peritoneum can produce local tamponade, and the patient presents with severe lower back or midabdominal pain. Overall, the mortality rate of ruptured AAA is 80%, with 50% of patients dead before they reach the hospital.

The risk of rupture is related to the size of the aneurysm: the annual rate of rupture is low if the aneurysm is smaller than 5 cm but is at least 10% to 20% for 6-cm aneurysms. The risk of rupture must be weighed against the surgical risk of elective repair, which traditionally required excision of the diseased aorta and replacement with a Dacron graft. The Society for Vascular Surgery and the American Association for Vascular Surgery (2003) recommend **elective repair of AAAs 5.5 cm or greater** in diameter or those expanding more than 0.5 cm per year. As for surveillance of AAAs, the current recommendations are that patients undergo some sort of imaging of the aneurysm (MRI, CT scan, or ultrasound study) at 3- to 12-month intervals, depending on the risk of rupture. Recently, endovascular grafts with stents have been used as a less invasive procedure with less risk than the traditional surgical repair, but the exact role of this procedure remains to be defined.

Comprehension Questions

6.1   A 59-year-old man complains of severe chest pain that radiates to his back. His brachial pulses appear unequal. He appears hemodynamically stable. On chest radiography, he has a widened mediastinum. Which of the following is the best next step?

A. Initiate thrombolytic therapy.
B. Obtain CT of chest with intravenous contrast.
C. Initiate aspirin and heparin.
D. Measure serial cardiac enzyme levels.

6.2   A 45-year-old woman with new-onset aortic regurgitation is found to have aortic dissection of the ascending aorta and aortic arch by echocardiography. She is relatively asymptomatic. Which of the following is the best management?

A. Oral atenolol therapy and monitor the dissection
B. Angioplasty
C. Surgical correction
D. Oral warfarin (Coumadin) therapy

6.3   A healthy 75-year-old man undergoing an ultrasound examination for suspected gallbladder disease is found incidentally to have a 4.5-cm abdominal aneurysm of the aorta. Which of the following is the best management for this patient?
A. Surgical repair of the aneurysm
B. Serial ultrasound examinations every 6 months
C. Urgent MRI
D. Beta-agonist therapy

6.4   A 45-year-old man is concerned because his father died of a ruptured abdominal aortic aneurysm. On evaluation, he is found to have a bicuspid aortic valve. Which of the following is the most accurate statement regarding his condition?
A. He is at risk for an aortic aneurysm of the ascending aorta.
B. He is at risk for an abdominal aortic aneurysm.
C. He is not at increased risk for aortic aneurysms.
D. He should have surgical correction of the aortic valve.

ANSWERS

6.1   **B.** A CT scan of the chest is a quick imaging test to confirm the aortic dissection. Thrombolytic therapy or anticoagulation can worsen the process.

6.2   **C.** Surgery is urgently required in the event of aortic root or other proximal (type A) dissections. Unrecognized and hence untreated aortic dissection can quickly lead to exsanguination and death.

6.3   **B.** When an AAA reaches 5.5 cm or greater, surgery usually is indicated because the risk of rupture is increased. For asymptomatic aneurysms smaller than 5 cm, the 5-year risk of rupture is less than 1% to 2%, so serial noninvasive monitoring is an alternative strategy.

6.4   **C.** Risk factors for AAA include smoking, hypertension, and peripheral vascular disease. A bicuspid aortic valve is usually asymptomatic and does not place the patient at risk for aortic aneurysms.

Clinical Pearls

➤ Hypertension is an underlying factor that predisposes to aortic dissection in the majority of cases. Other patients at risk include those with Marfan syndrome, congenital aortic anomalies, or otherwise normal women in the third trimester of pregnancy.

➤ Urgent surgical repair is indicated for type A (ascending) aortic dissections. Uncomplicated, stable, type B (transverse or descending) aortic dissections can be managed medically.

➤ Medical therapy for aortic dissection includes intravenous beta-blockers such as metoprolol or labetalol to lower cardiac contractility, arterial pressure, and shear stress, thus limiting propagation of the dissection.

➤ Anticoagulation or thrombolytic therapy usually is contraindicated in aortic dissection.

➤ Aortic dissection may be complicated by rupture, occlusion of any branch artery of the aorta, or retrograde dissection with hemopericardium and cardiac tamponade.

➤ The risk of rupture of abdominal aortic aneurysms increases with size. Aneurysms larger than 5.5 cm should undergo elective surgical repair; those smaller than 5 cm can be monitored with serial ultrasonography or other imaging procedure.

➤ Chest pain in the face of a widened mediastinum on chest X-ray should suggest aortic dissection.

REFERENCES

Brewster DC, Cronenwett JL, Hallett JW Jr, et al. Guidelines for the treatment of abdominal aortic aneurysm. *J Vasc Surg*. 2003;37:1106-1117.

Creager MA, Loscalzo J. Diseases of the aorta. In: Fauci AS, Braunwald E, Kasper DL, eds. *Harrison's Principles of Internal Medicine*. 17th ed. New York, NY: McGraw-Hill; 2008:1563-1568.

Erbel R, Alfonso F, Boileau C, et al. Diagnosis and management of aortic dissection. *Eur Heart J*. 2001;22:1642-1681.

Powell JT, Greenhalgh RM. Clinical practice: small abdominal aortic aneurysms. *N Engl J Med*. 2003;348:1895-1901.

Case 7

A 32-year-old man infected with human immunodeficiency virus (HIV), whose last CD4 count is unknown, presents to the emergency room with a fever of 102.5°F. He was diagnosed with HIV infection approximately 3 years ago when he presented to his doctor with oral thrush. He was offered highly active antiretroviral therapy (HAART) and stayed on this regimen until approximately 10 months ago, when he lost his job and insurance and could no longer pay for the drugs and discontinued all treatment. He has felt more "run down" recently. For the last 2 to 3 weeks he has had fever and a nonproductive cough, and he has felt short of breath with mild exertion, such as when cleaning his house. On examination his blood pressure is 134/82 mm Hg, pulse 110 bpm, and respiratory rate 28 breaths per minute. His oxygen saturation on room air at rest is 89% but drops to 80% when he walks 100 feet, and his breathing becomes quite labored. His lungs are clear to auscultation, but white patches cover his buccal mucosa. Otherwise, his examination is unremarkable. Laboratory testing shows a leukocyte count of 2800 cells/mm^3. Serum lactic (acid) dehydrogenase (LDH) is 540 IU/L. His chest radiograph is shown in Figure 7–1.

➤ What is the most likely diagnosis?

➤ What is your next step?

➤ What other diagnoses should be considered?

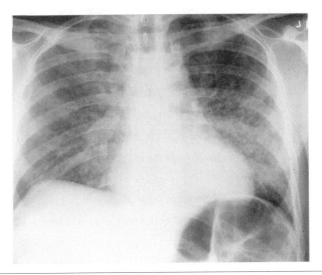

Figure 7–1. Chest radiograph. *Reproduced, with permission, from Walzer P. Pneumocystis carinii infection. In: Braunwald E, Fauci AS, Kasper KL, et al, eds.* Harrison's Principles of Internal Medicine. *15th ed. New York, NY: McGraw-Hill; 2001:1183.*

ANSWERS TO CASE 7:

HIV and Pneumocystis Pneumonia

Summary: A 32-year-old man with known HIV infection but unknown CD4 count presents with subacute onset of fever, dry cough, and gradually worsening dyspnea. He is not undergoing any antiretroviral therapy or taking prophylactic medications. Diffuse bilateral pulmonary infiltrate is seen on chest X-ray, and he is tachypneic and hypoxemic. The presence of oral thrush suggests that he is immunosuppressed. His leukocyte count is decreased, and his LDH level is elevated.

➤ **Most likely diagnosis:** Acquired immunodeficiency syndrome (AIDS) and probable *Pneumocystis* pneumonia (PCP).[1]

➤ **Next step:** The next step is to stabilize the patient, who is tachypneic and hypoxic but is in only mild distress and is hemodynamically stable. Therefore, there is time to further evaluate him. An arterial blood gas measurement can be obtained to quantify his degree of hypoxemia, as it will impact the treatment.

---

[1]As of 2002, the organism has been renamed *Pneumocystis jirovecii.* The abbreviation PCP remains for *Pneumocystis carinii* pneumonia.

➤ **Other diagnoses to be considered:** In patients with AIDS, other opportunistic infections must be considered. Other respiratory infections, such as tuberculosis (TB), atypical mycobacteria, cryptococcosis, and disseminated histoplasmosis, must be considered. In addition, HIV-infected patients are susceptible to the usual causes of community-acquired pneumonias: *Streptococcus pneumoniae*, mycoplasma, and viruses such as influenza.

ANALYSIS

Objectives

1. Understand the natural history of HIV infection.
2. Know the types of opportunistic infections that typically affect HIV-infected patients at various levels of immunocompromise.
3. Be familiar with respiratory infections in patients with AIDS.
4. Be familiar with indications for antiretroviral therapy and for prophylactic medications against opportunistic infections.

Considerations

This individual with HIV, currently not taking antiviral medications or any antibiotic prophylaxis, presents with subacute dyspnea and cough. His lack of sputum production and **elevated LDH** level is suggestive of PCP. The presence of oral thrush suggests a CD4 count less than 250. If the CD4 count is less than 200 cells/mm^3, then PCP seems the most likely explanation for his symptoms and chest X-ray findings. Obtaining an arterial blood gas measurement will provide information about prognosis and help guide therapy. Arterial oxygen concentration less than 70 mm Hg or alveolar-arterial gradient (A-a) more than 35 mm Hg suggests a worse prognosis and corticosteroids may be helpful, followed by treatment with trimethoprim-sulfamethoxazole (TMP-SMX).

APPROACH TO
HIV infections

DEFINITIONS

PNEUMOCYSTIS JIROVECII (Formerly Pneumocystis Carinii): A fungus which causes pneumonia in immunocompromised patients, especially those with HIV and CD4 counts less than 200 cells/mm^3.

AIDS: A CD4 count less than 200 cells/mm^3 or diagnosis of an AIDS defining illness in a patient who is HIV positive.

CLINICAL APPROACH

When evaluating a patient with HIV and suspected opportunistic infection, it is essential to know or estimate the patient's level of immunodeficiency. This is reflected by the CD4 (T4) cell count. Normal CD4 levels in adults range from 600 to 1500 cells/mm^3. As levels decline to less than 500 cells/mm^3, immune function is compromised, and patients become increasingly susceptible to unusual infections or malignancies.

Approximately 30% of patients first infected with HIV will develop an **acute HIV syndrome** characterized by sudden onset of a mononucleosis-like illness with fever, headaches, lymphadenopathy, pharyngitis, and sometimes a macular rash. The rest of the patients remain asymptomatic and have a clinically **latent period** of 8 to 10 years, on average, before the clinical manifestations of immunocompromise appear. As CD4 levels decline, various opportunistic infections appear. At CD4 levels less than **500**, patients are susceptible to infections, such as recurrent pneumonias, tuberculosis (TB), vaginal candidiasis, and herpes zoster. At CD4 levels less than **200**, patients are significantly immunocompromised and develop infections with organisms that rarely cause significant illness in immunocompetent hosts, such as *Pneumocystis jirovecii* (formerly *Pneumocystis carinii*), toxoplasmosis, cryptococcosis, histoplasmosis, or cryptosporidiosis. At CD4 levels less than **50**, patients are severely immunocompromised and are susceptible to disseminated infection with histoplasmosis and *Mycobacterium avium*–intracellulare complex (MAC) as well as development of cytomegalovirus (CMV) retinitis, colitis, and esophagitis, or primary central nervous system (CNS) lymphoma. The Centers for Disease Control and Prevention (CDC) has published a list of clinical conditions which define progression to AIDS in patient who is HIV positive, so called AIDS-defining conditions (see Table 7-1).

Pneumocystis pneumonia **(PCP)** remains the **most common opportunistic infection affecting AIDS patients** but often is very difficult to diagnose. The clinical presentation ranges from fever without respiratory symptoms, to mild, persistent, **dry cough,** to significant hypoxemia and respiratory compromise. In addition, the radiographic presentation can be highly variable, ranging from a near-normal chest film to a diffuse bilateral infiltrate, to large cysts or blebs (but almost never causes pleural effusion). The blebs can rupture, causing spontaneous pneumothorax. PCP often is suspected when patients present with subacute onset of fever and respiratory symptoms, but the diagnosis should usually be confirmed. **Definitive diagnosis can be established by use of Giemsa or silver stain** to visualize the cysts but usually requires induction of sputum using aerosolized hypertonic saline to induce cough or bronchoalveolar lavage to obtain a diagnostic specimen. **Elevated LDH** level often is used as an indirect marker for PCP, although it is nonspecific and may also be elevated in disseminated histoplasmosis or lymphoma. It is useful as a negative predictor because **patients with an LDH level less than 220 IU/L are very unlikely to have PCP.** Similarly, if patients have a CD4 count more than 250 cells/mm^3

Table 7–1 AIDS-DEFINING ILLNESSES

Bacterial infections, multiple or recurrent

Candidiasis of bronchi, trachea, or lungs

Candidiasis of esophagus

Cervical cancer, invasive

Coccidioidomycosis, disseminated or extrapulmonary

Cryptococcosis, extrapulmonary

Cryptosporidiosis, chronic intestinal (>1-mo duration)

Cytomegalovirus disease (other than liver, spleen, or nodes), onset at age >1 mo

Cytomegalovirus retinitis (with loss of vision)

Encephalopathy, HIV related

Herpes simplex: chronic ulcers (>1-mo duration) or bronchitis, pneumonitis, or
  esophagitis (onset at age >1 mo)

Histoplasmosis, disseminated or extrapulmonary

Isosporiasis, chronic intestinal (>1-mo duration)

Kaposi sarcoma

Lymphoid interstitial pneumonia or pulmonary lymphoid hyperplasia complex

Lymphoma, Burkitt (or equivalent term)

Lymphoma, immunoblastic (or equivalent term)

Lymphoma, primary, of brain

Mycobacterium avium complex or *Mycobacterium kansasii,* disseminated or
  extrapulmonary

Mycobacterium tuberculosis of any site, pulmonary, disseminated, or extrapulmonary

Mycobacterium, other species or unidentified species, disseminated or extrapulmonary

Pneumocystis jirovecii pneumonia

Pneumonia, recurrent

Progressive multifocal leukoencephalopathy

Salmonella septicemia, recurrent

Toxoplasmosis of brain, onset at age >1 mo

Wasting syndrome attributed to HIV

or if they were taking PCP prophylaxis with TMP-SMX, the diagnosis of PCP should be considered highly unlikely.

The level of oxygenation of PCP patients by arterial blood gas is useful because it may affect prognosis and therapy. Patients with arterial P_{O_2} less than **70 mm Hg or A-a gradient less than 35 mm Hg** have significant disease and have an **improved prognosis** if **prednisone is given in conjunction with antimicrobial therapy**. After prednisone is given to patients with hypoxia, the usual treatment for PCP is TMP-SMX. Patients who are allergic to sulfa can be treated with alternative regimens, including pentamidine or clindamycin with primaquine.

Many other respiratory infections are possible and should be considered in patients with AIDS. Diagnosis can be suggested by chest radiography. Diffuse interstitial infiltrates are seen with PCP, disseminated histoplasmosis, *Mycobacterium tuberculosis,* and *Mycobacterium kansasii.* Patchy infiltrates and pleural-based infiltrates can be seen with TB and cryptococcal lung disease. Cavitary lesions can be seen with TB, PCP, and coccidiomycosis. Clinical history should also be considered. Because the **most common causes of pneumonia in AIDS patients are the same organisms that cause pneumonia in immunocompetent hosts,** acute onset of fever and productive cough, with a pulmonary infiltrate, is most consistent with **community-acquired pneumonia.** A more indolent or chronic history of cough and weight loss, especially in a patient who has a high-risk background (prison, homeless, immigrant), should raise the question of **tuberculosis.** In patients with CD4 count more than 200 cells/mm^3, the radiographic appearance of TB is likely to be similar to that of other hosts, for example, bilateral apical infiltrate with cavitation; in those with CD4 count less than 200 cells/mm^3, the radiographic appearance is extremely variable. Because TB involves both the alveoli and the pulmonary circulation, patients with TB rarely are hypoxic with minimal infiltrate on chest X-ray (although this is relatively common in PCP). Patients with suspected pulmonary TB should be placed in respiratory isolation until it is assured they are not spreading airborne tuberculous infection. A negative PPD (purified protein derivative [tuberculin]) does not rule out tuberculosis in an immunocompromised host. Diagnosis and treatment of TB is discussed in Case 31. In HIV patients, **M *kansasii*** can cause pulmonary disease and radiographic findings identical to those of M *tuberculosis.*

Several other opportunistic infections in AIDS deserve mention. **Cerebral toxoplasmosis** is the **most common CNS mass lesion in AIDS patients.** It typically presents with headache, seizures, or focal neurologic deficits, and it is seen on CT or MRI scan, usually as multiple enhancing lesions, often located in the basal ganglia. Presumptive diagnosis often is made based on the radiologic appearance, supported by serologic evidence of infection. The major alternative diagnosis for CNS mass lesions is **CNS lymphoma.** This diagnosis is considered if there is a single mass lesion or if the lesions do not regress after 2 weeks of empiric toxoplasmosis therapy with sulfadiazine with pyrimethamine. If this is the case, historically, the next diagnostic step has been stereotactic brain biopsy. However, recent evidence indicates that examination of the cerebrospinal fluid (CSF) for **Epstein-Barr virus DNA** is a useful strategy because it is present in more than 90% of cases of patients with **CNS lymphoma.**

Another CNS complication that requires a high index of suspicion is **cryptococcal meningitis.** It is a chronic indolent infection, which often presents with vague symptoms of mood or personality changes, headaches, or visual disturbance. If the diagnosis is considered, one can screen for evidence of cryptococcal infection by a serum cryptococcal antigen or perform a lumbar puncture. The CSF frequently shows a lack of inflammatory response (ie, normal white blood cell [WBC] count), but the patient often presents with elevated intracranial pressures. Diagnosis can be confirmed by demonstrating the yeast by India ink stain, by fungal culture, or by measuring the level of cryptococcal antigen from CSF. Treatment of cryptococcal meningitis requires induction with intravenous amphotericin B plus flucytosine, then chronic suppression with oral fluconazole. At times, frequent lumbar punctures with removal of large volumes of CSF are required to treat the intracranial hypertension, and CSF shunts may be required.

At very low CD4 counts (<50 cells/mm^3), patients with AIDS are also susceptible to **CMV** infections. This can be manifested as viremia with persistent fever and constitutional symptoms, retinitis that can lead to blindness, esophagitis that can cause severe odynophagia, colitis, and necrotizing adrenalitis, which occasionally destroys sufficient adrenal tissue to produce clinical adrenal insufficiency. Therapy for severe CMV infections includes intravenous ganciclovir, foscarnet, or cidofovir.

Mycobacterium avium–**intracellulare** complex (MAC) is one of the most frequent opportunistic infections occurring in patients with very low CD4 counts. The most frequent presentations are disseminated infection with persistent fevers, weight loss, and constitutional symptoms, as well as gastrointestinal (GI) symptoms such as abdominal pain or chronic watery diarrhea. It often is diagnosed by obtaining a mycobacterial blood culture. Treatment with clarithromycin and ethambutol and rifabutin is required for weeks in an attempt to clear the bacteremia.

Because of the frequency and severity of common opportunistic infections, **antimicrobial prophylaxis** is routinely given as a patient's immune status declines. With CD4 counts less than 200 cells/mm^3, PCP prophylaxis should be given as one double-strength tablet of TMP-SMX three times per week. When counts fall to less than 100 cells/mm^3 and patients have a positive toxoplasma serology, toxoplasmosis can be prevented by increasing to daily dosing of TMP-SMX. If CD4 levels are less than 50 cells/mm^3, MAC prophylaxis consists of clarithromycin 500 mg daily or azithromycin 1200 mg weekly. Prophylaxis can be discontinued if HAART is started and the patient's CD4 levels recover.

HAART includes a combination at least three drugs consisting of a "base" of a nonnucleoside analog reverse transcriptase inhibitor or a protease inhibitor along with a "backbone" of two nucleoside analog reverse transcriptase inhibitors. HAART is very potent and has dramatically revolutionized the treatment of HIV patients, producing suppression of viral replication and allowing a patient's CD4 count to recover. However, initiation of HAART likely is not practical in acutely ill patients because the medications are not easy to take and often cause side effects that can be confused with the underlying disease process. Additionally, within 1 to 2 weeks of starting HAART, improvement in the immune system can actually cause worsening symptoms as a result of host responses, termed the "immune reconstitution syndrome." Therefore, it is better to wait until the acute illness has resolved and to initiate antiretroviral therapy after the patient has recovered, in consultation with an infectious diseases expert, when reliable follow-up has been assured.

Comprehension Questions

7.1   A 32-year-old woman with a 5-year history of HIV infection is noted to have a CD4 count of 100 cells/mm^3. She is admitted to the hospital with a 2-week history of fever, shortness of breath, and a dry cough. Which of the following diagnostic tests would most likely confirm the diagnosis?
       A. Silver stain of the sputum
       B. Gram stain of the sputum showing gram-positive diplococci
       C. Acid-fast smear of the sputum
       D. Serum cryptococcal antigen

7.2   Which of the following is the most likely organism to cause pneumonia in a patient with AIDS?
       A. *Pneumocystis jirovecii*
       B. *Mycobacterium tuberculosis*
       C. *Histoplasmosis capsulatum*
       D. *Streptococcus pneumoniae*

7.3   A 44-year-old woman infected with HIV is noted to have a CD4 count of 180 cells/mm^3. Which of the following is recommended as a useful prophylactic agent in this patient at this point?
       A. Fluconazole
       B. Azithromycin
       C. Trimethoprim-sulfamethoxazole
       D. Ganciclovir

7.4   A 36-year-old woman with HIV is admitted with new-onset seizures. The CT scan of the head reveals multiple ring enhancing lesions of the brain. Which of the following is the best therapy for the likely condition?
       A. Rifampin, isoniazid, ethambutol
       B. Ganciclovir
       C. Penicillin
       D. Sulfadiazine with pyrimethamine

ANSWERS

7.1   **A.** The fever, dry cough, and dyspnea is consistent with PCP, which is diagnosed by silver stain of the sputum, which often requires bronchoalveolar lavage to obtain.

7.2   **D.** The same organisms that cause community-acquired pneumonia in immunocompetent individuals are causative in HIV patients. Additionally, HIV patients are susceptible to other opportunistic infections, such as *Pneumocystis*.

7.3   **C.** When the CD4 count falls to less than 200 cells/mm³, trimethoprim-sulfamethoxazole (Bactrim) prophylaxis is generally initiated to prevent PCP. Prophylaxis against *Mycobacterium avium*–intracellulare complex usually is started when the CD4 count is less than 50 cells/mm³, and toxoplasmosis prophylaxis usually is started when the CD4 count is less than 100 cells/mm³.

7.4   **D.** The most common cause of a mass lesion of the brain in an HIV patient is toxoplasmosis, which is treated with sulfadiazine with pyrimethamine.

Clinical Pearls

➤ *Pneumocystis* pneumonia typically has a subacute presentation with fever and a dry cough, almost always in patients with a CD4 count less than 200 cells/mm³. Patients often have a diffuse bilateral infiltrate on chest X-ray and an elevated serum lactic acid dehydrogenase level.

➤ Pulmonary tuberculosis should always be considered in acquired immunodeficiency syndrome (AIDS) patients with respiratory symptoms and suggestive history; its radiographic presentation may be atypical.

➤ The most common causes of pneumonia in AIDS patients are the same as those in immunocompetent patients, that is, community-acquired organisms such as *Streptococcus pneumoniae*.

➤ In patients with CD4 counts less than 200 cells/mm3, trimethoprim-sulfamethoxazole (Bactrim) prophylaxis is effective in preventing Pneumocystis pneumonia and in preventing toxoplasmosis when the CD4 count is less than 100 cells/mm3. When the CD4 is less than 50 cells/mm³, clarithromycin or azithromycin can prevent *Mycobacterium avium*–intracellulare complex.

➤ Highly active antiretroviral therapy is effective in reducing viral replication, increasing CD4 counts, and restoring immunocompetence but generally should not be initiated during an acute illness.

REFERENCES

Fauci AS, Lane HC. HIV disease: AIDS and related disorders. In: Kasper DL, Braunwald E, Fauci AS, et al, eds. *Harrison's Principles of Internal Medicine*. 17th ed. New York, NY: McGraw-Hill; 2008:1137-1204.

Gray F, Chretien F, Vallat-Decouvelaere AV, et al. The changing pattern of HIV neuropathology in the HAART era. *J Neuropathol Exp Neurol*. 2003;62:429-440.

Smulian AG, Walzer PD. Pneumocystis infection. In: Fauci AS, Braunwald E, Kasper DL, eds. *Harrison's Principles of Internal Medicine*. 17th ed. New York, NY: McGraw-Hill; 2008:1267-1269.

Thomas CF, Limper AH. Pneumocystis pneumonia. *N Engl J Med*. 2004;350:2487-2498.

Wolff AJ, O'Donnell AE. Pulmonary manifestations of HIV infection in the era of highly active antiretroviral therapy. *Chest*. 2001;120:1888-1893.

Case 8

A 58-year-old man presents to the emergency room complaining of severe pain in his left foot that woke him from sleep. He has a history of chronic stable angina, hypercholesterolemia, and hypertension, for which he takes aspirin, atenolol, and simvastatin. He has experienced pain in both calves and feet with walking for several years, and the pain has gradually progressed so that he can now only walk 100 feet before he has to stop because of pain. He occasionally has experienced mild pain in his feet at night, but the pain usually gets better when he sits up and hangs his feet off the bed. This time, the pain was more severe and did not improve, and he now feels like the foot is numb and he cannot move his toes.

On physical examination, he is afebrile, with heart rate 72 bpm and blood pressure 125/74 mm Hg. Head and neck examination are significant for a right carotid bruit. His chest is clear to auscultation; his heart rhythm is regular with a nondisplaced apical impulse, an S_4 gallop, and no murmurs. His abdomen is benign, with no tenderness or masses. He has bilateral femoral bruits, and palpable femoral and popliteal pulses bilaterally. His pedal pulses are diminished, but they are present on the right but absent on the left. The left distal leg and foot are pale and cold to touch, with very slow capillary refill.

➤ What is the most likely diagnosis?

➤ What is your next step?

ANSWERS TO CASE 8:

Limb Ischemia (Peripheral Vascular Disease)

Summary: A 58-year-old man presents to the emergency room with severe pain and numbness of his left foot. He has angina and a carotid bruit suggesting systemic atherosclerotic disease. He previously had symptoms of bilateral calf claudication but now has sudden onset of pain, pallor, and pulselessness in the left foot.

➤ **Most likely diagnosis:** Acute limb ischemia, either thrombotic arterial occlusion or embolism from a distant source.

➤ **Next step:** Angiogram of the lower extremity.

ANALYSIS

Objectives

1. Understand the clinical presentation of a patient with atherosclerotic peripheral vascular disease, including acute limb ischemia.
2. Know the evaluation and medical management of peripheral vascular disease.
3. Understand the indications for extremity revascularization.

Considerations

This patient has diffuse atherosclerotic vascular disease, including coronary artery disease, carotid disease, and peripheral vascular disease. His **history of calf pain with walking, but resolution with rest, is classic for claudication.** Recently, the perfusion of his left leg likely was worsening, requiring his waking up and dangling his leg to enable blood flow and to help the pain. **Rest pain is a warning sign of possible critical limb vascular insufficiency.** The patient complains of sudden onset of **pain, pallor, and pulselessness**, indicative of acute arterial occlusion. His limb ischemia may result from acute arterial occlusion caused by an embolus, usually arising from a dislodged thrombus from the heart, or a previously diseased proximal artery. Depending on the level of occlusion, the patient may require urgent arterial thromboembolectomy, or possibly arteriography, to first determine the arterial anatomy and define the best mode of revascularization.

APPROACH TO
Peripheral Vascular Disease

DEFINITIONS

ANKLE-BRACHIAL INDEX (ABI): Ratio of ankle to brachial systolic blood pressure, determined using Doppler ultrasound flow.

CLAUDICATION SYNDROME: Calf pain that increases with walking or leg exertion in a predictable manner and resolves with rest.

CLINICAL APPROACH

Although atherosclerosis is a systemic disease, clinicians often focus on the coronary circulation and are less attentive to the extremities. Yet atherosclerotic peripheral arterial disease (PAD) is estimated to affect up to 16% of Americans 55 years and older and may exist without clinically recognized coronary or cerebrovascular disease. Furthermore, PAD confers the same risk of cardiovascular death as in persons with a prior myocardial infarction or stroke. **The most important risk factors** for PAD are **cigarette smoking and diabetes mellitus.** Hypertension, dyslipidemia, and elevated homocysteine levels also play significant roles.

Diagnosis

The most common symptom associated with chronic arterial insufficiency caused by PAD is **intermittent claudication**, characterized by pain, ache, a sense of fatigue, or other discomfort that occurs in one or both legs during exercise, such as walking, and is relieved with rest. It is ischemic pain and occurs distal to the site of the arterial stenosis, most commonly in the calves. The symptoms often are progressive and may severely limit a patient's activities and reduce the patient's functional status. An individual with proximal stenosis, such as aortoiliac disease, may complain of exertional pain in the buttocks and thighs. Severe occlusion may produce **rest pain**, which often occurs at night and may be relieved by sitting up and dangling the legs, using gravity to assist blood flow to the feet.

On physical examination, palpation of the **peripheral pulses may be diminished** or absent below the level of occlusion; **bruits** may indicate accelerated blood flow velocity and turbulence at the sites of stenosis. Bruits may be heard in the abdomen with aortoiliac stenosis and in the groin with femoral artery stenosis. **Elevation of the feet** above the level of the heart in the supine patient often induces **pallor in the soles**. If the legs are then placed in the dependent position, they frequently develop rubor as a result of reactive hyperemia.

Chronic arterial insufficiency may cause **hair loss on the legs and feet**, thickened and brittle toenails, and shiny atrophic skin. Severe ischemia may produce ulcers or gangrene.

When PAD is suspected, the test most commonly used to evaluate for arterial insufficiency is the **ankle-brachial index (ABI)**. Systolic blood pressures are measured by Doppler ultrasonography in each arm and in the dorsalis pedis and posterior tibial arteries in each ankle. Normally, blood pressures in the large arteries of the legs and arms are similar. In fact, blood pressures in the legs often are higher than in the arms because of an artifact of measurement, so the normal ratio of ankle to brachial pressures is more than 1. Patients with claudication typically have ABI values ranging from 0.41 to 0.90, and those with critical leg ischemia have less than or equal to 0.40. Further evaluation with exercise treadmill testing can clarify the diagnosis when symptoms are equivocal, can allow for assessment of functional limitations (eg, maximal walking distance), and can evaluate for concomitant coronary artery disease.

Management

The goals of therapy include reductions in cardiovascular morbidity and mortality, improvement in quality of life by decreasing symptoms of claudication and eliminating rest pain, and preservation of limb viability.

The first step in managing patients with PAD is risk factor modification. Because of the likelihood of coexisting atherosclerotic vascular disease such as coronary artery disease, patients with **symptomatic PAD** have an estimated **mortality** rate of **50% in 10 years**, most often as a consequence of cardiovascular events. **Smoking** is, by far, the **single most important risk factor** impacting both claudication symptoms and overall cardiovascular mortality. Besides slowing the progression to critical leg ischemia, **tobacco cessation reduces the risk of fatal or nonfatal myocardial infarction by as much as 50%,** more than any other medical or surgical intervention. In addition, treatment of hypercholesterolemia, control of hypertension and diabetes, and use of antiplatelet agents such as aspirin or clopidogrel all have been shown to improve cardiovascular health and may have an effect on peripheral arterial circulation. Carefully supervised exercise programs can improve muscle strength and prolong walking distance by promoting the development of collateral blood flow.

Specific medications for improving claudication symptoms have been used, with some benefit. Pentoxifylline, a substituted xanthine derivative that increases erythrocyte elasticity, has been reported to decrease blood viscosity, thus allowing improved blood flow to the microcirculation; however, results from clinical trials are conflicting, and the benefit of pentoxifylline, if present, appears small. A newer agent, cilostazol, a phosphodiesterase inhibitor with vasodilatory and antiplatelet properties, has been approved by the Food and Drug Administration (FDA) for treatment of claudication. It has been shown in randomized controlled trials to improve maximal walking distance. Figure 8–1 shows an algorithm for management of PAD.

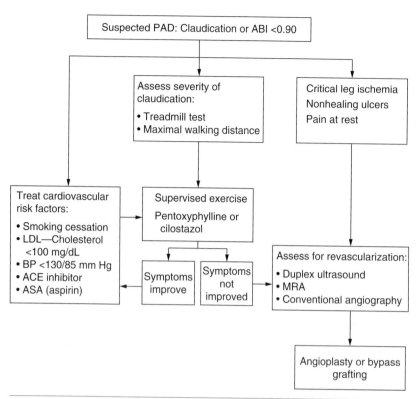

Figure 8–1. Algorithm for management of peripheral arterial disease. *Data from Hiatt W. Medical treatment of peripheral arterial disease and claudication.* N Engl J Med. 2001;344:1608-1621.

Patients with **critical leg ischemia**, defined as **ABI** less than **0.40, severe or disabling claudication, rest pain**, or **nonhealing ulcers**, should be **evaluated for a revascularization procedure**. This can be accomplished by percutaneous angioplasty, with or without placement of intraarterial stents, or surgical bypass grafting. Angiography (either conventional or magnetic resonance arteriography) should be performed to define the flow-limiting lesions prior to any vascular procedure. Ideal candidates for arterial revascularization are those with discrete stenosis of large vessels; diffuse atherosclerotic and small-vessel disease respond poorly.

Less common causes of chronic peripheral arterial insufficiency include thromboangiitis obliterans, or **Buerger disease**, which is an inflammatory condition of small- and medium-size arteries that may affect the upper or lower extremities and is found almost exclusively in smokers, especially males younger than 40 years. **Fibromuscular dysplasia** is a hyperplastic disorder **affecting medium and small arteries that usually occurs in women.** Generally, the renal or carotid arteries are involved, but when the arteries to the limbs are affected, the clinical symptoms are identical to those of atherosclerotic PAD. **Takayasu**

arteritis is an inflammatory condition, seen primarily in younger women, that usually affects branches of the aorta, most commonly the subclavian arteries, and causes **arm claudication and Raynaud phenomenon,** along with constitutional symptoms such as **fever** and **weight loss.**

Patients with chronic peripheral arterial insufficiency who present with sudden unremitting pain may have an **acute arterial occlusion,** most commonly the result of **embolism** or **in situ thrombosis. The heart is the most common source of emboli**; conditions that may cause cardiogenic emboli include atrial fibrillation, dilated cardiomyopathy, and endocarditis. Artery-to-artery embolization of atherosclerotic debris from the aorta or large vessels may occur spontaneously or, more often, after an intravascular procedure, such as arterial catheterization. Emboli tend to lodge at the bifurcation of two vessels, most often in the femoral, iliac, popliteal, or tibioperoneal arteries. Arterial thrombosis may occur in atherosclerotic vessels at the site of stenosis or in an area of aneurysmal dilation, which may also complicate atherosclerotic disease.

Patients with acute arterial occlusion may present with a number of signs, which can be remembered as **"six P's:" pain, pallor, pulselessness, paresthesias, poikilothermia (coolness), and paralysis.** The first five signs occur fairly quickly with acute ischemia; paralysis will develop if the arterial occlusion is severe and persistent.

Rapid restoration of arterial supply is mandatory in patients with an **acute arterial occlusion that threatens limb viability.** Initial management includes anticoagulation with heparin to prevent propagation of the thrombus. The affected limb should be placed below the horizontal plane without any pressure applied to it. Conventional arteriography usually is indicated to identify the location of the occlusion and to evaluate potential methods of revascularization. Surgical removal of an embolus or arterial bypass may be performed, particularly if a large proximal artery is occluded. A balloon catheter may also be attempted to remove the clot. Alternatively, a catheter can be used to deliver intraarterial thrombolytic therapy directly into the thrombus. In comparison with systemic fibrinolytic therapy, localized infusion is associated with fewer bleeding complications.

Comprehension Questions

8.1   A 49-year-old smoker with hypertension, diabetes, and hypercholesterolemia comes to the office complaining of pain in his calves when he walks 2 to 3 blocks. Which of the following therapies might offer him the greatest benefit in symptom reduction and in overall mortality?

A. Aspirin
B. Limb revascularization procedure
C. Cilostazol
D. Smoking cessation
E. Pravastatin

For Questions 8.2–8.4, match the most likely cause (A–E) of arterial insufficiency to the patient described:

A. Cholesterol embolism
B. Fibromuscular dysplasia
C. Thromboangiitis obliterans (Buerger disease)
D. Takayasu aortitis
E. Psychogenic pain

8.2   A 31-year-old male smoker with resting pain in his legs and a nonhealing foot ulcer.

8.3   A 21-year-old woman with fever, fatigue, and unequal pulses and blood pressures in her arms.

8.4   A 62-year-old man with livedo reticularis and three blue toes, including one with gangrene following cardiac catheterization.

8.5   A 67-year-old woman is noted to have significant peripheral vascular disease. She is evaluated by the cardiovascular surgeon but *not* felt to be a surgical candidate. Which of the following conditions is likely to be present in this patient?
A. Diffuse atherosclerotic disease
B. Leg pain at rest
C. Symptoms that do not improve with pharmacologic management
D. Nonhealing ulcers of the ankle

ANSWERS

8.1   **D.** Tobacco cessation is the most important intervention to improve cardiovascular morbidity and mortality in high-risk patients, such as those with PAD, and to improve claudication symptoms. Cilostazol may help with claudication symptoms but will not affect cardiovascular mortality. Aspirin, angiotensin-converting enzyme (ACE) inhibitor, and beta-hydroxy-beta-methylglutaryl coenzyme A (HMG-CoA) reductase inhibitors are important adjuncts for risk-factor modification and for relief of symptoms, but their benefits pale in comparison to smoking cessation.

8.2   **C.** Thromboangiitis obliterans, or Buerger disease, is a disease of young male smokers and may cause symptoms of chronic arterial insufficiency in either legs or arms.

8.3   **D.** Takayasu aortitis is associated with symptoms of inflammation such as fever, and most often affects the subclavian arteries, producing stenotic lesions that may cause unequal blood pressures, diminished pulses, and ischemic pain in the affected limbs.

8.4   **A.** Embolism of cholesterol and other atherosclerotic debris from the aorta or other large vessels to small vessels of skin or digits may complicate any intraarterial procedure.

8.5   **A.** Surgical therapy is reserved for severe symptoms after exercise and pharmacologic agents are used, and quality of life is impaired. Pain at rest, lack of symptoms for medical therapy, nonhealing ulcers, or gangrene are some of those indications. Duplex ultrasound can help to discern whether the patient is a potential surgical candidate. Arteriography may also be performed. Diffuse atherosclerotic disease is a contraindication for surgery since bypass would not help in the face of significant and widespread disease.

Clinical Pearls

➤ Smoking cessation is the single most important intervention for athero-sclerotic peripheral vascular disease. Other treatments include pentoxi-fylline or cilostazol, regular exercise, and cardiovascular risk factor modification.

➤ Revascularization by angioplasty or bypass grafting may be indicated for patients with debilitating claudication, ischemic rest pain, or tissue necrosis.

➤ Acute arterial occlusion that threatens limb viability is a medical emergency and requires immediate anticoagulation and investigation with conventional arteriography.

➤ Acute severe ischemia of an extremity causes the "six P's": pain, pallor, pulselessness, paresthesias, poikilothermia, and paralysis. Chronic incomplete arterial occlusion may result only in exertional pain or fatigue, pallor on elevation of the extremity, and rubor on dependency.

REFERENCES

Creager M, Loscalzo J. Vascular disease of the extremities. In: Kasper DL, Braunwald E, Fauci AS, et al, eds. *Harrison's Principles of Internal Medicine.* 17th ed. New York, NY: McGraw-Hill; 2008:1568-1575.

Hankey GJ, Normal PE, Eikelboom JW, et al. Medical treatment of peripheral arterial disease. *JAMA.* 2006; 295:547.

Hirsch AT, Haskal ZJ, Hertzer NR, et al. ACC/AHA 2005 practice guidelines for the management of patients with peripheral arterial disease. *Circulation.* 2006;113:e463.

Katzen BT. Clinical diagnosis and prognosis of acute limb ischemia. *Rev Cardiovasc Med.* 2002;3(Suppl 2):S2-S6.

Case 9

A 56-year-old man comes into your office as a new patient. Seven years ago at a work-related health screening, he was diagnosed with hypertension and hypercholesterolemia. At that time, he saw a physician who prescribed a diuretic and encouraged him to lose some weight and to diet and exercise. Since that time, the patient has not sought medical attention. During the past 2 months, he has been experiencing occasional headaches, which he attributes to increased stress at work. He denies chest pain, shortness of breath, dyspnea on exertion, or paroxysmal nocturnal dyspnea. He smokes one pack of cigarettes per day and has done so since he was 15 years old. He typically drinks two glasses of wine with dinner. On examination, the patient is obese, and you calculate his body mass index (BMI) as 30 kg/m². His blood pressure is 168/98 mm Hg in the right arm and 170/94 mm Hg in the left arm. His blood pressure did not change with changes in position. His heart rate is 84 bpm. He has no thyromegaly or lymphadenopathy. Funduscopic examination reveals narrowing of the arteries, arteriovenous *nicking*, and flame-shaped hemorrhages with cotton wool exudates. Cardiac examination reveals that his point of maximal impulse is displaced 2 cm left of the midclavicular line. There is an S_4 gallop. No murmurs are auscultated. Lung and abdomen examinations are normal.

➤ What are your next steps?

ANSWER TO CASE 9:
Hypertension, Outpatient

Summary: A 56-year-old hypertensive man is being evaluated as a new patient. His blood pressures are in the range of 170/95 mm Hg. Funduscopic examination reveals hypertensive retinopathy. His point of maximal impulse is displaced laterally, suggesting cardiomegaly, and a fourth heart sound is consistent with a thickened, noncompliant ventricle. In addition, he has multiple cardiovascular risk factors, including his age, obesity, and smoking.

> ➤ **Next steps:** (1) Laboratory evaluation to evaluate renal function such as electrolytes, creatinine, and urinalysis, evaluation of other cardiovascular risk factors such as serum glucose and lipid profile, and a baseline ECG to assess for target organ damage. (2) Start the patient on a two-drug antihypertensive regimen that includes a thiazide diuretic. (3) Recommend lifestyle changes, most importantly tobacco cessation.

ANALYSIS

Objectives

1. Understand the initial evaluation of a patient with hypertension.
2. Be familiar with the most common antihypertensive medications, and indications and cautions regarding their usage.
3. Be familiar with the various causes of secondary hypertension and when to pursue these diagnoses.

Considerations

This is a 56-year-old man with severe hypertension, who has evidence, on physical examination, of hypertensive end-organ damage, that is, hypertensive retinopathy and left ventricular hypertrophy as well as multiple risk factors for atherosclerotic disease. The most likely diagnosis is essential hypertension, but secondary causes still must be considered. Although you have measured his blood pressure (BP) only once in your office, he has been told before that he is hypertensive, and he already appears to have end-organ damage of hypertension. His blood pressure is above 160/100 mm Hg, which places him in **stage II hypertension, which warrants starting him on two-drug therapy without further delay.** One of the drugs should be a thiazide diuretic.

APPROACH TO
Hypertension

DEFINITIONS

ESSENTIAL HYPERTENSION: Also known as idiopathic or primary hypertension. It has no known cause, yet it comprises approximately 95% of all cases of hypertension.

LIFESTYLE MODIFICATION: A cornerstone in the treatment of hypertension, consisting of regular aerobic activity, weight loss, decreased salt intake, and increased intake of fruit and vegetables, while decreasing the amount of total fat, especially saturated fat, in the diet. Alcohol consumption should be moderated, no more than two glasses of wine per day for men and one glass per day for women.

PREHYPERTENSION: Blood pressures 120 to 139/80 to 89 mm Hg

STAGE I HYPERTENSION: Blood pressures 140 to 159/90 to 99 mm Hg

STAGE II HYPERTENSION: Blood pressures more than 160/100 mm Hg

SECONDARY HYPERTENSION: Elevated arterial blood pressure with a known underlying cause, such as renal artery stenosis or primary aldosteronism. Prevalence is approximately 5% to 10% of all cases of hypertension.

CLINICAL APPROACH

Initial Evaluation and Management

Hypertension can first be staged, to guide the intensity of medical intervention, by measuring blood pressures on two or more occasions. Underlying causes of hypertension must then be considered. Essential or idiopathic hypertension is the most common form of hypertension, comprising 90% to 95% of cases, but approximately 5% to 10% of cases of hypertension are caused by secondary causes (Table 9–1). To identify the secondary (and potentially reversible) causes of hypertension, the clinician must be aware of the clinical and laboratory manifestations of the processes. A secondary cause of hypertension, and thus more extensive testing, is indicated when patients have any of the following clinical features: age of onset before 25 years or after 55 years, presenting with malignant hypertension, requiring three or more antihypertensive medications, hypertension that has suddenly become uncontrolled, a rising creatinine level with the use of angiotensin-converting enzyme (ACE) inhibitors, or overt clinical signs of a secondary cause (Table 9–2).

Table 9–1 SECONDARY CAUSES OF HYPERTENSIONTY

Renal Diseases
- Parenchymal (glomerulonephritis, polycystic renal disease, diabetic nephropathy)
- Renovascular

Endocrine
- Primary aldosteronism
- Cushing syndrome
- Pheochromocytoma
- Hyperthyroidism
- Growth hormone excess (acromegaly)
- Oral contraceptives

Miscellaneous
- Coarctation of the aorta
- Increased intravascular volume (posttransfusion)
- Hypercalcemia
- Medications (sympathomimetics, glucocorticoids)

Other Cardiac Risk Factors and Evaluation for Target Organ Damage

Cardiovascular risk factors and hypertensive target organ damage should be identified. The major risk factors of cardiovascular disease are age, cigarette smoking, dyslipidemia, diabetes mellitus, obesity, kidney disease, and a family history of premature cardiovascular disease. Target organ damage of hypertension includes cardiomyopathy, nephropathy, and retinopathy. A complete history and physical examination, including funduscopic examination, auscultation of the major arteries for bruits, palpation of the abdomen for enlarged kidneys, masses, or an enlarged abdominal aorta, evaluation of the lower extremities for edema and perfusion, and a neurologic examination

Table 9–2 CLUES TO RENOVASCULAR HYPERTENSION

Epigastric or flank bruits
Accelerated or malignant hypertension
Severe hypertension in individuals younger than 25 years or older than 55 years
Sudden development or worsening of hypertension at any age
Hypertension with unexplained impairment of kidney function
Hypertension refractory to appropriate (three) drug regimen
Extensive occlusive disease in the peripheral circulation
Coronary and cerebral vascular disease

Table 9–3 BASIC TESTS FOR INITIAL EVALUATION OF HYPERTENSION
Urinalysis for protein, blood, glucose, and microscopic examination
Hemoglobin or hematocrit; leukocyte count
Serum potassium
Serum calcium and phosphate
Serum creatinine or blood urea nitrogen
Fasting glucose
Total, HDL and LDL, cholesterol; triglycerides
Electrocardiogram
Consider thyroid-stimulating hormone

should be standard. Some initial laboratory testing is also indicated (Table 9–3). Counseling patients on lifestyle changes is important at any blood pressure level and includes weight loss, limitation of alcohol intake, increased aerobic physical activity, reduced sodium intake, cessation of smoking, and reduced intake of dietary saturated fat and cholesterol.

Therapy

Initial therapy should be based on the stage or degree of hypertension. For all patients with hypertension, lifestyle modifications should be instituted. For those with **prehypertension** (blood pressure 120-139/80-89 mm Hg), lifestyle modifications are the only interventions indicated unless they have another comorbid condition, such as heart failure or diabetes, which necessitates use of an antihypertensive. Patient with **stage I hypertension** (blood pressure 140-159/90-99 mm Hg) should be started on a single antihypertensive agent, whereas those with **stage II hypertension** (blood pressure >160/100 mm Hg) usually will need at least two antihypertensives in combination.

For most patients, a low dose of the initial drug of choice should be administered slowly, titrating upward at a schedule dependent on the patient's age, needs, and responses. The **target blood pressure typically is 135/85 mm Hg, unless the patient has diabetes or renal disease, in which case the target would be lower than 130/80 mm Hg.** A long-acting formulation that provides 24-hour efficacy is preferred over short-acting agents for better compliance and more consistent blood pressure control. The list of oral and hypertensive drugs is extensive (Table 9–4). Because they are associated **with a decrease in mortality in all types of patients, thiazide diuretics** should be considered in all patients with hypertension who do not have compelling contraindications to this class of drugs. Both thiazide diuretics and beta-blockers should be used first in patents with uncomplicated hypertension, unless there are specific compelling indications to use other drugs. In diabetics, ACE inhibitors are

Table 9–4 PARTIAL LISTING OF ANTIHYPERTENSIVE AGENTS

CATEGORY	AGENTS	MECHANISMS OF ACTION	SIDE EFFECTS	CONTRAINDICATIONS/ CAUTIONS
Diuretic	Thiazide diuretic: **Hydrochlorothiazide, chlorthalidone**	Sodium diuresis, volume depletion, possible lower peripheral vascular resistance	Hypokalemia, hyponatremia, carbohydrate intolerance, hyperuricemia, hyperlipidemia	Diabetes mellitus, gout, hypokalemia
	Loop diuretic: **Furosemide**	**Hypokalemia,** hyperglycemia, hypocalcemia, rash, hyperuricemia	Gout, hypokalemia	
	Potassium sparing spironolactone	Competitive inhibitor of aldosterone, causing renal sodium loss	**Hyperkalemia,** gynecomastia, diarrhea	Renal failure
Antiadrenergic	**Clonidine**	Stimulation of alpha-2 vasomotor center of brain	Postural hypotension, drowsiness, dry mouth, **rebound hypertension** with abrupt withdrawal	History of medication non-compliance
	Beta-blocker: **Metoprolol, atenolol**	Block sympathetic effect of heart and kidneys (renin)	**Bronchospasm,** hyperlipidemia, gastrointestinal symptoms, depression, erectile dysfunction	Asthma, 2nd- or 3rd-degree heart block
	Alpha-beta blocker: **Carvedilol**	Same as beta-blockers and also direct vasodilation	Similar to beta-blockers	Similar to beta-blockers

Table 9–4 PARTIAL LISTING OF ANTIHYPERTENSIVE AGENTS (CONTINUED)

CATEGORY	AGENTS	MECHANISMS OF ACTION	SIDE EFFECTS	CONTRAINDICATIONS/ CAUTIONS
Vasodilator	**Hydralazine**	Arterial vasodilation, produces reflex tachycardia	Headache, tachycardia, angina, lupus-like syndrome	Severe coronary artery disease
	Nitroprusside	Direct arterial and venous dilator	Weakness, fatigue, nausea, muscle twitching, **cyanide toxicity**	
ACE inhibitor	Lisinopril, captopril, enalapril, etc	Inhibit conversion of angiotensin I to angiotensin II (powerful vasoconstrictor)	Leukopenia, pancytopenia, hypotension, **cough**, angioedema, urticarial rash, **hyperkalemia**, acute renal failure	Renal failure, bilateral renal artery stenosis, pregnancy
Angiotensin receptor antagonist	**Losartan, valsartan, candesartan**	Competitive inhibition of the angiotensin II receptor	Similar to ACE inhibitors but no cough or angioedema	Pregnancy, bilateral renal artery stenosis
Calcium channel antagonist	Dihydropyridines: **Amolidipine, nifedipine**	Blockade of L-channels, reducing intracellular calcium and causing vasodilation	Tachycardia, flushing, gastrointestinal side effects, hyperkalemia, **edema**	Heart failure, significant heart block
	Non-dihydropyridine: **Diltiazem, verapamil**	Similar to dihydropyridines	**Heart block**, constipation,	Heart failure, 2nd- or 3rd-degree heart block

Data from Fauci AS, Braunwald E, Kasper DL. Harrison's Principles of Internal Medicine. 17th ed. New York, NY: McGraw-Hill; 2008:1560.

typically the first-line agent with thiazide diuretics added if the blood pressure is uncontrolled, realizing that the thiazide may exacerbate hyperglycemia. Thus, **ACE inhibitors are the agents of choice in hypertensive patients with diabetes or heart failure.** Most patients ultimately need more than one drug to control their blood pressure. It is critical to tailor the treatment to the patient's personal, financial, lifestyle, and medical factors, and to periodically review compliance and adverse effects.

Selected Causes of Secondary Hypertension

The most common cause of secondary hypertension is renal disease (renal parenchymal or renal vascular). Renal artery stenosis is caused by atherosclerotic disease with hemodynamically significant blockage of the renal artery in older patients or by fibromuscular dysplasia in younger adults. Table 9–2 summarizes the clues to renal vascular hypertension. The clinician must have a high index of suspicion, and further testing may be indicated, for instance, in an individual with diffuse atherosclerotic disease. Potassium level may be low or borderline low in patients with renal artery stenosis caused by secondary hyperaldosteronism. A captopril-enhanced radionuclide renal scan often is helpful in establishing the diagnosis; other diagnostic tools include magnetic resonance angiography and spiral computed tomography. Surgical or angioplastic correction of the vascular occlusion may be considered.

Polycystic kidney disease is inherited as an autosomal dominant trait. The classic clinical findings are positive family history of polycystic kidney disease, bilateral flank masses, flank pain, elevated blood pressure, and hematuria. Other causes of chronic renal disease very commonly lead to hypertension.

Other causes of secondary hypertension include **primary hyperaldosteronism,** which typically will cause hypertension and hypokalemia. Anabolic steroids, sympathomimetic drugs, tricyclic antidepressants, nonsteroidal anti-inflammatory agents, and illicit drugs, such as cocaine, as well as licit ones, such as caffeine and tobacco, are included in possible secondary causes of hypertension.

Obstructive sleep apnea is another fairly common cause of hypertension. The cause of obstructive sleep apnea is a critical narrowing of the upper airway that occurs when the resistance of the upper airway musculature fails against the negative pressure generated by inspiration. In most patients, this is a result of a reduced airway size that is congenital or perhaps complicated by obesity. These patients frequently become hypoxic and hypercarbic multiple times during sleep, which, among other things, eventually can lead to systemic vasoconstriction, systolic hypertension, and pulmonary hypertension.

Hyperthyroidism may also cause hypertension. The patient will have a widened pulse pressure with increased systolic blood pressure and decreased diastolic blood pressure, as well as a hyperdynamic precordium. The patient may have warm skin, tremor, and thyroid gland enlargement or a palpable thyroid nodule. A low level of serum thyroid-stimulating hormone (TSH) and elevated levels of thyroid hormones (such as free T_4) are diagnostic.

Glucocorticoid excess states, including **Cushing syndrome,** and iatrogenic (treatment with glucocorticoids) states usually present with, thinning of the extremities with truncal obesity, round moon face, supraclavicular fat pad, purple striae, acne, and possible psychiatric symptoms. An excess of corticosteroids can cause secondary hypertension because many glucocorticoid hormones have mineralocorticoid activity. Dexamethasone suppression testing of the serum cortisol level aids in the diagnosis of Cushing syndrome.

Coarctation of the aorta is a congenital narrowing of the aortic lumen and usually is diagnosed in younger patients by finding hypertension along with discordant upper and lower extremity blood pressures. Coarctation of the aorta can cause leg claudication, cold extremities, and diminished or absence of femoral pulses as a result of decreased blood pressure in the lower extremities.

Carcinoid syndrome is caused by overproduction of serotonin. Carcinoid tumors arise from the enterochromaffin cells located in the gastrointestinal tract and in the lungs. Clinical manifestations include cutaneous flushing, headache, diarrhea, and bronchial construction with wheezing. Carcinoid syndrome is also accompanied by hypertension.

Pheochromocytoma is a catecholamine-releasing tumor that typically produces hypertension. Clinical manifestations include headaches, palpitations, diaphoresis, and chest pain. Other symptoms include anxiety, nervousness, tremor, pallor, malaise, and, occasionally nausea and/or vomiting. Symptoms typically are paroxysmal and associated with hypertension. Patients with pheochromocytoma may have orthostatic hypotension. Thus, in the evaluation of newly diagnosed hypertension, orthostatic blood pressure measurements may be helpful.

Comprehension Questions

9.1   A 30-year-old woman is noted to have blood pressures in the 160/100 mm Hg range. She also has increased obesity, especially around her abdomen, with striae. She has been bruising very easily and has hirsutism. Which of the following is the most likely diagnosis?

A. Hyperthyroidism
B. Coarctation of the aorta
C. Cushing syndrome
D. Pheochromocytoma

9.2   A 45-year-old man is diagnosed with idiopathic hypertension based on two blood pressures of 150/100 and 156/102. Which of the following would most likely provide prognostic information regarding this patient?
       A. Vascular biopsy
       B. End-organ effects from hypertension, such as left ventricular hypertrophy
       C. Patient's enrollment in a clinical trial
       D. Measurement of serum homocysteine levels

9.3   A 34-year-old woman is noted to be diagnosed with stage I hypertension and after an evaluation is noted to have no complications. Which of the following antihypertensive agents are generally considered first-line agents for this individual?
       A. Thiazide diuretics
       B. Angiotensin-receptor blockers
       C. Alpha-blocking agents
       D. Nitrates
       E. Vasodilators such as hydralazine

9.4   A 45-year-old man with type II diabetes is noted to have blood pressures of 145/90 and 150/96 mm Hg on two separate occasions. Which of the following is the best initial therapy for this patient?
       A. Hydrochlorothiazide
       B. ACE inhibitor
       C. Beta-blocker
       D. Beta-blocker and hydrochlorothiazide

ANSWERS

9.1   **C.** The central obesity, abdominal striae, hirsutism, and easy bruisability are consistent with Cushing syndrome, a disease of adrenal steroid overproduction.

9.2   **B.** Prognosis in hypertension depends on the patient's other cardiovascular risks and observed end-organ effects from the hypertension.

9.3   **A.** Thiazide diuretics and beta-blockers are generally considered first-line agents for uncomplicated hypertension because of their effect in reducing cardiovascular mortality and their cost-effectiveness.

9.4   **B.** For diabetics, in general, the anti-hypertensive agent of choice is the ACE inhibitor. If the blood pressure is uncontrolled then a thiazide diuretic may be added. The patient will have survival advantage with the ACE inhibitor.

Clinical Pearls

➤ In general, the diagnosis of hypertension requires two or more blood pressure measurements on at least two visits.

➤ Cardiovascular disease risk evaluation consists of identifying target organ dysfunction and cardiovascular risk factors, such as diabetes and hyperlipidemia.

➤ Most patients with hypertension have essential hypertension, but secondary causes of hypertension should be evaluated when clinically indicated.

➤ Renal diseases, including renovascular hypertension, are the most common causes of secondary hypertension.

➤ Lifestyle modifications consisting of dietary, exercise, and stress relief measures are the cornerstone of hypertension control and lower cardiovascular risk.

➤ Consider diuretics and beta-blockers as first-line agents in patients with uncomplicated hypertension, unless there are compelling indications for using other drugs.

REFERENCES

Chobanian AV, Aram GL, Bakris GL, Black HR. The seventh report of the Joint National Committee on Prevention, Detection, Evaluation, and Treatment of High Blood Pressure. The JNC 7 report. JAMA. 2003;289:2560-2572.

Kotchen TA. Hypertensive vascular disease. In: Kasper DL, Braunwald E, Fauci AS, et al, eds. Harrison's Principles of Internal Medicine. 17th ed. New York, NY: McGraw-Hill; 2008: 1549-1562.

Case 10

A 39-year-old man is brought to the emergency room by ambulance after he was found wandering in the street in a disoriented state. He is confused and agitated, and further history is obtained from his wife. She reports that for the last several months he has been complaining of intermittent headaches and palpitations, and he had experienced feelings of lightheadedness and flushed skin when playing basketball. Three weeks ago, he was diagnosed with hypertension and was started on clonidine twice per day. He took the clonidine for 2 weeks, but because the drug made him feel sedated, he was instructed by his physician 5 days ago to stop the clonidine and to begin metoprolol twice daily. On examination, he is afebrile, with heart rate 110 bpm, respiratory rate 26 breaths per minute, oxygen saturation 98%, and blood pressure 215/132 mm Hg, equal in both arms. He is agitated and diaphoretic, and he is looking around the room but does not appear to recognize his wife. His pupils are dilated but reactive, and he has papilledema and scattered retinal hemorrhages. He has no thyromegaly. Heart, lung, and abdominal examinations are normal. His pulses are bounding and equal in his arms and legs. He moves all of his extremities well, his reflexes are brisk and symmetric, and he is slightly tremulous. A noncontrast computed tomography (CT) of the head is read as negative for hemorrhage. Laboratory studies include a normal leukocyte count and a hemoglobin level of 16.5 g/dL. Serum sodium level is 139 mEq/L, potassium 4.7 mEq/L, chloride 105 mEq/L, HCO_3 29 mEq/L, blood urea nitrogen (BUN) 32 mg/dL, and creatinine 1.3 mg/dL. Urinalysis is normal, and a urine drug screen is negative. Lumbar puncture is performed, and the cerebrospinal fluid (CSF) has no cells and normal protein and glucose.

➤ What is the most likely diagnosis?

➤ What is the underlying etiology?

➤ What is the next step?

ANSWERS TO CASE 10:

Hypertensive Encephalopathy/Pheochromocytoma

Summary: A 39-year-old man recently diagnosed with hypertension is now in the emergency room in an acute confusional state and with critically elevated blood pressures. He has been having episodes of palpitations, headaches, and lightheadedness. His medication was recently changed from clonidine to metoprolol. His examination is significant for dilated pupils, papilledema, and bounding peripheral pulses. The urine drug screen is negative. The CT scan of the head is normal, and CSF studies show no evidence of hemorrhage or infection.

> **Most likely diagnosis:** Hypertensive encephalopathy.

> **Possible etiology:** Pheochromocytoma.

> **Next step:** Admit to the intensive care unit (ICU), immediately lower blood pressure with a parenteral agent, and closely monitor arterial pressure.

ANALYSIS

Objectives

1. Learn the definition and management of hypertensive emergencies and urgencies.
2. Understand the relationship between systemic blood pressure and cerebral blood flow.
3. Know how to diagnose and medically treat a patient with a pheochromocytoma.

Considerations

This is a relatively young man with severely elevated blood pressures who presents with **altered mental status**. Use of illicit drugs, such as cocaine and amphetamines, must be considered, but this patient's drug screen was negative. **Hypertensive encephalopathy**, a symptom complex of **severely elevated blood pressures, confusion, increased intracranial pressure, and/or seizures**, is a diagnosis of exclusion, meaning other causes for the patient's acute mental decline, such as stroke, subarachnoid hemorrhage, meningitis, or mass lesions, must be ruled out. Knowing the specific etiology of the patient's hypertension is not necessary to treat his encephalopathy; urgent blood pressure lowering is indicated. However, it is not necessary, and **may be harmful, to *normalize* the blood pressure too quickly,** because it may cause cerebral hypoperfusion. **Parenteral medications should be used to lower the diastolic**

blood pressure to 100 to 110 mm Hg. The patient has tachycardia, hypertension, diaphoresis, dilated pupils, and a slight tremor, all signs of a hyperadrenergic state. Pheochromocytoma must be considered as a possible underlying etiology of his hypertension. His antihypertensive medication changes may also be contributory—perhaps clonidine rebound.

APPROACH TO
Hypertensive Emergencies

DEFINITIONS

MEN IIA: Multiple endocrine neoplasia syndromes which can occur in families. Type IIa includes pheochromocytoma, medullary thyroid cancer, and hyperparathyroidism.

MEN IIB: Pheochromocytoma, medullary thyroid cancer, and mucosal neuromas.

CLINICAL APPROACH

Hypertensive crises are critical elevations in blood pressure, which usually are classified as either hypertensive emergencies or urgencies. The presence of **acute** end-organ damage constitutes a **hypertensive emergency**, whereas the absence of such complications is considered **hypertensive urgency**. Examples of acute end-organ damage include hypertensive encephalopathy, myocardial ischemia or infarction associated with markedly elevated blood pressure, aortic dissection, and pulmonary edema secondary to acute left ventricular failure.

Hypertensive emergencies require immediate reduction in blood pressure over a few hours, typically with intravenous medications and close monitoring in an intensive care unit. Hypertensive urgencies also require prompt medical attention, but the blood pressure can be lowered over 1 to 2 days and can be monitored in the outpatient setting for patients with reliable follow-up.

Hypertensive crises are uncommon but occur most often in patients with an established history of so-called essential hypertension, that is, hypertension without an apparent underlying cause. A crisis may be precipitated by use of sympathomimetic agents, such as cocaine, or by conditions that produce excess sympathetic discharge, such as clonidine withdrawal. Hypertensive crises also result from underlying diseases that cause hypertension, such as renovascular disease (eg, renal artery stenosis), renal parenchymal disease (eg, glomerulonephritis), and pheochromocytoma.

Although the pathophysiology is not completely understood, abrupt rises in vascular resistance are met with endothelial compensation by the release of vasodilator molecules such as nitric oxide. If the increase in arterial pressure persists, the endothelial response is overwhelmed and decompensates, leading to a further rise in pressure and endothelial damage and dysfunction.

Cerebral blood flow is a good example of vascular compensation by vasodilation or vasoconstriction in response to changes in arterial pressure (Figure 10–1). In normotensive adults, cerebral blood flow remains relatively constant over a range of mean arterial pressures between 60 and 120 mm Hg because cerebral vasoconstriction limits excessive cerebral perfusion. As the mean arterial pressure increases beyond the normal range of cerebral autoregulation, there is cerebrovascular endothelial dysfunction and increased permeability of the blood-brain barrier, leading to vasogenic edema and the formation of microhemorrhages. Patients then manifest symptoms of hypertensive encephalopathy, such as lethargy, confusion, headaches, or vision changes. Typical imaging findings on magnetic resonance imaging (MRI) include posterior leukoencephalopathy, usually in the parietooccipital regions, which may or may not be seen on CT scanning. Without therapy, the condition can lead to seizures, coma, and death.

The **definition of hypertensive emergency does not require numerical thresholds** of arterial pressure but **is based on end-organ effects**. Autoregulation failure can occur in previously normotensive individuals at blood pressures as low as 160/100 mm Hg; however, individuals with long-standing hypertension frequently develop adaptive mechanisms (eg, cerebral arterial autoregulation) and may not show clinical manifestations until the blood pressure rises to above 220/110 mm Hg. Thus, **emergent treatment of hypertensive encephalopathy** (and indeed all hypertensive emergencies) should **focus on the symptoms** rather than the numbers. In fact, it may be

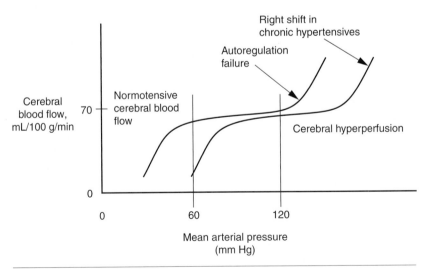

Figure 10–1. Cerebral blood flow autoregulation. Cerebral blood flow is fairly constant over a range of blood pressures. Chronic hypertensive patients have an adaptive mechanism that shifts the curve to the right.

dangerous to "normalize" the blood pressure of patients with chronic hypertension. As a consequence of the right shift in the autoregulation curve, these "normal" blood pressures may lead to decreased perfusion to the brain, resulting in infarction, or similar renal or coronary hypoperfusion, and ischemic injury. Usually, a reasonable goal is reduction of mean arterial pressures by no more than 25% or to a diastolic blood pressure of 100 to 110 mm Hg over a period of minutes to hours.

Treatment of **hypertensive emergencies usually necessitates parenteral medication without delay**; direct blood pressure monitoring with an arterial catheter often is necessary. One of the most commonly used medications for treating hypertensive emergencies is **sodium nitroprusside**. It has the advantage of nearly instantaneous onset of action, and its dose can be easily titrated for a smooth reduction in blood pressure. However, its metabolite may accumulate, resulting in cyanide or thiocyanate toxicity when it is given for more than 2 to 3 days. Certain clinical situations may favor the use of other medications. Intravenous loop diuretics and vasodilators such as nitroglycerin decrease the preload (central venous pressure) in acute pulmonary edema. Myocardial ischemia or infarction is treated with intravenous nitroglycerin to improve coronary perfusion and beta-blockers to reduce blood pressure, heart rate, and myocardial oxygen demand. Patients with aortic dissection benefit from medications that reduce the shear forces affecting the aorta, which will help limit propagation of the dissection. A useful technique in treating these individuals is the use of intravenous nitroprusside to lower the arterial blood pressure and a beta-blocker to blunt reflex tachycardia. Alternatively, intravenous labetalol, a combined alpha- and beta-blocker, alone can be used. Patients presenting with acute cerebral infarction generally should not have acute blood pressure lowering because of the possibility of worsening cerebral ischemia.

The vast majority of hypertension has no discernible cause, so-called *essential hypertension*. Some patients have secondary causes, such as renal artery stenosis, hyperaldosteronism, aortic stenosis, or pheochromocytoma. A history of paroxysmal hypertension with headaches, palpitations, and hyperadrenergic state (flushing, dilated pupils, diaphoresis) suggests the diagnosis of **pheochromocytoma;** pheochromocytomas are catecholamine-producing tumors that arise from chromaffin cells of the adrenal medulla. Other symptoms may include episodic anxiety, tremor, and orthostatic hypotension caused by volume contraction from pressure-induced natriuresis. Although uncommon, accounting for only 0.01% to 0.1% of hypertensive individuals, these tumors have important therapeutic considerations.

The diagnosis is established by measuring increased concentrations of catecholamines or their metabolites in either urine or plasma. Usually, **a 24-hour urine collection** is assayed for **metanephrines, vanillylmandelic acid (VMA), and unconjugated, or "free," catecholamines**. After the biochemical tests document the excess catecholamines, the next step is to locate the tumor for surgical removal. Approximately 90% of pheochromocytomas are in the adrenal gland, usually identified by computed tomography or magnetic resonance imaging. If the initial imaging is unrevealing, scintigraphic localization with ^{123}I-metaiodobenzylguanidine (^{123}I-MIBG) or an octreotide (somatostatin-analogue) scan is indicated, because this radioisotope is preferentially taken up in catecholamine-producing tumors.

The treatment of choice for these tumors is surgical resection, but it is critical to reverse the acute and chronic effects of the excess catecholamines prior to excision. Alpha-adrenergic blocking agents, such as phenoxybenzamine, an irreversible, long-acting agent, started 1 week prior to surgery helps to prevent hypertensive exacerbations, which are especially worrisome during surgery. To expand the commonly seen contracted blood volume, a liberal salt diet is initiated. **Sometimes, a beta-blocking agent is started, but only after alpha-blockade is established.** The products of pheochromocytomas stimulate both the alpha- and beta-adrenergic receptors; thus, using a beta-blocker alone may worsen the hypertension because of unopposed alpha-adrenergic stimulation. Also, beta-blockade may result in acute pulmonary edema, especially in the presence of cardiomyopathy secondary to chronic catecholamine exposure.

Less than 10% of pheochromocytomas are familial, and these tend to be bilateral. One should consider screening for the presence of the *RET* protooncogene seen in multiple endocrine neoplasia type II (MEN II) or the *VHL* gene for von Hippel-Lindau syndrome, or screening family members for these diseases as well as for familial pheochromocytoma and neurofibromatosis.

Comprehension Questions

10.1 A 30-year-old man with chronic hypertension presents at the clinic having run out of his medication, clonidine. He has no complaints and has a blood pressure of 200/104 mm Hg. Which of the following is the best management?
   A. Admit in the hospital and initiate intravenous nitroprusside
   B. Restart the clonidine and recheck the blood pressure in 24 to 48 hours
   C. Change to an angiotensin-converting enzyme (ACE) inhibitor
   D. Refer to a social worker and do not prescribe an antihypertensive agent

10.2 An 80-year-old woman without a history of hypertension undergoes surgery for a hip fracture. Her blood pressure on postoperative day 1 is 178/110 mm Hg. She is asymptomatic except for hip pain. Which of the following is the best next step?
   A. Transfer the patient to the intensive care unit, obtain cardiac enzyme levels, and lower the blood pressures to the 140/90 mm Hg range.
   B. Control the pain and monitor the blood pressure.
   C. Start the patient on a beta-blocker and monitor the blood pressure.
   D. Restrict visitors and turn down television, alarms, and other noise.

10.3   A 61-year-old man with coronary artery disease complains of progressive orthopnea and pedal edema. He is hospitalized with a blood pressure of 190/105 mm Hg. Cardiac enzyme levels and electrocardiogram (ECG) are normal. Intravenous furosemide has been administered. Which of the following is the best next step?
   A. Prescribe a beta-blocker to decrease myocardial oxygen demands
   B. Start intravenous dopamine
   C. Observe
   D. Start an ACE inhibitor

10.4   A 58-year-old woman with aphasia and right-arm weakness of 8 hours' duration is seen in the emergency room. Her blood pressure is 162/98 mm Hg. Which of the following is the best next step?
   A. Normalize the blood pressure with beta-blockade
   B. Admit to ICU with sodium nitroprusside
   C. Normalize the blood pressure with an ACE inhibitor
   D. Observe the blood pressure

ANSWERS

10.1   **B.** This man has a hypertensive urgency—elevated blood pressures without end-organ symptoms, perhaps due to clonidine rebound. The appropriate treatment is initiation of blood pressure medication and reassessment in 24 to 48 hours.

10.2   **B.** Elevated blood pressures without symptoms may occur acutely after surgery, particularly as a consequence of postoperative pain. Generally, this hypertension, unless markedly elevated, does not need to be treated and can lead to orthostatic hypotension when the patient gets out of bed.

10.3   **D.** Elevated blood pressures may exacerbate congestive heart failure and must be treated. Generally, beta-blockers are avoided when patients are volume overloaded because beta-blockers decrease myocardial contractility, exacerbating the decreased ejection fraction. ACE inhibition reduces afterload and is used to treat acute heart failure.

10.4   **D.** In general, hypertension should not be acutely decreased unless markedly elevated in an individual suspected of having a stroke because of the concern for cerebral hypoperfusion and worsening brain ischemia.

Clinical Pearls

> A hypertensive emergency is defined as an episode of elevated blood pressure associated with acute end-organ damage or dysfunction and requires immediate lowering of the blood pressure.

> Asymptomatic patients with elevated blood pressure usually can be started back on an oral regimen and reassessed as outpatients in 24 to 48 hours.

> The cerebral autoregulation curve of individuals with chronic hypertension is shifted to the right. Nevertheless, marked elevations in mean arterial pressure can exceed the ability of cerebral vessels to constrict, causing hyperperfusion, cerebral edema, and hypertensive encephalopathy.

> Pheochromocytomas may cause paroxysmal blood pressure elevations, in association with episodic headaches, palpitations, and diaphoresis.

> Preoperative blood pressure control in pheochromocytoma can be achieved with the use of alpha-blockers such as phenoxybenzamine. Beta-blockers used alone can, paradoxically, increase blood pressure because of unopposed alpha-adrenergic effects.

REFERENCES

Dluhy RG, Lawrence JE, Williams GH. Endocrine hypertension. In: Larsen PR, Kronenberg HM, Melmed S, Polonsky KS, eds. *Williams' Textbook of Endocrinology.* 10th ed. Philadelphia, PA: WB Saunders; 2003:555-562.

Kotchen TA. Hypertensive vascular disease. In: Fauci AS, Braunwald E, Kasper DL, eds. *Harrison's Principles of Internal Medicine.* 17th ed. New York, NY: McGraw-Hill; 2008:1549-1562.

Neumann HP. Pheochromocytoma. In: Fauci AS, Braunwald E, Kasper DL, eds. *Harrison's Principles of Internal Medicine.* 17th ed. New York, NY: McGraw-Hill; 2008:2269-2275.

Pacak K, Linehan WM, Eisenhofer G, et al. Recent advances in the diagnosis, localization, and treatment of pheochromocytoma. *Ann Intern Med.* 2001;134:315-329.

Vaughan CJ, Delanty N. Hypertensive emergencies. *Lancet.* 2000;356:411-417.

Case 11

A 28-year-old man comes to your office complaining of a 5-day history of nausea, vomiting, diffuse abdominal pain, fever to 101°F, and muscle aches. He has lost his appetite, but he is able to tolerate liquids and has no diarrhea. He has no significant medical history or family history, and he has not traveled outside the United States. He admits to having 12 different lifetime sexual partners, denies illicit drug use, and he drinks alcohol occasionally, but not since this illness began. He takes no medications routinely, but he has been taking acetaminophen, approximately 30 tablets per day for 2 days for fever and body aches since this illness began. On examination, his temperature is 100.8°F, heart rate 98 bpm, and blood pressure 120/74 mm Hg. He appears jaundiced, his chest is clear to auscultation, and his heart rhythm is regular without murmurs. His liver percusses 12 cm, and is smooth and slightly tender to palpation. He has no abdominal distention or peripheral edema. Laboratory values are significant for a normal complete blood count, creatinine 1.1 mg/dL, alanine aminotransferase (ALT) 3440 IU/L, aspartate aminotransferase (AST) 2705 IU/L, total bilirubin 24.5 mg/dL, direct bilirubin 18.2 mg/dL, alkaline phosphatase 349 IU/L, serum albumin 3.0 g/dL, and prothrombin time 14 seconds.

➤ What is the most likely diagnosis?

➤ What is the most important immediate diagnostic test?

ANSWERS TO CASE 11:

Acute Viral Hepatitis, Possible Acetaminophen Hepatotoxicity

Summary: A 28-year-old man complains of nausea, vomiting, diffuse abdominal pain, fever, and myalgias. He has had 12 different lifetime sexual partners and currently is taking acetaminophen. He appears icteric and has a low-grade fever and tender hepatomegaly. Results of his laboratory studies are consistent with severe hepatocellular injury and somewhat impaired hepatic function.

➤ **Most likely diagnosis:** Acute hepatitis, either viral infection or toxic injury, possibly exacerbated by acetaminophen use.

➤ **Most important immediate diagnostic test:** Acetaminophen level, because acetaminophen toxicity may greatly exacerbate liver injury but is treatable.

ANALYSIS

Objectives

1. Understand the use of viral serologic studies for diagnosing hepatitis A, B, and C infections.
2. Know the prognosis for acute viral hepatitis and recognize fulminant hepatic failure.
3. Know measures to prevent hepatitis A and B infections.
4. Understand the use of the acetaminophen nomogram and the treatment of acetaminophen hepatotoxicity.

Considerations

This patient has an acute onset of hepatic injury and systemic symptoms that predate his acetaminophen use. The markedly elevated hepatic transaminase and bilirubin levels are consistent with viral hepatitis or possibly toxic injury. This patient denied intravenous drug use, which would be a risk factor for hepatitis B and C infections. His sexual history is a possible clue. The degree and pattern of transaminase (ALT and AST) elevation can provide some clues to help differentiate possible etiologies. Transaminase levels more than 1000 IU/L are seen in conditions that produce extensive hepatic necrosis, such as toxic injury, viral hepatitis, and ischemia ("shock liver"). Patients with alcoholic hepatitis almost always has levels less than 500 IU/L and often have an AST/ALT ratio of 2:1. In this case, it is important to consider the possibility of acetaminophen toxicity, both because the condition can produce fatal liver failure and because an effective antidote is available. By obtaining a serum

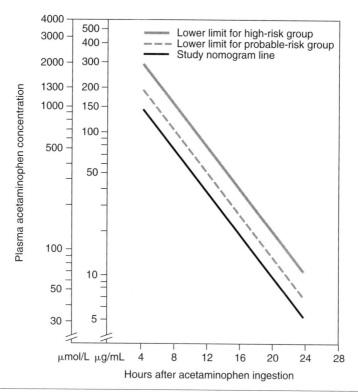

Figure 11–1. Acetaminophen nomogram. *Reproduced, with permission, from Dienstag JL, Isselbacher KJ. Poisoning and drug overdose. In: Braunwald E, Fauci AS, Kasper DL, et al. eds.* Harrison's Principles of Internal Medicine. *15th ed. New York, NY: McGraw-Hill; 2001:2602.*

acetaminophen level and knowing the time of his last ingestion, these data can be plotted on a nomogram (Figure 11–1) to help predict acetaminophen-related liver damage and the possible need for *N*-acetylcysteine.

APPROACH TO

Suspected Hepatitis

DEFINITIONS

HEPATITIS: An inflammation of the liver. At least six forms of hepatitis have been identified, referred to as hepatitis A, B, C, D, E, and G.

CHRONIC HEPATITIS: A syndrome that is defined clinically by evidence of liver disease for at least 6 consecutive months.

CLINICAL APPROACH

VIRAL HEPATITIS

Most cases of acute hepatitis are caused by infection with one of five viruses: hepatitis A, B, C, D, or E. They can produce virtually indistinguishable clinical syndromes, although it is unusual to observe acute hepatitis C. Affected individuals often complain of a prodrome of nonspecific constitutional symptoms, including fever, nausea, fatigue, arthralgias, myalgias, headache, and sometimes pharyngitis and coryza. This is followed by the onset of visible jaundice caused by hyperbilirubinemia, with tenderness and enlargement of the liver, and dark urine caused by bilirubinuria. The clinical course, and prognosis then vary based on the type of virus causing the hepatitis.

Hepatitis A and **E** both are very contagious and transmitted by fecal-oral route, usually by contaminated food or water where sanitation is poor, and in daycare by children. **Hepatitis A** is found worldwide and is the **most common cause of acute viral hepatitis in the United States. Hepatitis E** is much less common and is found in Asia, Africa, Central America, and the Caribbean. Both hepatitis A and E infections usually lead to self-limited illnesses and generally resolve within weeks. Almost all patients with hepatitis A recover completely and have no long-term complications. A few may have fulminant disease resulting in liver failure. Most patients with hepatitis E also have uncomplicated courses, but some patients, particularly pregnant women, have been reported to develop severe hepatic necrosis and fatal liver failure.

Hepatitis B is the second most common type of viral hepatitis in the United States, and it is **usually sexually transmitted**. It also may be acquired parenterally, such as by intravenous drug use, and during birth from chronically infected mothers. The outcome depends on the age at which the infection was acquired. Up to 90% of infected newborns develop chronic hepatitis B infection, which places the affected infant at significant risk of hepatocellular carcinoma later in adulthood. For individuals infected later in life, approximately 95% of patients will recover completely without sequelae. Between 5% and 10% of patients will develop chronic hepatitis, which may progress to cirrhosis. A chronic carrier state may be seen in which the virus continues to replicate, but it does not cause irreversible hepatic damage in the host.

Hepatitis C is transmitted **parenterally by blood transfusions or intravenous drug use**, and rarely by sexual contact. The mode of transmission is unknown in approximately 40% of cases. It is uncommonly diagnosed as a cause of acute hepatitis, often producing subclinical infection, but is frequently diagnosed later as a cause of chronic hepatitis.

Hepatitis D is a defective RNA virus that requires the presence of the hepatitis B virus to replicate. It can be acquired as a coinfection simultaneously with acute hepatitis B or as a later superinfection in a person with a chronic hepatitis B infection. Patients afflicted with chronic hepatitis B virus who then become infected with hepatitis D may suffer clinical deterioration; in 10% to 20% of these cases, individuals develop severe fatal hepatic failure.

Fortunately, in most cases of acute viral hepatitis, patients recover completely, so the treatment is generally supportive. However, **fulminant hepatic failure** as a result of massive hepatic necrosis may progress over a period of weeks. This usually is caused by infection by the hepatitis B and D viruses, or is drug-induced. This syndrome is characterized by rapid progression of encephalopathy from confusion or somnolence to coma. Patients also have worsening coagulopathy as measured by increasing prothrombin times, rising bilirubin levels, ascites and peripheral edema, hypoglycemia, hyperammonemia, and lactic acidosis. Fulminant hepatitis carries a poor prognosis (the mortality for comatose patients is 80%) and often is fatal without an emergency liver transplant.

Diagnosis

Clinical presentation does not reliably establish the viral etiology, so serologic studies are used to establish a diagnosis. Anti–hepatitis A immunoglobulin M (IgM) establishes an acute hepatitis A infection. Anti–hepatitis C antibody is present in acute hepatitis C, but the test result may be negative for several weeks. The hepatitis C RNA assay, which becomes positive earlier in the disease course, often aids in the diagnosis. Acute hepatitis B infection is diagnosed by the presence of hepatitis B surface antigen (HBsAg) in the clinical context of elevated serum transaminase levels and jaundice. HBsAg later disappears when the antibody (anti-HBs) is produced (Figure 11–2). There is

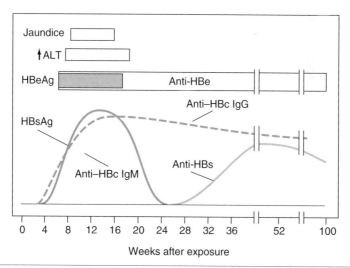

Figure 11–2. Serologic markers in acute hepatitis B infection. *Reproduced, with permission, from Deinstag JL, Isselbacher KJ. Acute viral hepatitis. In: Braunwald E, Fauci AS, Kasper DL, et al. eds. Harrison's Principles of Internal Medicine. 16th ed. New York, NY: McGraw-Hill; 2005:1825.*

often an interval of a few weeks between the disappearance of HBsAg and the appearance of anti-HBsAb. This period is referred to as the "window period." During this interval, the presence of anti–hepatitis B core antigen IgM (anti–HBc IgM) is indicative of an acute hepatitis B infection. Hepatitis B precore antigen (HBeAg) represents a high level of viral replication. It is almost always present during acute infection, but its persistence after 6 weeks of illness is a sign of chronic infection and high infectivity. Persistence of HBsAg or HBeAg is a marker for chronic hepatitis or a chronic carrier state; elevated versus normal serum transaminase levels distinguish between these two entities, respectively.

Prevention

The efficacy of the hepatitis A vaccine for hepatitis A (available in two doses given 6 months apart) exceeds 90%. It is indicated for individuals planning to travel to endemic areas. Postexposure prophylaxis with hepatitis A immunoglobulin, along with the first injection of the vaccine, should be given to household and intimate contacts within 2 weeks of exposure. The hepatitis B vaccine (given in three doses over 6 months) provides effective immunity in more than 90% of patients. It is recommended for health-care workers, as well as for universal vaccination of infants in the United States. Hepatitis B immunoglobulin (HBIg) is given after exposure, such as a needle-stick injury from an infected patient, or to a newborn of infected mothers. The first inoculation of the vaccine usually is given concurrently. There is no immunization and no proven postexposure prophylaxis for persons exposed to hepatitis C. **Interferon treatment** may be used in individuals with hepatitis B or C infection, and lamivudine is used to treat patients with chronic hepatitis B.

ACETAMINOPHEN HEPATITIS

Acetaminophen-induced hepatocellular injury may result after a single, large ingestion, as in a suicide attempt, or by chronic use of over-the-counter acetaminophen-containing preparations for treatment of pain or fever. **Hepatic toxicity** most often occurs after an acute ingestion of **10 g or more**, but lower doses may cause injury in patients with preexisting liver disease, particularly in those who abuse alcohol. Acetaminophen is metabolized in the liver by the cytochrome P450 enzyme system, which produces a toxic metabolite; this metabolite is detoxified by binding to glutathione. Potential hepatic injury is greater when P450 activity is augmented by drugs such as ethanol or phenobarbital, or when less glutathione is available, as in alcoholism, malnutrition, or AIDS (acquired immunodeficiency syndromes). Acetaminophen levels are measured between 4 and 24 hours after an acute ingestion and plotted on a **nomogram** to predict possible hepatotoxicity and determine if treatment is necessary (Figure 11–1). Sometimes, empiric therapy is started even before labs results return.

If acetaminophen levels are above the level that predisposes to hepatic injury, treatment is started with gastric decontamination with charcoal and administration of **N-acetylcysteine**, which provides cysteine to replenish glutathione stores. N-Acetylcysteine should be started within the first 10 hours to prevent liver damage and is continued for 72 hours. Meanwhile, the patient should not receive any medications that are known to be hepatotoxic.

Comprehension Questions

11.1   A 25-year-old medical student is stuck with a hollow needle during a procedure performed on a patient known to have hepatitis B and C viral infection, but who is HIV negative. The student's baseline laboratory studies include serology: HBsAg negative, anti-HBsAb positive, anti-HBc IgG negative. Which of the following regarding this medical student's hepatitis status is true?

A. Prior vaccination with hepatitis B vaccine
B. Acute infection with hepatitis B virus
C. Prior infection with hepatitis B virus
D. The student was vaccinated for hepatitis B but is not immune

11.2   What postexposure prophylaxis should the student described in Question 11.1 receive?

A. Hepatitis B immunoglobulin (HBIg)
B. Oral lamivudine
C. Intravenous immunoglobulin (IVIG)
D. Reassurance

11.3   In a suicide attempt, an 18-year-old adolescent female takes 4 g of acetaminophen, approximately 8 hours previously. Her acetaminophen level is 30 µg/mL. Which of the following is the best next step to be performed for this patient?

A. Immediately start N-acetylcysteine
B. Observation
C. Alkalinize the urine
D. Administer intravenous activated charcoal

ANSWERS

11.1   **A.** This student's serology is most consistent with vaccination and not prior infection. Like all health-care workers, the student should have been vaccinated against the hepatitis B virus, which induces anti–HBs IgG antibody, which is thought to be protective. Not all people receiving the vaccine develop an adequate antibody titer; if none were detected, it would indicate the need for revaccination. Patients with prior hepatitis B infection will also likely have anti–HBsAb but will also have anti–HBc IgG. Acute infection would be signified by the presence of either HBsAg or anti–HBc IgM.

11.2   **D.** No postexposure prophylaxis is definitively indicated. The student has detectable protective antibody levels against the hepatitis B virus, and if the levels are judged to be adequate, the student is protected against infection. Oral lamivudine is a treatment for chronic hepatitis B infection and is part of an antiretroviral prophylaxis if the patient was HIV positive. There is no effective prophylaxis for hepatitis C exposure.

11.3   **B.** The serum acetaminophen level of 30 μg/mL, with last ingestion 8 hours previously, is plotted on the nomogram and falls below the "danger zone" of possible hepatic injury. Thus, this patient should be observed. Sometimes, patients will take more than one medication so that serum and/or urine drug testing may be worthwhile. Gastrointestinal activated charcoal, not intravenous charcoal, is used for other ingestions.

Clinical Pearls

➤ The three most common causes of acute hepatitis with elevated transaminase levels exceeding 1000 IU/L are viral infection, toxic exposure, and ischemic injury.

➤ The large majority of adults with acute hepatitis B viral infection recover completely, but 5% to 10% develop chronic hepatitis.

➤ Fulminant hepatic failure, characterized by the rapid development of hepatic encephalopathy, coagulopathy, peripheral edema, and ascites, usually is fatal unless a liver transplant is performed.

➤ Prevention of hepatitis B viral infection hinges on long-term immunity with a highly effective recombinant vaccine and short-term postexposure prophylaxis with hepatitis B immunoglobulin (HBIg).

➤ The likelihood of toxic acetaminophen injury and the need for treatment can be predicted from a nomogram based on serum level and the time since last ingestion.

REFERENCES

Bass NM. Toxic and drug-induced liver disease. In: Cecil RL, Bennett JC, Goldman L, eds. *Cecil's Textbook of Medicine*. 21st ed. Philadelphia, PA: WB Saunders; 2000: 781-782.

Deinstag JL. Acute viral hepatitis. In: Kasper DL, Braunwald E, Fauci AS, et al. eds. *Harrison's Principles of Internal Medicine*. 17th ed. New York, NY: McGraw-Hill; 2008:1932-1949.

Dienstag JL. Toxic and drug-induced hepatitis. In: Kasper DL, Braunwald E, Fauci AS, et al. eds. *Harrison's Principles of Internal Medicine*. 17th ed. New York, NY: McGraw-Hill; 2008:1949-1955.

Luis S, Marsano MD. Hepatitis. *Prim Care Clin Office Pract*. 2003;30:81-107.

Case 12

A 38-year-old woman presents to your office for evaluation of menstrual irregularity. She states that her periods started when she was 12 years old, and they have been fairly regular ever since, coming once every 28 to 30 days. She has had three previous uncomplicated pregnancies and deliveries. However, approximately 9 months ago, her cycles seemed to lengthen, and for the last 3 months she has not had a period at all. She stopped breast-feeding 3 years ago, but over the last 3 months she noticed that she could express a small amount of milky fluid from her breasts. She had a bilateral tubal ligation after her last pregnancy, and she has no other medical or surgical history. She takes no medications except multivitamins. Over the last year or so, she thinks she has gained about 10 lb, and she feels as if she has no energy despite adequate sleep. She has noticed some mild thinning of her hair and slightly more coarse skin texture. She denies headaches or visual changes. Her physical examination, including pelvic and breast examinations, are normal. She is not obese or hirsute. You elicit slight whitish nipple discharge. Her pregnancy test is negative.

➤ What is the most likely diagnosis?

➤ What is the most likely etiology for the condition?

ANSWERS TO CASE 12:
Oligomenorrhea Caused by Hypothyroidism and Hyperprolactinemia

Summary: A 38-year-old woman complains of oligomenorrhea and now secondary amenorrhea, along with galactorrhea. She previously had regular menses and three uncomplicated pregnancies and deliveries. She had a bilateral tubal ligation after her last pregnancy, but she has no other medical or surgical history, and she takes no medications that might cause galactorrhea. She has experienced weight gain, fatigue, mild thinning of her hair, and slightly more coarse skin. She denies headaches or visual changes, which might suggest a pituitary adenoma. Her physical examination, including pelvic and breast examinations, are normal. She is not obese or hirsute. You can elicit slight whitish nipple discharge.

➤ **Most likely diagnosis:** Oligomenorrhea and galactorrhea due to hypothyroidism.

➤ **Most likely etiology:** In this patient with symptoms of weight gain, fatigue, thinning hair, and galactorrhea in the setting of previously normal menses, hypothyroidism is the most likely diagnosis.

ANALYSIS

Objectives

1. Understand the differential diagnosis of secondary amenorrhea and the approach to the investigation of possible hormonal causes.
2. Understand the interactions of the hormones involved in the hypothalamic-pituitary-gonadal axis.
3. Recognize the clinical features and diagnostic evaluation of hypothyroidism.
4. Be familiar with the treatment of hypothyroidism.

Considerations

This 38-year-old woman presents with oligomenorrhea, weight gain, fatigue, and galactorrhea despite having previously normal menses and discontinuing breast-feeding 3 years ago. Her history of fatigue, weight gain, and hair loss suggest a systemic cause of her symptoms, specifically hypothyroidism. However, her normal physical examination with lack of myxedema or bradycardia, normal reflexes, normal cognition, and nondisplaced point of maximal impulse suggest mild hypothyroidism. Lack of virilization or obesity does not exclude polycystic ovarian syndrome, but their absence makes this diagnosis less likely. Hypothyroidism alone could attribute to galactorrhea, because hypothyroidism can be associated with hyperprolactinemia. Although prolactinomas can also cause galactorrhea as well as secondary amenorrhea, the lack of visual disturbance in this patient is reassuring.

A variety of other disorders could lead to the symptoms exhibited by this woman (eg, hypopituitarism, adrenal insufficiency). The definitive workup, aside from a thorough history and physical examination, invariably will include laboratory studies. To make informed and cost-effective choices, a carefully formulated stepwise approach should be undertaken by the physician.

APPROACH TO
Oligomenorrhea

DEFINITIONS

AMENORRHEA: *Primary*—Absence of menarche by the age of 16 years regardless of the presence or absence of secondary sex characteristics. *Secondary*—Absence of menstruation for 3 or more months in women with normal past menses.

GALACTORRHEA: Any white discharge from the nipple that is persistent and looks like milk.

OLIGOMENORRHEA: Menses occurring at infrequent intervals of more than 40 days or fewer than nine menses per year.

POLYCYSTIC OVARIAN SYNDROME: Syndrome characterized by infertility, hirsutism, obesity, and amenorrhea or oligomenorrhea.

CLINICAL APPROACH

The assessment of oligomenorrhea is similar to the workup for secondary amenorrhea with the understanding that secondary amenorrhea is present when a normally menstruating woman stops having periods for 3 consecutive months or more. **The most common cause of both symptoms, and the easiest to exclude in the office, is pregnancy.** A negative in-office pregnancy test should be confirmed with a serum beta–human chorionic gonadotropin (hCG). Primary amenorrhea is present when the first menses has not appeared in a girl by the age of 16 years and is generally caused by a variety of genetic or congenital defects and is commonly associated with disorders of puberty. Given this patient's age and history, primary amenorrhea is not a consideration; thus, a diagnostic pathway for secondary amenorrhea/oligomenorrhea should be undertaken.

Problems of the Hypothalamic-Pituitary-Ovarian Axis

Excluding pregnancy and problems in the genital outflow tract, disorders of the hypothalamic-pituitary-ovarian axis account for the largest number of cases of oligomenorrhea and amenorrhea. Disorders of the hypothalamus account for the largest percentage of abnormality (>45%); these include problems of nutrition (rapid weight loss/anorexia), excessive exercise, stress, and infiltrative diseases (eg, craniopharyngioma, sarcoidosis, histiocytosis). The largest single cause of oligomenorrhea is polycystic ovarian syndrome (PCOS), accounting for 30% of all cases. The PCOS was once thought to be a disease originating in the ovary; however, it now is known that **PCOS is a much more complicated neuroendocrine disorder** with evidence of **estrogenization,** as well as **insulin resistance.** Other important causes of amenorrhea include diseases of the pituitary, specifically neoplasms (eg, prolactinomas, functioning or nonfunctioning adenomas), which account for 18% of cases. Empty sella syndrome, caused by cerebrospinal fluid (CSF) herniation into the pituitary fossa, and Sheehan syndrome, caused by severe obstetric hemorrhage and/or maternal hypotension at delivery, are important causes of atrophy and ischemia of the pituitary. If suspected, they should be investigated by magnetic resonance imaging (MRI). Finally, disorders such as premature ovarian failure (loss of all functional ovarian follicles before age 40 years), diseases of the thyroid, and adult-onset adrenal hyperplasia should be considered and investigated if supported by history and physical examination with the appropriate laboratory studies (Table 12–1).

Table 12–1 DIFFERENTIAL DIAGNOSIS OF OLIGOMENORRHEA*

	HISTORY	LABORATORY	THERAPY
Polycystic ovarian syndrome	Irregular menses since menarche, obesity, hirsutism	Slightly elevated testosterone, elevated LH/FSH	Oral contraceptive agent
Hypothyroidism	Fatigue, cold intolerance	Elevated TSH	Thyroxine replacement
Hyperprolactinemia	Headache, bitemporal hemianopsia, galactorrhea, medications, hypothyroidism	Elevated prolactin level	Depends on etiology
Ovarian failure	Hot flushes, hypoestrogenemia	Elevated FSH and LH	Replacement of hormones
Sheehan syndrome	Postpartum hemorrhage, unable to breast-feed	Low pituitary hormones (FSH, TSH, ACTH)	Replacement of pituitary hormones

Abbreviations: ACTH, adrenocorticotropic hormone; FSH, follicle-stimulating hormone; LH, luteinizing hormone; TSH, thyroid-stimulating hormone.
*Pregnancy must always be suspected with oligomenorrhea or amenorrhea.

The history and physical examination will narrow the range of possible causes. In this patient, the history of fatigue, weight gain, and galactorrhea, along with previously normal menses and a normal physical examination, place hypothyroidism at the top of the list. Because of the lack of headaches or visual field changes, a prolactinoma is less likely; however, a prolactin level that is very high would direct investigation toward this entity, given the history of galactorrhea. In the workup of secondary amenorrhea, these two diagnoses are the easiest to start with because the tests are minimally invasive and relatively inexpensive, and the treatment is straightforward.

Hypothyroidism

Hypothyroidism is defined as the insufficient production of thyroid hormone. Secondary hypothyroidism as a result of dysfunction of hypothalamic and pituitary hormone secretion are much less common but should be suspected in a patient with a history suggestive of Sheehan syndrome or with symptoms or signs of a tumor in the region of the sella. **Ninety-five percent of cases of hypothyroidism** are caused by **primary thyroid gland failure**, resulting in insufficient thyroid hormone production. In the United States, **the most common cause of hypothyroidism is lymphocytic (Hashimoto) thyroiditis**, in which cytotoxic antibodies are produced, which leads to thyroid atrophy and fibrosis. The next most common cause is surgical or radioactive iodine treatment for hyperthyroidism, or Graves disease. **Worldwide, iodine deficiency** is the **most common cause of goitrous (enlarged thyroid) hypothyroidism**, but in the United States, this is rare.

Most hypothyroid patients present with vague and nonspecific symptoms. **Elderly** individuals may be suspected of having **dementia or depression** when the cause is really hypothyroidism. In general, symptoms of fatigue, weight gain, muscle cramping, cold intolerance, hair thinning, menstrual changes, or carpal tunnel syndrome are common and should prompt an investigation of thyroid function. In severe, prolonged hypothyroidism, a syndrome termed **myxedema**, may develop. These patients present with dull facies, swollen eyes, and doughy extremities from the accumulation of hydrophilic polysaccharides in the dermis, sparse hair, and a thickened tongue. They may have an enlarged heart, nonmechanical intestinal obstruction (ileus), and a delayed relaxation phase of their deep tendon reflexes. Without treatment, they may become stuporous and hypothermic, especially if challenged with an intercurrent illness. This is a life-threatening emergency with a high mortality, even when managed aggressively with intravenous levothyroxine.

When testing outpatients for hypothyroidism, measurement of the **serum thyroid-stimulating hormone (TSH)** level is the most sensitive and useful test. Because almost all cases of hypothyroidism are caused by thyroid gland failure, the normal pituitary response is to markedly increase the TSH levels in an attempt to stimulate the failing gland. Falling levels of thyroid hormone produce logarithmic increases in the TSH concentration. Measurements of the thyroid hormone level can also be performed, but one needs to remember that almost all thyroxine (T_4) circulates bound to protein, but it is the free fraction that is able to diffuse into cells and become active. So, one can either measure the free T_4 directly in some laboratories, or it can be **estimated by using the triiodothyronine (T_3) uptake,** which is a measure of available protein binding, to calculate the free thyroxine index (FTI). When there is **excess** thyroid-binding globulin (TBG), as in pregnancy or oral contraceptive use, T_4 **levels will be high (as a consequence of the large amount of carrier protein),** but T_3 **uptake will be low** (value varies inversely with amount of TBG present). Conversely, when there is a low level of TBG, as in a hypoproteinemic patient with nephrotic syndrome, the T_4 level will necessarily also be low (not much carrier protein), but the T_3 uptake will be high. An easy way to remember this is by like vector analysis: when T_4 and T_3 **uptake both are high, the patient really is hyperthyroid; when they both are low, the patient is hypothyroid.** However, when they vary in opposite directions, for example, high T_4 with low T_3 uptake, they "cancel each other out," that is, it is a protein-binding abnormality as described above.

In mild cases, or "subclinical hypothyroidism," the TSH level is mildly elevated, but the measured free T_4 or FTI is within the normal range (although probably lower than what it would be if the patient were really euthyroid). Patients may be asymptomatic or report the vague and subtle symptoms of hypothyroidism, such as fatigue. About half of such patients will progress to overt hypothyroidism within 5 years. They often have some **derangement of cholesterol metabolism, such as elevated total and low-density lipoprotein (LDL) cholesterol**. Thyroid hormone replacement can be prescribed in an attempt to relieve symptoms or possibly to reduce cardiovascular risk.

In overt hypothyroidism, the TSH level is markedly elevated, and a low free T_4 or free thyroxine index (low T_4, low T_3 uptake) is also seen. The T_3 levels can be normal, because the elevated TSH levels may induce hypersecretion of T_3 from the gland. Elevated cholesterol levels are also common.

The overwhelming majority of patients with hypothyroidism can be treated with once-daily dosing of synthetic levothyroxine, which is biochemically identical to the natural hormone. **Levothyroxine is relatively inexpensive, has a long half-life (6-7 days), allowing once-daily** dosing, and gives a predictable response. Older thyroid preparations, such as desiccated thyroid extract, are available but are not favored because they have a high content of T_3, which is rapidly absorbed and can produce tachyarrhythmias, and the T_4 content is less predictable. In **older patients and in those with known cardiovascular disease, dosing should start at a low level,** such as 25 to 50 µg/d, and increased at similar increments once every 4 to 6 weeks to an average dose of 1.7 to 2.1 µg/kg body weight. Overly rapid replacement with the sudden increase in metabolic rate can overwhelm the coronary or cardiac reserve. Depending on the cause of hypothyroidism and the amount of residual gland function, individual patient needs will vary widely. The **TSH level will take 6 to 8 weeks to readjust to a new dosing level,** so follow-up laboratory testing should be scheduled accordingly.

Comprehension Questions

12.1   A 42-year-old woman presents to your office for her annual physical. On examination, you note neck fullness. When you palpate her thyroid, it is enlarged, smooth, rubbery, and nontender. The patient is asymptomatic. You send her for thyroid function testing: her T_4, free T_4, and T_3 are normal, but her TSH is slightly elevated. Which of the following is the most likely diagnosis?
A. Iodine deficiency
B. Thyroid cancer
C. Hashimoto thyroiditis
D. Graves disease
E. Multinodular goiter

12.2   Which of the following laboratory tests could be performed to confirm your diagnosis of the patient in Question 12.1?
A. Repeat thyroid function tests
B. Thyroid ultrasound
C. Nuclear thyroid scan
D. Antithyroid antibody tests
E. Complete blood count with differential

12.3   A 19-year-old gymnast active in national competition is brought to your office by her mother because the daughter's menses have ceased for the last 3 months. Prior to this, she was always regular. She denies excess dieting, although she does work out with her team 3 hours daily. Her physical examination is normal except for her body mass index (BMI) of 20 kg/m². Which of the following laboratory tests should be ordered first?
A. Thyroid function tests
B. Complete blood count
C. Luteinizing hormone (LH)/follicle-stimulating hormone (FSH)
D. Prolactin
E. Beta-hCG

12.4   A 35-year-old woman who was diagnosed with hypothyroidism 4 weeks
        ago presents to your office complaining of persistent feelings of fatigue
        and sluggishness. After confirming your diagnosis with a measurement
        of the TSH, you started her on levothyroxine 50 µg daily. She has been
        reading about her diagnosis on the Internet and wants to try desiccated
        thyroid extract instead of the medicine you gave her. On examination,
        she weighs 175 lb, her heart rate is 64 bpm at rest, and her blood pres-
        sure is normal. Which of the following is the best next step?
        A. Tell her that this delay in resolution of symptoms is normal and
           schedule a follow-up visit with her in 2 months.
        B. Change her medication, as requested, to thyroid extract and titrate.
        C. Increase her dose of levothyroxine and have her come back in
           4 weeks.
        D. Tell her to start a multivitamin with iron to take with her levothy-
           roxine.

ANSWERS

12.1   **C.** Hashimoto thyroiditis is the most common cause of hypothy-
        roidism with goiter in the United States. It is most commonly found
        in middle-aged women, although it can be seen in all age groups.
        Patients can present with a rubbery, nontender goiter that may have
        "scalloped" borders. Iodine deficiency is exceedingly uncommon in
        the United States because of iodized salt. Graves disease is a hyper-
        thyroid condition. Patients with multinodular goiter usually are
        euthyroid. Patients with thyroid cancer usually are euthyroid and
        have a history of head and neck irradiation.

12.2   **D.** Hashimoto thyroiditis is an autoimmune disease of the thyroid.
        Several different autoantibodies directed toward components of the
        thyroid gland will be present in the patient's serum; however, of these,
        antithyroperoxidase antibody almost always is detectable (also called
        antimicrosomal antibody). These antibodies are the markers, not the
        cause, of gland destruction. On thyroid biopsy, lymphocytic infiltra-
        tion and fibrosis of the gland are pathognomonic. The presence of
        these autoantibodies predicts progressive gland failure and the need
        for hormone replacement. None of the other tests will be helpful.

12.3   **E.** In a young woman with oligomenorrhea, pregnancy should always
        be the first diagnosis considered. Urine pregnancy tests are easily per-
        formed in the office and are highly sensitive. Serum beta-hCG can
        be measured to confirm a negative test. In this patient, the next most
        likely diagnosis is hypothalamic hypogonadism, secondary to her
        strenuous exercise regimen. These young women are at risk for osteo-
        porosis and should be counseled on adequate nutrition and offered
        combined oral contraceptives if the amenorrhea persists.

12.4   **C.** Levothyroxine is the preferred replacement hormone for hypothyroidism. The amount of hormone batch to batch and the patient dose response are believed to be more predictable than with other forms of hormone replacement, such as thyroid extract, which is made from desiccated beef or pork thyroid glands. There is no evidence that the natural hormone replacement is superior to the synthetic form. The dose of levothyroxine should be titrated to relief of symptoms, as well as to normalization of the TSH. Other medications, especially iron-containing vitamins, should be taken at different times than levothyroxine because they may interfere with absorption.

Clinical Pearls

➤ The most common causes of oligomenorrhea are disorders of the hypothalamic-pituitary-gonadal axis, such as polycystic ovarian syndrome and hypothyroidism.

➤ Hypothyroidism is a cause of hyperprolactinemia. Both hypothyroidism and hyperprolactinemia may cause hypothalamic dysfunction, leading to menstrual irregularities.

➤ The most common cause of hypothyroidism is primary thyroid gland failure as a result of Hashimoto thyroiditis.

➤ A low free T_4 or free thyroxine index and a high thyroid-stimulating hormone characterize primary hypothyroidism.

➤ Synthetic levothyroxine (T_4) replacement is the treatment of choice for hypothyroidism; in older patients, you need to "start low and go slow."

➤ The goal of therapy is to normalize the thyroid-stimulating hormone level in primary hypothyroidism and to relieve symptoms.

REFERENCES

Carr BR, Bradshaw KD. In: Kasper DL, Braunwald E, Fauci AS, et al. eds. Disturbances of menstruation. *Harrison's Principles of Internal Medicine*. 16th ed. New York, NY: McGraw-Hill; 2005:2198-2213.

Cooper DS. Subclinical hypothyroidism. *N Engl J Med*. 2001;345:260-265.

Jameson JL, Weetman AP. Disorders of the thyroid gland. In: Kasper DL, Braunwald E, Fauci AS, et al. eds. *Harrison's Principles of Internal Medicine*. 17th ed. New York, NY: McGraw-Hill; 2008:2224-2247.

Ladenson PW, Singer PA, Ain KB, et al. American Thyroid Association guidelines for detection of thyroid dysfunction. *Arch Intern Med*. 2000;160:1573-1575.

Case 13

A 49-year-old woman presents to the emergency room complaining of a 4-week history of progressive abdominal swelling and discomfort. She has no other gastrointestinal symptoms, and she has a normal appetite and normal bowel habits. Her medical history is significant only for three pregnancies, one of which was complicated by excessive blood loss, requiring a blood transfusion. She is happily married for 20 years, exercises, does not smoke, and drinks only occasionally. On pointed questioning, however, she does admit that she was "wild" in her youth, and she had snorted cocaine once or twice at parties many years ago. She does not use drugs now. She was HIV negative at the time of the birth of her last child.

On examination, her temperature is 100.3°F, heart rate 88 bpm, and blood pressure 94/60 mm Hg. She is thin, her complexion is sallow, her sclerae are icteric, her chest is clear, and her heart rhythm is regular with no murmur. Her abdomen is distended, with mild diffuse tenderness, hypoactive bowel sounds, shifting dullness to percussion, and a fluid wave. She has no peripheral edema. Laboratory studies are normal except for Na 129 mEq/L, albumin 2.8 mg/dL, total bilirubin 4 mg/dL, prothrombin time 15 seconds, hemoglobin 12 g/dL with mean cell volume (MCV) 102 fL, and platelet count 78,000/mm^3.

➤ What is the most likely diagnosis?

➤ What is your next step?

ANSWERS TO CASE 13:
Cirrhosis, Probable Hepatitis C–Related

Summary: A 49-year-old woman presents with new-onset abdominal swelling. Her history reveals a blood transfusion with postpartum hemorrhage and cocaine use. On examination, her temperature is 100.3°F, heart rate 88 bpm, and blood pressure 94/60 mm Hg. Her sclerae are icteric. Her abdomen is distended, with mild diffuse tenderness, shifting dullness to percussion, and a fluid wave, consistent with ascites. She has no peripheral edema. Laboratory studies show the following levels: Na 129 mmol/L, albumin 2.8 mg/dL, prothrombin time 15 seconds, hemoglobin 12 g/dL with MCV 102 fL, and platelet count 78,000/mm^3.

> **Most likely diagnosis:** Ascites caused by portal hypertension as a complication of hepatic cirrhosis.

> **Next step:** Perform a paracentesis to evaluate the ascitic fluid to try to determine its likely etiology as well as evaluate for the complication of spontaneous bacterial peritonitis.

ANALYSIS

Objectives

1. Know the causes of chronic hepatitis, especially hepatitis C virus (HCV).
2. Learn the complications of chronic hepatitis, such as cirrhosis and portal hypertension.
3. Understand the utility of the serum-ascites albumin gradient (SAAG) to differentiate causes of ascites.
4. Know how to diagnose spontaneous bacterial peritonitis.

Considerations

This 49-year-old woman had been in good health until recently, when she noted increasing abdominal swelling and discomfort, indicative of ascites. The physical examination is consistent with ascites with the fluid wave and shifting dullness. Her icterus suggests liver disease as the etiology of the ascites. Her laboratory studies are significant for hypoalbuminemia and coagulopathy (prolonged prothrombin time), indicating probable impaired hepatic synthetic function and advanced liver disease. She does have prior exposures, most notably a blood transfusion, which put her at risk for hepatitis viruses, especially hepatitis C. Currently, she also has a low-grade fever and mild abdominal tenderness, both signs of infection. Bacterial infection of the ascitic fluid must be considered, because untreated cases have a high mortality.

Although the large majority of patients with ascites and jaundice have cirrhosis, other etiologies of the ascites must be considered, including malignancy. Thus, paracentesis using a needle introduced through the skin into the peritoneal cavity can be used to assess for infection as well as to seek an etiology of the ascites.

APPROACH TO
Chronic Hepatitis

DEFINITIONS

ASCITES: Abnormal accumulation (>25 mL) of fluid within the peritoneal cavity.

CHRONIC HEPATITIS: Evidence of hepatic inflammation and necrosis for at least 6 months.

CIRRHOSIS: Histologic diagnosis reflecting irreversible chronic hepatic injury, which includes extensive fibrosis and formation of regenerative nodules.

PORTAL HYPERTENSION: Increased pressure gradient (>10 mm Hg) in the portal vein, usually resulting from resistance to portal flow and most commonly caused by cirrhosis.

SPONTANEOUS BACTERIAL PERITONITIS: Bacterial infection of ascitic fluid without any intra-abdominal source of infection. Occurs in 10% to 20% of cirrhotic patients with ascites.

CLINICAL APPROACH

Chronic hepatitis is diagnosed when patients have evidence of hepatic inflammation and necrosis (usually found by elevated transaminases) for at least 6 months. The **most common causes of chronic hepatitis are viral infections,** such as **hepatitis B and C, alcohol use, chronic exposure to other drugs or toxins, and autoimmune hepatitis.** Less common causes are inherited metabolic disorders, such as hemochromatosis, Wilson disease, or α_1-antitrypsin deficiency. Table 13–1 lists the diagnostic markers for these disorders.

Hepatitis C infection is most commonly acquired through percutaneous exposure to blood. It also can be transmitted through exposure to other body fluids, although this method is less effective. Risk factors for acquisition of hepatitis C include intravenous drug use, sharing of straws to snort cocaine, hemodialysis, blood transfusion, tattooing, and piercing. In contrast to hepatitis B, sexual transmission is rare. Vertical transmission from mother to child is uncommon but occurs more often when the mother has high viral titers or is HIV positive.

Table 13–1 CAUSES OF CHRONIC HEPATITIS

CAUSE	TEST
Hepatitis C	Anti-HCV Ab, presence of HCV RNA
Hepatitis B	Persistent HBsAg, presence of HBeAg
Autoimmune	ANA, anti-LKM (liver kidney microsome)
Hemochromatosis	High transferrin saturation (>50%), high ferritin
Wilson disease	Low serum ceruloplasmin
α_1-antitrypsin deficiency	Low α_1-antitrypsin enzyme activity

Abbreviations: ANA, antinuclear antibody; HBeAg, hepatitis B e antigen; HbsAg, hepatitis B surface antigen.

Most patients diagnosed with hepatitis C are asymptomatic, and report no prior history of acute hepatitis. The clinician must have a high index of suspicion and offer screening to those individuals with risk factors for infection. To date, the best methods for detecting infection include the enzyme-linked immunosorbent assay (ELISA) test, which detects anti-HCV antibody (Ab), or the polymerase chain reaction (PCR) to detect HCV RNA. Approximately 70% to 80% of all patients infected with hepatitis C will develop chronic hepatitis in the 10 years following infection. Within 20 years, 20% of those will develop cirrhosis. Among those with cirrhosis, 1% to 4% annually may develop hepatocellular carcinoma. Therapy is directed toward reducing the viral load to prevent the sequelae of end-stage cirrhosis, liver failure, and hepatocellular carcinoma. Currently, the **treatment of choice for chronic hepatitis C is combination therapy with pegylated alpha-interferon and ribavirin**. Trials have demonstrated a sustained response (undetectable viral levels) in up to 75% to 80% of those with favorable HCV genotypes (types 2 and 3). However, the therapy has many side effects, such as influenzalike symptoms and depression with interferon, and hemolysis with ribavirin. The goal of interferon therapy for hepatitis C is preventing the complications of chronic hepatitis.

Cirrhosis is the end result of chronic hepatocellular injury that leads to both **fibrosis and nodular regeneration**. With ongoing hepatocyte destruction and collagen deposition, the liver shrinks in size and becomes nodular and hard. Alcoholic cirrhosis is one of the most common forms of cirrhosis encountered in the United States. It is related to chronic alcohol use, but there appears to be some hereditary predisposition to the development of fibrosis, and the process is enhanced by concomitant infection with hepatitis C. Clinical symptoms are produced by the hepatic dysfunction as well as by portal hypertension, which is produced by increased resistance to portal blood flow, producing portal hypertension, and sometimes to resultant portosystemic shunting (Table 13–2). Loss of functioning hepatic mass leads to jaundice as well as impaired synthesis of albumin (leading to edema) and of clotting factors (leading to coagulopathy). Fibrosis and increased sinusoidal resistance lead to portal hypertension and its complications, such as esophageal varices, ascites, and hypersplenism. Portosystemic shunting via natural collaterals or iatrogenic shunts causes hepatic encephalopathy. Portal hypertension causes caput medusa and hemorrhoids. Decreased liver production of steroid hormone binding globulin (SHBG) leads to an increase in unbound

Table 13–2 COMPLICATIONS OF CIRRHOSIS

DISORDER	DIAGNOSIS	CLINICAL PRESENTATION	TREATMENT
Portal hypertension	Diagnosis is made by the appearance of the features described earlier, and evaluation of portal blood flow using Doppler ultrasonography	Clinical features are related to portal hypertension and its sequelae: ascites, splenomegaly, hypersplenism, encephalopathy, and bleeding varices	Nonselective beta-blockers such as propranolol lower portal pressure; during acute variceal hemorrhage, Sandostatin or octreotide causes splanchnic vasoconstriction
Ascites	Made by finding free peritoneal fluid on physical examination or on an imaging study	Abdominal distention, sometimes with peripheral edema	Sodium restriction, spironolactone; loop diuretics; large-volume paracentesis
Spontaneous bacterial peritonitis	Diagnosis can be made when the ascitic fluid contains > 250 polymorphonuclear neutrophils/mm^3 and confirmed with a positive culture; the most common organisms are *Escherichia coli*, *Klebsiella*, other enteric flora, enterococci, and pneumococci	Abdominal pain, distention, fever, decreased bowel sounds, or sometimes few abdominal symptoms but worsening encephalopathy	IV antibiotics, such as cefotaxime or ampicillin/sulbactam

estrogen manifested by spider angiomata, palmar erythema, and gynecomastia in men. Hepatic encephalopathy is characterized by mental status changes, asterixis, and elevated ammonia levels.

The most common cause of ascites is portal hypertension as a consequence of cirrhosis. The pathogenesis involves a combination of decreased effective circulatory blood volume because of portal hypertension (underfill theory), inappropriate renal sodium retention leading to expansion of plasma volume (overfill theory), and decreased plasma oncotic pressure. When not caused by portal hypertension, ascites may be a result of exudative causes such as infection (eg, tuberculous peritonitis) or malignancy. The patient usually presents with abdominal swelling and demonstration of free fluid by physical examination or imaging procedures such as ultrasonography.

It is important to try to determine the cause of ascites in order to look for reversible causes and for serious causes, such as malignancy, and to guide therapy. Ascitic fluid is obtained by paracentesis and examined for protein, albumin, cell count with differential, and culture. The first step in trying to determine the cause of ascites (Table 13–3) is to determine whether it is caused by portal hypertension or by an exudative process by calculating the SAAG:

Serum-ascites albumin gradient = serum albumin − ascitic albumin.

The **treatment of ascites usually consists of dietary sodium restriction coupled with diuretics.** Loop diuretics are often combined with spironolactone to provide effective diuresis and to maintain normal potassium levels. **Spontaneous bacterial peritonitis** is a relatively common complication of ascites, thought to be caused by translocation of gut flora into the peritoneal fluid. Symptoms include fever and abdominal pain, but often there is paucity of signs and symptoms. Diagnosis is established by paracentesis and finding more than

---

Table 13–3 DIFFERENTIAL DIAGNOSIS OF ASCITES BASED ON SAAG*

High gradient >1.1 g/dL: Portal hypertension
- Cirrhosis
- Portal vein thrombosis
- Budd-Chiari syndrome
- Congestive heart failure
- Constrictive pericarditis

Low gradient <1.1 g/dL: Nonportal hypertension
- Peritoneal carcinomatosis
- Tuberculous peritonitis
- Pancreatic ascites
- Bowel obstruction or infarction
- Serositis, eg, as in lupus
- Nephrotic syndrome

*SAAG: Serum-ascites albumin gradient = serum albumin − ascitic albumin.

250 polymorphonuclear neutrophils/mm^3 or by a positive culture. Culture of ascitic fluid often fails to yield the organism. However, fluid cultures, when positive, usually reveal a single organism, most often gram-negative enteric flora but occasionally enterococci or pneumococci. This is in contrast to secondary peritonitis, for example, as a consequence of intestinal perforation, which usually is polymicrobial. Empiric therapy includes coverage for gram-positive cocci and gram-negative rods, such as intravenous ampicillin and gentamicin, or a third-generation cephalosporin or a quinolone antibiotic.

Comprehension Questions

For the following questions choose the one cause (A-G) that is probably responsible for the patient's presentation:

A. Wilson disease
B. Hematochromatosis
C. Primary biliary cirrhosis
D. Sclerosing cholangitis
E. Autoimmune hepatitis
F. Alcohol-induced hepatitis
G. Viral hepatitis

13.1 A 15-year-old adolescent female with elevated liver enzymes and a positive antinuclear antibody (ANA)

13.2 A 56-year-old man with brittle diabetes, tan skin, and a family history of cirrhosis

13.3 A 35-year-old man with ulcerative colitis

13.4 A 56-year-old woman who presented with complaints of pruritus and fatigue

13.5 A 32-year-old man with Kayser-Fleischer rings, dysarthria, and spasticity

ANSWERS

13.1 **E.** Idiopathic or autoimmune hepatitis is a less-well-understood cause of hepatitis that seems to be caused by autoimmune cell-mediated damage to hepatocytes. A subgroup of these patients includes young women with positive ANAs and hypergammaglobulinemia who may have other symptoms and signs of systemic lupus erythematosus.

13.2   **B.** Hemochromatosis is a genetic disorder of iron metabolism. Progressive iron overload leads to organ destruction. Diabetes mellitus, cirrhosis of the liver, hypogonadotrophic hypogonadism, arthropathy, and cardiomyopathy are among the more common end-stage developments. Skin deposition of iron leads to "bronzing" of the skin, which could be mistaken for a tan. Diagnosis is made early in the course of disease by demonstrating elevated iron stores but can be made through liver biopsy with iron stains. Genetic testing is available. Therapy involves phlebotomy to remove excess iron stores.

13.3   **D.** Sclerosing cholangitis is an autoimmune destruction of both the intrahepatic and extrahepatic bile ducts and often is associated with inflammatory bowel disease, most commonly ulcerative colitis. Patients present with jaundice or symptoms of biliary obstruction; cholangiography reveals the characteristic beading of the bile ducts.

13.4   **C.** Primary biliary cirrhosis is thought to be an autoimmune disease leading to destruction of small- to medium-size bile ducts. Most patients are women between the ages of 35 and 60 years, who usually present with symptoms of pruritus and fatigue. An alkaline phosphatase level elevated two to five times above the baseline in an otherwise asymptomatic patient should raise suspicion for the disease. No specific therapy is available.

13.5   **A.** Wilson disease is an inherited disorder of copper metabolism. The inability to excrete excess copper leads to deposition of the mineral in the liver, brain, and other organs. Patients can present with fulminant hepatitis, acute nonfulminant hepatitis, or cirrhosis, or with bizarre behavioral changes as a result of neurologic damage. Kayser-Fleischer rings develop when copper is released from the liver and deposits in Descemet membrane of the cornea.

Clinical Pearls

➤ The most common causes of cirrhosis are alcohol use, hepatitis B and C, and autoimmune disorders.

➤ Hepatitis C is most commonly contracted through blood exposure and rarely through sexual contact. Most patients are asymptomatic until they develop complications of chronic liver disease.

➤ A serum ascites albumin gradient more than 1.1 g/dL suggests that ascites is caused by portal hypertension, as occurs in cirrhosis.

➤ Treatment of cirrhotic ascites requires sodium restriction and, usually, diuretics, such as spironolactone and furosemide.

➤ Spontaneous bacterial peritonitis is infection of the ascitic fluid characterized by more than 250 polymorphonuclear cells/mm^3, sometimes with a positive monomicrobial culture.

REFERENCES

Bacon BR. Cirrhosis and its complications. In: Kasper DL, Braunwald E, Fauci AS, et al. eds. *Harrison's Principles of Internal Medicine*. 17th ed. New York, NY: McGraw-Hill; 2008:1971-1980.

Dienstag JL. Chronic hepatitis. In: Kasper DL, Braunwald E, Fauci AS, et al. eds. *Harrison's Principles of Internal Medicine*. 17th ed. New York, NY: McGraw-Hill; 2008:1955-1969.

Gines P, Cardenas A, Arroyo, V. et al. Management of cirrhosis and ascites. *N Engl J Med*. 2004;350:1646-1654.

Liang TJ. Shortened therapy for hepatitis C virus genotype 2 or 3—is less more? *N Engl J Med*. 2007;357:176-178.

Strader DB, Wright T, Thomas DL, et al. AASLD guideline: Diagnosis, management, and treatment of hepatitis C. *Hepatology*. 2004;39:1147-1171.

Case 14

A 42-year-old Hispanic woman presents to the emergency department complaining of 24 hours of severe, steady epigastric abdominal pain, radiating to her back, with several episodes of nausea and vomiting. She has experienced similar painful episodes in the past, usually in the evening following heavy meals, but the episodes always resolved spontaneously within an hour or two. This time the pain did not improve, so she sought medical attention. She has no medical history and takes no medications. She is married, has three children, and does not drink alcohol or smoke cigarettes.

On examination, she is afebrile, tachycardic with a heart rate of 104 bpm, blood pressure 115/74 mm Hg, and shallow respirations of 22 breaths per minute. She is moving uncomfortably on the stretcher, her skin is warm and diaphoretic, and she has scleral icterus. Her abdomen is soft, mildly distended with marked right upper quadrant and epigastric tenderness to palpation, hypoactive bowel sounds, and no masses or organomegaly appreciated. Her stool is negative for occult blood. Laboratory studies are significant for a total bilirubin (9.2 g/dL) with a direct fraction of 4.8 g/dL, alkaline phosphatase 285 IU/L, aspartate aminotransferase (AST) 78 IU/L, alanine aminotransferase (ALT) 92 IU/L, and elevated amylase level 1249 IU/L. Her leukocyte count is 16,500/mm^3 with 82% polymorphonuclear cells and 16% lymphocytes. A plain film of the abdomen shows a nonspecific gas pattern and no pneumoperitoneum.

➤ What is the most likely diagnosis?

➤ What is the most likely underlying etiology?

➤ What is your next diagnostic step?

ANSWERS TO CASE 14:
Pancreatitis, Gallstones

Summary: A 42-year-old woman with a prior history consistent with symptomatic cholelithiasis now presents with epigastric pain and nausea for 24 hours,
much longer than would be expected with uncomplicated biliary colic. Her
symptoms are consistent with acute pancreatitis. She also has hyperbilirubinemia and an elevated alkaline phosphatase level, suggesting obstruction of
the common bile duct caused by a gallstone, which is the likely cause of her
pancreatitis.

➤ **Most likely diagnosis:** Acute pancreatitis.

➤ **Most likely etiology:** Choledocholithiasis (common bile duct stone).

➤ **Next diagnostic step:** Right upper quadrant abdominal ultrasonography.

ANALYSIS

Objectives

1. Know the causes, clinical features, and prognostic factors in acute pancreatitis.
2. Learn the principles of treatment and complications of acute pancreatitis.
3. Know the complications of gallstones.
4. Understand the medical treatment of a patient with biliary sepsis and the
   indications for endoscopic retrograde cholangiopancreatography (ERCP)
   or surgical intervention.

Considerations

This 42-year-old woman complained of episodes of mild right upper quadrant
abdominal pain with heavy meals in the past. These prior episodes were short-
lived. This is very consistent with biliary colic. However, this episode is different in severity and location of pain (now radiating straight to her back and
accompanied by nausea and vomiting). The elevated amylase level confirms
the clinical impression of acute pancreatitis. She likely has acute pancreatitis
caused by a stone in the common bile duct. Biliary obstruction is suggested by
the elevated bilirubin level. She is moderately ill but is hemodynamically stable and has only one prognostic feature to predict mortality—her elevated
white blood cell (WBC) count (Table 14–1). She likely can be managed on a
hospital ward without the need for intensive care.

Table 14–1 RANSON CRITERIA FOR SEVERITY OF PANCREATITIS

Initial
- Age >55 years
- WBC >16,000/mm³
- Serum glucose >200
- Serum lactate dehydrogenase (LDH) >350 IU/L
- AST >250 IU/L

Within 48 hours of admission
- Hematocrit drop >10 points
- Blood urea nitrogen (BUN) rise >5 mg/dL after intravenous hydration
- Arterial Po$_2$ <60 mm Hg
- Serum calcium <8 mg/dL
- Base deficit >4 mEq/L
- Estimated fluid sequestration of >6 L

Data from: Ranson JH. Etiological and prognostic factors in human acute pancreatitis: a review. *Am J Gastroenterol.* 1982;77:633.

APPROACH TO
Acute Pancreatitis

DEFINITIONS

ACUTE PANCREATITIS: An inflammatory process in which pancreatic enzymes are activated and cause autodigestion of the gland.

PANCREATIC PSEUDOCYST: Cystic space within the pancreas not lined by epithelial cells, often associated with chronic pancreatitis.

CLINICAL APPROACH

Acute pancreatitis can be caused by many processes, but in the United States, **alcohol use is the most common cause**, and episodes are often precipitated by binge drinking. The next most common cause is biliary tract disease, usually due to passage of a gallstone into the common bile duct. Hypertriglyceridemia is another common cause and occurs when serum triglyceride levels are more than 1000 mg/dL, as is seen in patients with familial dyslipidemias or diabetes (etiologies are given in Table 14–2). When patients appear to have "idiopathic" pancreatitis, that is, no gallstones are seen on ultrasonography and no other predisposing factor can be found, biliary tract disease is still the most likely cause—either biliary sludge (microlithiasis) or sphincter of Oddi dysfunction.

Table 14–2 CAUSES OF ACUTE PANCREATITIS

Biliary tract disease (eg, gallstones)
Alcohol use
Drugs (eg, the antiretroviral didanosine [ddI], pentamidine, thiazides,
    furosemide, sulfonamides, azathioprine, L-asparaginase)
Surgical manipulation of the gland or ERCP
Hypertriglyceridemia/hypercalcemia
Infections such as mumps or cytomegalovirus
Trauma such as blunt abdominal trauma

Abdominal pain is the cardinal symptom of pancreatitis and often is severe, typically in the **upper abdomen with radiation to the back**. The pain often is relieved by sitting up and bending forward, and is exacerbated by food. Patients **commonly experience nausea and vomiting** that is precipitated by oral intake. They **may have low-grade fever** (if temperature is >101°F, one should suspect infection) and often are volume depleted because of the vomiting, inability to tolerate oral intake, and because the inflammatory process may cause third spacing with sequestration of large volumes of fluid in the peritoneal cavity.

The most common test used to diagnose pancreatitis is an **elevated serum amylase level**. It is released from the inflamed pancreas within hours of the attack and remains elevated for 3 to 4 days. Amylase undergoes renal clearance, and after serum levels decline, its level remains elevated in the urine. **Amylase is not specific to the pancreas,** however, and can be elevated as a consequence of many other abdominal processes, such as **gastrointestinal ischemia with infarction or perforation; even just the vomiting** associated with pancreatitis can cause elevated amylase of **salivary origin.** Elevated **serum lipase level,** also seen in acute pancreatitis, is **more specific than is amylase to pancreatic origin and remains elevated longer than does amylase.** When the diagnosis is uncertain or when complications of pancreatitis are suspected, computed tomographic **(CT) imaging of the abdomen is highly sensitive** for showing the inflammatory changes in patients with moderate to severe pancreatitis.

Treatment of pancreatitis is mainly supportive and includes "pancreatic rest," that is, **withholding food or liquids by mouth until symptoms subside** and adequate **narcotic analgesia, usually with meperidine. Intravenous fluids** are necessary for maintenance and to replace any deficits. In patients with severe pancreatitis who sequester large volumes of fluid in their abdomen as pancreatic ascites, sometimes prodigious amounts of parenteral fluid replacement are necessary to maintain intravascular volume. Patients with adynamic ileus and abdominal distention or protracted vomiting may benefit from nasogastric suction. When pain has largely subsided and the patient has bowel sounds, oral clear liquids can be started and the diet advanced as tolerated.

The large majority of patients with acute pancreatitis will recover spontaneously and have a relatively uncomplicated course. Several criteria have been developed in an attempt to identify the 15% to 25% of patients who will have a more complicated course. These include the Ranson (United States) and Glasgow/Imrie (United Kingdom) criteria, as well as the APACHE (Acute Physiology and Chronic Health Evaluation) II scoring system. When three or more of the following criteria are present, a severe course complicated by pancreatic necrosis can be predicted by Ranson criteria (Table 14–1). **The most common cause of early death in patients with pancreatitis is hypovolemic shock,** which is multifactorial: third spacing and sequestration of large fluid volumes in the abdomen, as well as increased capillary permeability. Others develop pulmonary edema, which may be noncardiogenic as a consequence of acute respiratory distress syndrome (ARDS), or cardiogenic as a consequence of myocardial dysfunction.

Pancreatic complications include a **phlegmon,** which is a solid mass of inflamed pancreas, often with patchy areas of necrosis. Sometimes, extensive areas of **pancreatic necrosis** develop within a phlegmon. Either necrosis or a phlegmon can become secondarily infected, resulting in **pancreatic abscess.** Abscesses typically develop 2 to 3 weeks after the onset of illness and should be suspected if there is fever or leukocytosis. If pancreatic abscesses are not drained, mortality approaches 100%. Pancreatic necrosis and abscess are the leading causes of death in patients after the first week of illness. A **pancreatic pseudocyst** is a cystic collection of inflammatory fluid and pancreatic secretions, which unlike true cysts do not have an epithelial lining. Most pancreatic pseudocysts resolve spontaneously within 6 weeks, especially if they are smaller than 6 cm. However, if they are causing pain, are large or expanding, or become infected, they usually require drainage. Any of these local complications of pancreatitis should be suspected if persistent pain, fever, abdominal mass, or persistent hyperamylasemia occurs.

Gallstones

Gallstones usually form as a consequence of precipitation of cholesterol microcrystals in bile. They are very common, occurring in 10% to 20% of patients older than 65 years. Patients often are asymptomatic. When discovered incidentally, they can be followed without intervention, as only 10% of patients will develop any symptoms related to their stones within 10 years. When patients do develop symptoms because of a stone in the cystic duct or Hartmann pouch, the typical attack of **biliary colic** usually has a sudden onset, often precipitated by a large or fatty meal, with severe steady pain in the right upper quadrant or epigastrium, lasting between 1 and 4 hours. They may have mild elevations of the alkaline phosphatase level and slight hyperbilirubinemia, but elevations of the bilirubin level over 3 g/dL suggest a common duct stone. The first diagnostic test in a patient with suspected gallstones usually is an **ultrasonogram.** The test is noninvasive and very sensitive for detecting stones in the gallbladder as well as intrahepatic or extrahepatic biliary duct dilation.

One of the most common complications of gallstones is **acute cholecystitis**, which occurs when a stone becomes impacted in the cystic duct, and edema and inflammation develop behind the obstruction. This is apparent ultrasonographically as gallbladder wall thickening and pericholecystic fluid, and is characterized clinically as a persistent right upper quadrant abdominal pain, with fever and leukocytosis. Cultures of bile in the gallbladder often yield enteric flora such as *Escherichia coli* and *Klebsiella*. If the diagnosis is in question, nuclear scintigraphy with a **hepatobiliary iminodiacetic acid (HIDA) scan** may be performed. The positive test shows visualization of the liver by the isotope, but nonvisualization of the gallbladder may indicate an obstructed cystic duct. Treatment of acute cholecystitis usually involves making the patient npo (nil per os), intravenous fluids and antibiotics, and early cholecystectomy within 48 to 72 hours.

Another complication of gallstones is **cholangitis**, which occurs when there is intermittent obstruction of the common bile duct, allowing reflux of bacteria up the biliary tree, followed by development of purulent infection behind the obstruction. If the patient is septic, the condition requires urgent decompression of the biliary tree, either surgically or by endoscopic retrograde cholangiography (ERCP), to remove the stones endoscopically after performing a papillotomy, which allows the other stones to pass.

Comprehension Questions

14.1   A 43-year-old man who is an alcoholic is admitted to the hospital with acute pancreatitis. He is given intravenous hydration and is placed NPO. Which of the following findings is a poor prognostic sign?

   A. His age
   B. Initial serum glucose level of 60 mg/dL
   C. Blood urea nitrogen (BUN) level rises 7 mg/dL over 48 hours
   D. Hematocrit drops 3%
   E. Amylase level of 1000 IU/L

14.2   A 37-year-old woman is noted to have gallstones on ultrasonography. She is placed on a low-fat diet. After 3 months she is noted to have severe right upper quadrant pain, fever to 102°F, and nausea. Which of the following is the most likely diagnosis?

   A. Acute cholangitis
   B. Acute cholecystitis
   C. Acute pancreatitis
   D. Acute perforation of the gallbladder

14.3   A 45-year-old man was admitted for acute pancreatitis, thought to be
a result of blunt abdominal trauma. After 3 months he still has epi-
gastric pain but is able to eat solid food. His amylase level is elevated
at 260 IU/L. Which of the following is the most likely diagnosis?
   A. Recurrent pancreatitis
   B. Diverticulitis
   C. Peptic ulcer disease
   D. Pancreatic pseudocyst

ANSWERS

14.1   **C.** When the BUN rises by 5 mg/dL after 48 hours despite IV hydration, it is a poor prognostic sign. Notably, the amylase level does not
correlate to the severity of the disease. An elevated serum glucose
would be a poor prognostic factor. A drop of hematocrit of at least
10% is a significant poor prognostic criteria.

14.2   **B.** Acute cholecystitis is one of the most common complications of
gallstones. This patient with fever, right upper quadrant pain, and a
history of gallstones likely has acute cholecystitis.

14.3   **D.** A pancreatic pseudocyst has a clinical presentation of abdominal
pain and mass and persistent hyperamylasemia in a patient with prior
pancreatitis.

Clinical Pearls

➤ The most common causes of acute pancreatitis in the United States are
alcohol consumption, gallstones, and hypertriglyceridemia.
➤ Acute pancreatitis usually is managed with pancreatic rest, intravenous
hydration, and analgesia, often with narcotics.
➤ Patients with pancreatitis who have zero to two of the Ranson criteria are
expected to have a mild course; those with three or more criteria can have
significant mortality.
➤ Pancreatic complications (phlegmon, necrosis, abscess, pseudocyst)
should be suspected if persistent pain, fever, abdominal mass, or persistent
hyperamylasemia occurs.
➤ Patients with asymptomatic gallstones do not require treatment; they can
be observed and treated if symptoms develop. Cholecystectomy is performed for patients with symptoms of biliary colic or for those with complications.
➤ Acute cholecystitis is best treated with antibiotics and then cholecystectomy, generally within 48 to 72 hours.

REFERENCES

Ahmed A, Cheung RC, Keefe EB. Management of gallstones and their complications. *Am Fam Physician*. 2000;61:1673-1680.

Greenberger NJ, Paumgartner G. Diseases of the gallbladder and bile ducts. In: Braunwald E, Fauci AS, Kasper KL, et al. eds. *Harrison's Principles of Internal Medicine*. 17th ed. New York, NY: McGraw-Hill; 2008:1991-2001.

Greenberger NJ, Toskes PP. Acute and chronic pancreatitis. In: Braunwald E, Fauci AS, Kasper KL, et al. eds. *Harrison's Principles of Internal Medicine*. 17th ed. New York, NY: McGraw-Hill; 2008:2005-2017.

Tenner S. Initial management of acute pancreatitis: critical issues during the first 72 hours. *Am J Gastroenterol*. 2004;99:2489-2494.

Case 15

A 72-year-old man is brought to the emergency room after fainting while in church. He had stood up to sing a hymn and then fell to the floor. His wife, who witnessed the episode, reports that he was unconscious for approximately 5 minutes. When he awakened, he was groggy for another minute or two, then seemed himself. No abnormal movements were noted. This has never happened to him before, but his wife does report that for the last several months he has had to curtail activities, such as mowing the lawn, because he becomes weak and feels lightheaded. His only medical history is osteoarthritis of his knees, for which he takes acetaminophen.

On examination, he is alert, talkative, and smiling. He is afebrile, his heart rate is regular at 35 bpm, and his blood pressure is 118/72 mm Hg, which remains unchanged on standing. He has contusions on his face, left arm, and chest wall, but no lacerations. His chest is clear to auscultation, and his heart rhythm is regular but bradycardic with a nondisplaced apical impulse. He has no focal deficits. Laboratory examination shows normal blood counts, renal function, and serum electrolyte levels, and negative cardiac enzymes. His ECG (electrocardiogram) is shown in Figure 15–1.

➤ What is the most likely diagnosis?

➤ What is your next step?

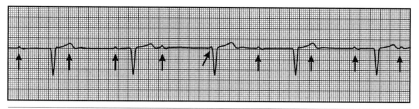

Figure 15–1. Electrocardiogram. *Reproduced, with permission, from Stead LG, Stead SM, Kaufman MS. First Aid for the Medicine Clerkship. 2nd ed. New York, NY: McGraw-Hill; 2006:46.*

ANSWERS TO CASE 15:

Syncope—Heart Block

Summary: A 72-year-old man presents with a witnessed syncopal episode, which was brief and not associated with seizure activity. He has experienced decreasing exercise tolerance recently because of weakness and presyncopal symptoms. He is bradycardic, with third-degree atrioventricular (AV) block on ECG. Arrows in Figure 15–1 point to P waves.

➤ **Most likely diagnosis:** Syncope as a consequence of third-degree AV block.

➤ **Next step:** Placement of temporary transcutaneous or transvenous pacemaker and evaluation for placement of a permanent pacemaker.

ANALYSIS

Objectives

1. Know the major causes of syncope and important historical clues to the diagnosis.
2. Understand the basic evaluation of syncope based on the history.
3. Recognize vasovagal syncope and carotid sinus hypersensitivity.
4. Be able to diagnose and know the management of first-, second-, and third-degree AV block.

Considerations

There are two major considerations to the management of this patient: the cause and the management of his AV block. He should be evaluated for myocardial infarction and structural cardiac abnormalities. If this evaluation is negative, he may simply have conduction system disease as a consequence of aging. Regarding temporary management, atropine or isoproterenol can be used when the conduction block is at the level of the AV node, but in this case, the heart rate is less than 40 bpm, and the QRS borderline is widened, suggesting the defect is below the AV node, in the bundles of His. A pacemaker likely is required.

APPROACH TO
Syncope

DEFINITIONS

SYNCOPE: A transient loss of consciousness and postural tone with subsequent spontaneous recovery.

VASOVAGAL SYNCOPE: Fainting due to excessive vagal tone causing impaired autonomic responses such as hypotension without appropriate rise in heart rate or vasomotor tone.

CLINICAL APPROACH

Syncope is a very common phenomenon, resulting in 5% to 10% of emergency room visits and resulting hospitalization. The causes are varied, but they all result in transiently diminished cerebral perfusion leading to loss of consciousness. The prognosis is quite varied, ranging from a benign episode in an otherwise young, healthy person with a clear precipitating event, such as emotional stress, to a more serious occurrence in an older patient with cardiac disease. In the latter situation, syncope has been referred to as "sudden cardiac death, averted." For that reason, higher risk patients routinely undergo hospitalization and sometimes extensive evaluation to determine the cause.

Traditionally, the etiologies of syncope have been divided into neurologic and cardiac. However, this probably is not a useful classification, because neurologic diseases are uncommon causes of syncopal episodes. Syncope is essentially never a result of transient ischemic attacks (TIAs), because syncope reflects global cerebral hypoperfusion, and TIAs are a result of regional ischemia. Vertebrobasilar insufficiency with resultant loss of consciousness is often discussed yet rarely seen in clinical practice. Seizure episodes are a common cause of transient loss of consciousness, and distinguishing seizure episodes from syncopal episodes based on history often is quite difficult. To further complicate matters, the same lack of cerebral blood flow that produced the loss of consciousness can lead to postsyncopal seizure activity. Seizures are best discussed elsewhere, so our discussion here is confined to syncope. **The only neurologic diseases that commonly cause syncope** are disturbances in **autonomic function** leading to **orthostatic hypotension as occurs in diabetes, parkinsonism, or idiopathic dysautonomia.** For patients in whom a definitive diagnosis of syncope can be ascertained, the causes usually are excess vagal activity, orthostatic hypotension, or cardiac disease—either arrhythmias or outflow obstructions. Table 15–1 lists the most common causes of syncope. By far, the most useful evaluation for diagnosing the cause of syncope is the patient's history. Because, by definition, the patient was unconscious, the patient

Table 15–1 CAUSES OF SYNCOPE

Cardiogenic

Cardiac arrhythmias
- Bradyarrhythmias
  - Sinus bradycardia, sinoatrial block, sinus arrest, sick sinus syndrome
  - Atrioventricular block
- Tachyarrhythmias
  - Supraventricular tachycardia with structural cardiac disease
  - Atrial fibrillation associated with the Wolff-Parkinson-White syndrome
  - Atrial flutter with 1:1 atrioventricular conduction
  - Ventricular tachycardia

Other cardiopulmonary etiologies
- Pulmonary embolism
- Pulmonary hypertension
- Atrial myxoma
- Myocardial disease (massive myocardial infarction)
- Left ventricular myocardial restriction or constriction
- Pericardial constriction or tamponade
- Aortic outflow tract obstruction (aortic valvular stenosis, hypertrophic obstructive cardiomyopathy)

Noncardiogenic

Vasovagal (vasodepressor, neurocardiogenic)
Postural (orthostatic) hypotension
- Drug induced (especially antihypertensive or vasodilator drugs)
- Peripheral neuropathy (diabetic, alcoholic, nutritional, amyloid)
- Idiopathic postural hypotension
- Neurologic disorder (Shy-Drager syndrome)
- Physical deconditioning
- Sympathectomy
- Acute dysautonomia (Guillain-Barré syndrome variant)
- Decreased blood volume (adrenal insufficiency, acute blood loss, etc)
- Carotid sinus hypersensitivity

Situational
- Cough
- Micturition
- Defecation
- Valsalva

may only be able to report preceding and subsequent symptoms, so finding a witness to describe the episode is extremely helpful.

Vasovagal syncope refers to excessive vagal tone causing impaired autonomic responses, that is, a fall in blood pressure without appropriate rise in heart rate or vasomotor tone. This is, by far, the **most common cause of syncope** and is the usual cause of a "fainting spell" in an otherwise healthy young person. Episodes often are precipitated by physical or emotional stress, or by a painful experience. There is usually a clear precipitating event by history and, often, prodromal symptoms such as nausea, yawning, or diaphoresis. The episodes are brief, lasting seconds to minutes, with a rapid recovery. Syncopal episodes also can be triggered by physiologic activities that increase vagal tone, such as **micturition**, defecation, or coughing in otherwise healthy people.

Carotid sinus hypersensitivity is also **vagally mediated**. This usually occurs in older men, and episodes can be triggered by turning the head to the side, by wearing a tight collar, or even by shaving the neck over the area. Pressure over one or both carotid sinuses causes excess vagal activity with resultant cardiac slowing and can produce sinus bradycardia, sinus arrest, or even AV block. Less commonly, carotid sinus pressure can cause a fall in arterial pressure without cardiac slowing. When recurrent syncope as a result of bradyarrhythmias occurs, a demand pacemaker is often required.

Patients with **orthostatic hypotension** typically report symptoms related to positional changes, such as rising from a seated or recumbent position, and **the postural drop in systolic blood pressure by more than 20 mm Hg** can be demonstrated on examination. This can occur because of hypovolemia (hemorrhage, anemia, diarrhea or vomiting, Addison disease) or with adequate circulating volume but impaired autonomic responses. The most common reason for this autonomic impairment probably is iatrogenic as a result of antihypertensive or other medications, especially in elderly persons. It also can be caused by autonomic insufficiency seen in diabetic neuropathy, in a syndrome of chronic idiopathic orthostatic hypotension in older men, or the primary neurologic conditions mentioned previously. Multiple events that all are unwitnessed or that occur only in periods of emotional upset suggest **factitious** symptoms.

Etiologies of **cardiogenic syncope** include rhythm disturbances and structural heart abnormalities. Certain structural heart abnormalities will cause obstruction of blood flow to the brain, resulting in syncope. These include aortic stenosis or hypertrophic obstructive cardiomyopathy (HOCM). Syncope due to cardiac outflow obstruction can also occur with massive pulmonary embolism and severe pulmonary hypertension. Syncope caused by cardiac outflow obstruction typically presents during or immediately after exertion. An echocardiogram often is obtained to elucidate such abnormalities.

Arrhythmias, usually bradyarrhythmias, are the most common cardiac cause of syncope. Sinus bradycardia most often due to degenerative sinoatrial node dysfunction and AV node blocks (see section on Heart Block) are bradyarrhythmic causes of syncope. Sick sinus syndrome (SSS) in elderly patients is one of the most common causes for pacemaker placement. Patients with SSS may experience sinus bradycardia or arrest, alternating with a supraventricular tachycardia, most often atrial fibrillation (tachycardia-bradycardia syndrome). Tachyarrhythmias such as atrial fibrillation or flutter, supraventricular tachycardia (SVT), ventricular tachycardia (VT), or ventricular fibrillation (VF) are more likely to produce palpitations than syncope. Often, the rhythm abnormality is apparent by routine ECG, or, if it occurs paroxysmally, it can be recorded using a 24-hour Holter monitor or an event monitor. Sometimes evaluation requires invasive electrophysiologic studies to assess sinus node or AV node function or to induce supraventricular or ventricular arrhythmias.

Heart Block

There are three types of AV node block, all based on ECG findings. **First-degree AV block** is a prolonged PR interval longer than 200 ms (>1 large box). This is a conduction delay in the AV node. Prognosis is good, and there is usually no need for pacing. **Second-degree AV block** comes in two types. Mobitz type I (Wenckebach) is a progressive **lengthening of the PR interval,** until a dropped beat is produced. The resulting P wave of the dropped beat is not followed by a QRS complex. This phenomenon is caused by abnormal conduction in the AV node and may be the result of inferior myocardial infarction. Prognosis is good, and there is generally no need for pacing unless the patient is symptomatic (ie, bradycardia, syncope, heart failure, asystole >3 seconds). On the other hand, **Mobitz type II produces dropped beats without lengthening of the PR interval.** This is usually caused by a block within the bundle of His. Permanent pacing is often indicated in these patients because the Mobitz type II AV block may later progress to complete heart block. **Third-degree AV block** is a complete heart block, where the sinoatrial (SA) node and AV node fire at independent rates. The atrial rhythm is faster than the ventricular escape rhythm. Permanent pacing is indicated in these patients, especially when associated with symptoms such as exercise intolerance or syncope.

Comprehension Questions

15.1   An 18-year-old adolescent female is brought to the emergency room because she fainted at a rock concert. She apparently recovered spontaneously, did not exhibit any seizure activity, and has no medical history. Her heart rate is 90 bpm and blood pressure 110/70 mm Hg. Neurologic examination is normal. The pregnancy test is negative. Which of the following is the most appropriate management?

A. Admit to hospital for cardiac evaluation.

B. Outpatient echocardiogram.

C. Twenty-four–hour Holter monitor.

D. Reassurance and discharge home.

15.2   A 67-year-old woman has diabetes and mild hypertension. She is noted to have some diabetic retinopathy, and she states that she cannot feel her legs. She has recurrent episodes of lightheadedness when she gets up in the morning. She comes in now because she had fainted this morning. Which of the following is the most likely cause of her syncope?

A. Carotid sinus hypersensitivity
B. Pulmonary embolism
C. Autonomic neuropathy
D. Critical aortic stenosis

15.3   A 74-year-old man with no prior medical problems faints while shaving. He has a quick recovery and has no neurologic deficits. His blood sugar level is normal, and ECG shows a normal sinus rhythm. Which of the following is the most useful diagnostic test of his probable condition?

A. Carotid massage
B. Echocardiogram
C. Computed tomographic (CT) scan of head
D. Serial cardiac enzymes

15.4   A 49-year-old man is admitted to the intensive care unit (ICU) with a diagnosis of an inferior myocardial infarction. His heart rate is 35 bpm and blood pressure 90/50 mm Hg. His ECG shows a Mobitz type I heart block. Which of the following is the best next step?

A. Atropine
B. Transvenous pacer
C. Lidocaine
D. Observation

ANSWERS

15.1   **D.** A young patient without a medical history and with no seizure activity is unlikely to have any serious problems.

15.2   **C.** This diabetic patient has evidence of microvascular disease, including peripheral neuropathy, and likely has autonomic dysfunction.

15.3   **A.** He likely has carotid hypersensitivity; thus, careful carotid massage (after auscultation to ensure no bruits are present) may be given in an attempt to reproduce the symptoms.

15.4   **A.** This patient's bradycardia is severe, probably a result of the inferior myocardial infarction. Atropine is the agent of choice in this situation. Mobitz type I block has a good prognosis (vs complete heart block), so transvenous pacing is not usually required.

Clinical Pearls

➤ Vasovagal syncope is the most common cause of syncope in healthy young people. It often has a precipitating event, prodromal symptoms, and an excellent prognosis.

➤ Carotid sinus hypersensitivity causes bradyarrhythmias in older patients with pressure over the carotid bulb and sometimes requires a pacemaker.

➤ Syncope caused by cardiac outflow obstruction, such as aortic stenosis, occurs during or after exertion.

➤ Syncope is a very common problem, affecting nearly one-third of the adult population at some point, but a specific cause is identified in less than half of cases.

➤ Permanent pacing usually is indicated for symptomatic bradyarrhythmias (eg, sick sinus syndrome), Mobitz II atrioventricular block, or third-degree heart block.

REFERENCES

Carlson MD. Syncope. In: Kasper DL, Braunwald E, Fauci AS, et al. eds. Harrison's Principles of Internal Medicine. 17th ed. New York, NY: McGraw-Hill; 2008:139-144.

Gregoratos G, Abrams J, Epstein AE, et al. ACC/AHA/NASPE 2002 guideline update for implantation of cardiac pacemakers and antiarrhythmia devices—summary article: a report of the American College of Cardiology/American Heart Association Task Force on practice guidelines (ACC/AHA/NASPE Committee to Update the 1998 Pacemaker Guidelines). J Am Coll Cardiol. 2002;40:1703-1709.

Kapoor WN. Syncope. N Engl J Med. 2000;343:1856-1862.

Tomaselli GF. The bradyarrhythmias. In: Kasper DL, Braunwald E, Fauci AS, et al. eds. Harrison's Principles of Internal Medicine. 17th ed. New York, NY: McGraw-Hill; 2008:1416-1424.

Case 16

A 28-year-old man comes to the emergency room complaining of 2 days of abdominal pain and diarrhea. He describes his stools as frequent, with 10 to 12 per day, small volume, sometimes with visible blood and mucus, and preceded by a sudden urge to defecate. The abdominal pain is crampy, diffuse, and moderately severe, and it is not relieved with defecation. In the past 6 to 8 months, he has experienced similar episodes of abdominal pain and loose mucoid stools, but the episodes were milder and resolved within 24 to 48 hours. He has no other medical history and takes no medications. He has neither traveled out of the United States nor had contact with anyone with similar symptoms. He works as an accountant and does not smoke or drink alcohol. No member of his family has gastrointestinal (GI) problems.

On examination, his temperature is 99°F, heart rate 98 bpm, and blood pressure 118/74 mm Hg. He appears uncomfortable, is diaphoretic, and is lying still on the stretcher. His sclerae are anicteric, and his oral mucosa is pink and clear without ulceration. His chest is clear, and his heart rhythm is regular, without murmurs. His abdomen is soft and mildly distended, with hypoactive bowel sounds and minimal diffuse tenderness but no guarding or rebound tenderness.

Laboratory studies are significant for a white blood cell (WBC) count of 15,800/mm^3 with 82% polymorphonuclear leukocytes, hemoglobin 10.3 g/dL, and platelet count 754,000/mm^3. The HIV (human immunodeficiency virus) assay is negative. Renal function and liver function tests are normal. A plain film radiograph of the abdomen shows a mildly dilated air-filled colon with a 4.5-cm diameter and no pneumoperitoneum or air/fluid levels.

➤ What is the most likely diagnosis?

➤ What is your next step?

ANSWERS TO CASE 16:
Ulcerative Colitis

Summary: A 28-year-old man comes in with a moderate to severe presentation of colitis, as manifested by crampy abdominal pain with tenesmus, low-volume bloody mucoid stool, and colonic dilatation on X-ray. He has no travel or exposure history to suggest infection. He reports a history of previous similar episodes, which suggests a chronic inflammatory rather than acute infectious process.

➤ **Most likely diagnosis:** Colitis, probably ulcerative colitis.

➤ **Next step:** Admit to the hospital, obtain stool samples to exclude infection, and begin therapy with corticosteroids.

ANALYSIS

Objectives

1. Know the typical presentation of inflammatory bowel disease (IBD).
2. Know the differences between Crohn disease and ulcerative colitis.
3. Know the treatment of IBD.

Considerations

Although the likelihood of infection seems low, it must be excluded, and it is necessary to check for infections with organisms such as *Entamoeba histolytica, Salmonella, Shigella,* and *Campylobacter,* as well as *Clostridium difficile, which* can occur in the absence of prior antibiotic exposure.. The main consideration in this case would be IBD versus infectious colitis. The absence of travel history, sick contacts, and the chronicity of the illness all point away from infection.

At the moment, the patient does not appear to have any life-threatening complication of colitis, such as perforation or toxic megacolon, but he must be monitored closely, and surgical consultation may be helpful. The combination of abdominal pain, bloody diarrhea, and the abdominal X-ray localizing the disease to the colon points to a "colitis."

APPROACH TO
Colitis

DEFINITIONS

COLITIS: Inflammation of the intestines typically the large intestines, although the small bowel can be affected.

INFLAMMATORY BOWEL DISEASE: Autoimmune forms of colitis primarily due to either Crohn disease or ulcerative colitis.

CLINICAL APPROACH

The differential diagnosis for colitis includes ischemic colitis, infectious colitis (C *difficile*, *E coli*, *Salmonella*, *Shigella*, *Campylobacter*), radiation colitis, and IBD (Crohn disease vs ulcerative colitis). Mesenteric ischemia usually is encountered in people older than 50 years with known atherosclerotic vascular disease or other cause of hypoperfusion. The pain usually is acute in onset following a meal and not associated with fevers. With an infectious etiology, patients often have engaged in foreign travel, the symptoms are acute, or the patients recently used antibiotics. Also, family members often have the same symptoms.

The IBD is most commonly diagnosed in young patients between the ages of 15 and 25 years. There is a second peak in the incidence of IBD (usually Crohn disease) between the ages of 60 and 70 years. The IBD may present with a low-grade fever. The chronic nature of this patient's disease (several months) is typical of IBD. Anemia may be present, either due to iron deficiency from chronic GI blood loss, or anemia of chronic disease. Patients with IBD may also report fatigue and weight loss.

Ulcerative colitis usually presents with grossly bloody stool, whereas symptoms of Crohn disease are much more variable, mainly chronic abdominal pain, diarrhea, and weight loss. Ulcerative colitis involves only the large bowel, whereas Crohn disease may affect any portion of the GI tract, typically the colon and terminal ileum. **Ulcerative colitis** always begins in the rectum and proceeds proximally in a **continuous** pattern; disease is **limited to the colon**. Crohn disease classically involves the terminal ileum but may occur anywhere in the GI tract from the mouth to the anus. Anal fissures and non-healing ulcers are often seen in Crohn disease. Additionally, the pattern of **Crohn disease** is **not contiguous** in the GI tract; classically, it has a patchy distribution that is often referred to as "skip lesions." Patients with Crohn may develop strictures caused by fibrosis from repeated inflammation which can lead to bowel obstruction, with crampy abdominal pain and nausea/vomiting. **Ulcerative colitis** is characterized by diarrhea and typically leads to bowel obstruction. The diagnosis usually is confirmed after colonoscopy with biopsy

Table 16–1 COMPARISON OF CROHN DISEASE VERSUS ULCERATIVE COLITIS

	CROHN DISEASE	ULCERATIVE COLITIS
Site of origin	Terminal ileum	Rectum
Pattern of progression	"Skip" lesions/irregular	Proximally contiguous
Thickness of inflammation	Transmural	Submucosa or mucosa
Symptoms	Crampy abdominal pain	Bloody diarrhea
Complications	Fistulas, abscess, obstruction	Hemorrhage, toxic megacolon
Radiographic findings	String sign on barium X-ray	Lead pipe colon on barium X-ray
Risk of colon cancer	Slight increase	Marked increase
Surgery	For complications such as stricture	Curative

of the affected segments of bowel and histologic examination. In ulcerative colitis, inflammation will be limited to the **mucosa and submucosa**, whereas in **Crohn disease**, the inflammation will be **transmural** (throughout all layers of the bowel). Tables 16–1 and 16–2 list further clinical features. Surgery is indicated for complications of Crohn disease, such as obstruction, fistulas, or perforation, but recurrent disease is common.

Crohn Disease Versus Ulcerative Colitis

The treatment of ulcerative colitis can be complex because the pathophysiology of the disease is incompletely understood. Management is aimed at reducing the inflammation. Most commonly, **sulfasalazine** and other 5-aminosalicylic acid (ASA) compounds such as **mesalamine** are used and are available in oral and rectal preparations. They are used in mid to moderate active disease and to induce remission, and in the maintenance of disease to reduce the frequency of flare-ups. **Corticosteroids** may be used (po, PR, or IV) to treat patients with moderate to severe disease. Once remission is achieved, the steroids should be tapered over 6 to 8 weeks and then discontinued if possible to minimize their side effects. Immune modulators are used for more severe, refractory disease. Such medications include 6-mercaptopurine, azathioprine, methotrexate, and the tumor necrosis factor (TNF) antibody infliximab. Anti-TNF therapy, such

Table 16–2 EXTRAINTESTINAL MANIFESTATIONS OF INFLAMMATORY BOWEL DISEASE

	CROHN DISEASE	ULCERATIVE COLITIS
Skin manifestations	Erythema nodosum: 15% Pyoderma gangrenosum: rare	Erythema nodosum: 10% Pyoderma gangrenosum: 1%-12%
Rheumatologic	Arthritis (polyarticular, asymmetric): common Ankylosing spondylitis: 10%	Arthritis: less common Ankylosing spondylitis: less common
Ocular	Uveitis: common (photophobia, blurred vision, headache)	Uveitis: common (photophobia, blurred vision, headache)
Hepatobiliary	Cholelithiasis fatty liver: common Primary sclerosing cholangitis: rare	Fatty liver: common Primary sclerosing cholangitis: uncommon but more often than Crohn
Urologic	Nephrolithiasis (10%-20%) after small bowel resection or ileostomy	

as **infliximab**, has been an important treatment of patients with Crohn disease who are refractory to steroids, and more recently has shown efficacy in ulcerative colitis. Patients receiving the potent immunomodulator infliximab are at increased risk of infection, including reactivation of latent tuberculosis.

Surgery is indicated for complications of ulcerative colitis. **Total colectomy** is performed in patients with **carcinoma, toxic megacolon, perforation, and uncontrollable bleeding**. Surgery is curative for ulcerative colitis if symptoms persist despite medical therapy. Two very important and potentially life-threatening complications of ulcerative colitis are toxic megacolon and colon cancer. **Toxic megacolon** occurs when the colon dilates to a diameter more than 6 cm. It usually is accompanied by **fever, leukocytosis, tachycardia, and evidence of serious toxicity, such as hypotension or altered mental status**. Therapy is designed to reduce the chance of perforation and includes IV fluids, nasogastric tube placed to suction, and placing the patient npo (nothing by mouth). Additionally, IV antibiotics are given in anticipation of possible perforation, and IV steroids are given to reduce inflammation. The most severe consequence of toxic megacolon is colonic perforation complicated by peritonitis or hemorrhage.

Patients with **ulcerative colitis** have a marked **increase in the incidence of colon cancer** compared to the general population. The risk of cancer increases over time and is related to disease duration and extent. It is seen both in patients with active disease and in patients whose disease has been in remission. Annual or biennial colonoscopy is advised in patients with ulcerative colitis, beginning 8 years after diagnosis of pancolitis, and random biopsies should be sent for evaluation. If colon cancer or dysplasia is found, a colectomy should be performed.

Comprehension Questions

16.1   A 32-year-old woman has a history of chronic diarrhea and gallstones and now has rectovaginal fistula. Which of the following is the most likely diagnosis?

A. Crohn disease
B. Ulcerative colitis
C. Systemic lupus erythematosus
D. Laxative abuse

16.2   A 45-year-old man with a history of ulcerative colitis is admitted to the hospital with 2 to 3 weeks of RUQ abdominal pain, jaundice, and pruritus. He has no fever and a normal WBC count. Endoscopic retrograde cholangiopancreatography (ERCP) shows multifocal strictures of the both intrahepatic and extrahepatic bile ducts with intervening segments of normal and dilated ducts. Which of the following is the most likely diagnosis?

A. Acute suppurative cholangitis
B. Cholangiocarcinoma
C. Primary sclerosing cholangitis (PSC)
D. Choledocholithiasis with resultant biliary strictures

16.3   A 25-year-old man is hospitalized for ulcerative colitis. He has now developed abdominal distention, fever, and transverse colonic dilation of 7 cm on X-ray. Which of the following is the best next step?

A. 5-ASA
B. Steroids
C. Antibiotics and prompt surgical consultation
D. Infliximab

16.4   A 35-year-old woman has chronic crampy abdominal pain and intermittent constipation and diarrhea, but no weight loss or gastrointestinal bleeding. Her abdominal pain is usually relieved with defection. Colonoscopy and upper endoscopy with biopsies are normal, and stool cultures are negative. Which of the following is the most likely diagnosis?

A. Infectious colitis
B. Irritable bowel syndrome
C. Crohn disease
D. Ulcerative colitis

ANSWERS

16.1   **A.** Fistulas are common with Crohn disease because of its transmural nature but are uncommon in ulcerative colitis. Gallstones are common in patients with Crohn disease due to ileal bile salt malabsorption and depletion, causing the formation of more cholesterol-rich lithogenic bile.

16.2   **C.** The ERCP shows the typical appearance for primary sclerosing cholangitis (PSC), which is associated with IBD in 75% of cases. Stone-induced strictures should be extrahepatic and unifocal. Cholangiocarcinoma is less common but may develop in 10% of patients with PSC.

16.3   **C.** With toxic megacolon, antibiotics and surgical intervention are often necessary and life-saving. Medical therapy is usually ineffective.

16.4   **B.** Irritable bowel syndrome is characterized by intermittent diarrhea and crampy abdominal pain often relieved with defecation, but no weight loss or abnormal blood in the stool. It is a diagnosis of exclusion once other conditions, such as inflammatory bowel disease and parasitic infection (eg, giardiasis), have been excluded.

Clinical Pearls

➤ Ulcerative colitis always involves the rectum and may extend proximally in a continuous distribution.

➤ Crohn disease most commonly involves the distal ileum, but it may involve any portion of the gastrointestinal tract and has "skip lesions."

➤ Because of transmural inflammation, Crohn disease often is complicated by fistula formation.

➤ Toxic megacolon is characterized by dilation of the colon along with systemic toxicity; failure to improve with medical therapy may require surgical intervention.

➤ Both ulcerative colitis and Crohn disease can be associated with extraintestinal manifestations, such as uveitis, erythema nodosum, pyoderma gangrenosum, arthritis, and primary sclerosing cholangitis.

REFERENCES

Banerjee S, Peppercorn MA. Inflammatory bowel disease. Medical therapy of specific clinical presentations. *Gastroenterol Clin North Am.* 2002;341:147-166.

Friedman S, Blumber RS. Inflammatory bowel disease. In: Fauci AS, Braunwald E, Kasper DL, eds. *Harrison's Principles of Internal Medicine.* 17th ed. New York, NY: McGraw-Hill; 2008:1886-1899.

Kornbluth A, Sachar DB. Ulcerative colitis practice guidelines in adults (update). *Am J Gastroenterol.* 2004;99:1371-1385.

Podolsky DK. Medical progress: inflammatory bowel disease. *N Engl J Med.* 2002;342:7.

Case 17

A 54-year-old man with a history of type 2 diabetes and coronary artery disease is admitted to the coronary care unit with worsening angina and hypertension. His pain is controlled with intravenous nitroglycerin, and he is treated with aspirin, beta-blockers to lower his heart rate, and angiotensin-converting enzyme (ACE) inhibitors to lower his blood pressure. Cardiac enzymes are normal. He undergoes coronary angiography, which reveals no significant stenosis. By the next day, his urine output has diminished to 200 mL over 24 hours. Examination at that time reveals that he is afebrile, his heart rate is regular at 56 bpm, and his blood pressure is 109/65 mm Hg. His fundus reveals dot hemorrhages and hard exudates, his neck veins are flat, his chest is clear, and his heart rhythm is normal with an S_4 gallop and no murmur or friction rub. His abdomen is soft without masses or bruits. He has no peripheral edema or rashes, with normal pulses in all extremities. Current laboratory studies include Na 140 mEq/L, K 5.3 mEq/L, Cl 104 mEq/L, CO_2 19 mEq/L, and blood urea nitrogen (BUN) 69 mg/dL. His creatinine (Cr) level has risen to 2.9 mg/dL from 1.6 mg/dL on admission.

➤ What is the patient's new clinical problem?

➤ What is your next diagnostic step?

ANSWERS TO CASE 17:

Acute Renal Failure

Summary: A 54-year-old diabetic male is receiving medical therapy consisting of oral aspirin, beta-blockers, ACE inhibitor, and intravenous nitroglycerin for treatment of his angina and hypertension. He undergoes coronary angiography, which reveals no significant stenosis. He is normotensive. His funduscopic examination shows dot hemorrhages and hard exudates, evidence of diabetic retinopathy. In this setting, the baseline elevated creatinine level on admission likely represents diabetic nephropathy as well. His creatinine level has risen to 2.9 mg/dL from 1.6 mg/dL on admission. By the next day, he has become oliguric.

> **New clinical problem:** Acute renal failure (ARF).

> **Next step:** Urinalysis and urine chemistries to determine whether the process is prenal or renal, or less likely postrenal.

ANALYSIS

Objectives

1. Be familiar with the common causes, evaluation, and prevention of ARF in hospitalized patients.
2. Know how to use urinalysis and serum chemistry values in the diagnostic approach of ARF so as to be able to categorize the etiology as prerenal, renal, or postrenal.
3. Be familiar with the management of hyperkalemia and indications for acute dialysis.

Considerations

A 54-year-old man with diabetes, retinopathy, and some preexisting kidney disease develops ARF in the hospital, as indicated by the elevated serum creatinine level to 2.9 mg/dL and BUN of 69 mg/dL. He has undergone several medical therapies and procedures, all of which might be potentially contributory: acute lowering of his blood pressure, an ACE inhibitor, radiocontrast media, and arterial catheterization with possible atheroemboli. The mortality rate associated with critically ill patients who develop ARF is high; thus, identifying and treating the underlying etiology of this patient's kidney failure and taking measures to protect the kidneys from further damage are essential.

APPROACH TO
Acute Renal Failure

DEFINITIONS

ACUTE RENAL FAILURE (ARF): Abrupt decline in glomerular filtration rate (GFR). True GFR is difficult to measure, so we rely on increases in serum creatinine levels to indicate a fall in GFR. Because creatinine is both filtered and secreted by the kidneys, changes in serum creatinine concentrations always lag behind and underestimate the decline in the GFR. In other words, **by the time the serum creatinine level rises, the GFR has already fallen significantly.**

ANURIA: Less than 50 mL of urine output in 24 hours. Acute obstruction, cortical necrosis, and vascular catastrophes such as aortic dissection should be considered in the differential diagnosis.

OLIGURIA: Less than 400 mL of urine output in 24 hours. Physiologically, it is the lowest amount of urine a person on a normal diet can make if he or she is severely dehydrated and does not retain uremic waste products. **Oliguria is a poor prognostic sign in ARF.** Patients with **oliguric renal failure have higher mortality rates** and less renal recovery than do patients who are nonoliguric.

UREMIA: Nonspecific symptoms of fatigue, weakness, nausea and early morning vomiting, itchiness, confusion, pericarditis, and coma attributed to the retention of waste products in renal failure but do not always correlate with the BUN level. A highly malnourished patient with renal failure may have a modestly elevated BUN and be uremic. Another patient may have a highly elevated BUN and be asymptomatic. Elevated BUN without symptoms is called **azotemia.**

CLINICAL APPROACH

The differential diagnosis of ARF proceeds from consideration of three basic pathophysiologic mechanisms: **prerenal failure, postrenal failure, and intrinsic renal failure.** Individuals with **prerenal failure** experience diminished GFR as a result of a marked **decreased renal blood perfusion** so that less glomerular filtrate is formed. Sometimes, the clinical presentation is straightforward, such as volume depletion from gastrointestinal fluid loss or hemorrhage; at other times, the presentation of patients with prerenal failure can be more confusing. For example, a patient with severe nephrotic syndrome may appear to be volume overloaded because of the massive peripheral edema present, while the effective arterial blood volume may be very low as a consequence of the severe hypoalbuminemia. Yet the mechanism of this individual's ARF is prerenal. Similarly, a patient with severe congestive heart failure may have prerenal failure because of a low cardiac ejection fraction, yet be fluid overloaded with peripheral and pulmonary edema. **The key is to assess "what the kidneys see" versus the remainder of the body.** Typically, the BUN:Cr ratio is more than 20 in prerenal failure. Medications such as aspirin, nonsteroidal anti-inflammatory drugs (NSAIDs), and ACE inhibitors can alter intrarenal blood flow and result in prerenal failure. Table 17–1 provides an abbreviated listing of the etiologies of prerenal failure.

Postrenal failure, also referred to as obstructive nephropathy, implies **blockage of urinary flow.** The site of obstruction can be anywhere along the urinary system, including the intratubular region (crystals), ureters (stones, extrinsic compression by tumor), bladder, or urethra. By far, the most common causes of obstructive nephropathy are ureteral obstruction due to malignancy, or prostatic obstruction due to benign or malignant hypertrophy. The patient's symptoms depend on whether or not both kidneys are involved, the degree of obstruction, and the time course of the blockage. This is usually diagnosed by seeing **hydronephrosis on renal ultrasound.**

Intrinsic renal failure is caused by disorders that injure the renal glomeruli or tubules directly. These include glomerulonephritis, tubulointerstitial nephritis, and acute tubular necrosis (ATN) from either ischemia or nephrotoxic drugs. Table 17–2 lists major causes of intrinsic ARF.

Evaluation of a patient with ARF starts with a detailed history and physical examination. Does the patient have signs or symptoms of a systemic disease, such as heart failure or cirrhosis, that could cause prerenal failure? Does the patient have symptoms of a disease, such as lupus, that could cause a glomerulonephritis? Did the patient receive something in the hospital that could cause ATN, such as intravenous contrast or an aminoglycoside? While in the operating room did the patient become hypotensive from sepsis or from hemorrhage that caused ischemic ATN? Is the patient receiving an antibiotic and now has allergic interstitial nephritis? In addition to the history and physical examination, **urinalysis and measurement of urinary electrolytes** are helpful in making the diagnosis.

Table 17–1 CAUSES OF PRERENAL ACUTE RENAL FAILURE

True volume depletion
- Gastrointestinal losses
- Renal losses (diuretics)

Reduced effective arterial blood volume
- Nephrotic syndrome
- Cirrhosis with portal hypertension
- Severe burns
- Sepsis
- Systemic inflammatory response syndrome (SIRS)

Medications
- ACE inhibitors
- NSAIDs

Decreased cardiac output
- Congestive heart failure
- Pericardial tamponade

Table 17–2 CAUSES OF INTRINSIC ACUTE RENAL FAILURE

Acute tubular necrosis

Nephrotoxic agents
- Aminoglycosides
- Radiocontrast
- Chemotherapy

Ischemic
- Hypotension
- Vascular catastrophe

Glomerulonephritis

Postinfectious

Vasculitis

Immune complex diseases (lupus, MPGN [mesangioproliferative glomerulonephritis] cryoglobulinemia)

Cholesterol emboli syndrome

Hemolytic uremic syndrome/thrombotic thrombocytopenic purpura

Tubulointerstitial nephritis

Medications (cephalosporins, methicillin, rifampin)

Infection (pyelonephritis, HIV)

Urinalysis

The urine findings based on testing with reagent paper and microscopic examination help with the diagnosis of ARF (Table 17–3). In **prerenal failure**, urinalysis usually reveals a **high specific gravity** and **normal microscopic findings**. Individuals with **postrenal failure** typically are **unable to concentrate the urine**, so the urine osmolality is equal to the serum osmolality (**isosthenuria**) and the **specific gravity is 1.010**. The **microscopic findings vary** depending on the cause of the obstruction: hematuria (crystals or stones), leukocytes (prostatic hypertrophy), or normal (extrinsic ureteral compression from a tumor). Urinalysis of various intrinsic renal disorders may be helpful. **Ischemic and nephrotoxic ATN** usually is associated with urine that is **isosthenuric,** often with **proteinuria,** and containing **"muddy brown" granular casts** on microscopy. In **glomerulonephritis,** the urine generally reveals moderate to severe **proteinuria,** sometimes in the nephrotic range, and **microscopic hematuria and red blood cell (RBC) casts.** Tubulointerstitial nephritis classically produces urine that is **isosthenuric** (the tubules are unable to concentrate the urine), with **mild proteinuria,** and on microscopy, reveals **leukocytes, white cell casts, and urinary eosinophils.**

Urinary Electrolytes

Measurement of urinary electrolytes and calculation of the fractional excretion of sodium (FE_{Na}) were devised to differentiate oliguric prerenal failure from oliguric ATN; they are of little use in other circumstances. FE_{Na} represents the

Table 17–3 EVALUATION OF ACUTE RENAL FAILURE

ETIOLOGY OF RENAL FAILURE	URINALYSIS	FE_{NA}	U_{NA}
Prerenal failure	Concentrated (high specific gravity) with normal sediment	<1%	<20 mEq/L
ATN	Isosthenuric with muddy brown granular casts	>1%	>20 mEq/L
Glomerulonephritis	Moderate to severe proteinuria with red blood cells and red blood cell casts	<1%	Variable
Interstitial nephritis	Mild to moderate proteinuria with red and white blood cells and white blood cell casts	>1%	>20 mEq/L
Postrenal failure	Variable depending on cause	<1% (early) >1% (later)	<20 mEq/L (early) >20 mEq/L (later)

Abbreviation: U_{Na}, Urinary concentraction of sodium

amount of sodium filtered by the kidneys that is not reabsorbed. The **kidneys of a healthy person on a normal diet** usually reabsorb more than 99% of the sodium that is filtered, with a corresponding FE_{Na} less than **1%.** Normally, the excreted sodium represents the dietary intake of sodium, maintaining sodium homeostasis. In prerenal failure, decreased renal perfusion leads to a diminished GFR; if the renal tubular function is intact, FE_{Na} remains less than 1%. Furthermore, because the patient has either true volume depletion or "effective" volume depletion, serum aldosterone will stimulate the kidneys to retain sodium, and the urinary sodium will be low (<20 mEq/L). On the other hand, in oliguric ATN, the renal failure is caused by tubular injury. Hence, there is **tubular dysfunction** with an associated **inability to reabsorb sodium,** leading to an FE_{Na} more than 2% and a **urinary sodium** more than **20 mEq/L.**

Measurements of FE_{Na} and urinary sodium are less helpful in other circumstances. For example, in nonoliguric ATN, the injury usually is less severe, so the kidneys still may maintain sodium reabsorption and be able to produce an FE_{Na} less than 1%. Diuretic medications, which interfere with sodium reabsorption, are often used in congestive heart failure or nephrotic syndrome. Although these patients may have prerenal failure, the use of diuretics will increase the urinary sodium and FE_{Na}. In acute glomerulonephritis, the kidneys often avidly resorb sodium, leading to very low urinary sodium levels and

FE_{Na}. Early in the course of postobstructive renal failure caused by ureteral obstruction, the afferent arteriole typically undergoes intense vasoconstriction, with consequent, low urinary sodium levels (Table 17–3).

The **indications for dialysis** in ARF include **fluid overload, such as pulmonary edema, metabolic acidosis, hyperkalemia, uremic pericarditis, severe hyperphosphatemia, and uremic symptoms**. Because of the risk of fatal cardiac arrhythmias, severe hyperkalemia is considered an emergency, best treated acutely medically and not with dialysis. An urgent electrocardiogram (ECG) should be performed on any patient with suspected hyperkalemia; if the classic peaked or "tented" T waves are present, intravenous calcium should be administered immediately. Although it will not lower the serum potassium level, the calcium will oppose the membrane effects of the high potassium concentration on the heart, allowing time for other methods to lower the potassium level. One of the most effective methods for treating hyperkalemia is administration of intravenous insulin (usually 10 units), along with 50 to 100 mL of 50% glucose solution to prevent hypoglycemia. Insulin drives potassium into cells, lowering levels within 30 minutes. Potassium also can be driven intracellularly with a beta-agonist, such as albuterol by nebulizer. In the presence of a severe metabolic acidosis, administration of intravenous sodium bicarbonate also promotes intracellular diffusion of potassium, albeit less effectively. All three therapies have only a transient effect on serum potassium levels, because the total body potassium balance is unchanged, and the potassium eventually leaks back out of the cells. Definitive treatment of hyperkalemia, removal of potassium from the body, is accomplished by one of three methods: (1) administration of a loop diuretic such as furosemide to increase urinary flow and excretion of potassium, or, if the patient does not make sufficient urine, (2) administration of sodium polystyrene sulfonate (Kayexalate), a cationic exchange resin that lowers potassium by exchanging sodium for potassium in the colon, or, finally, (3) emergency dialysis.

Comprehension Questions

17.1 A 63-year-old woman with a history of cervical cancer treated with hysterectomy and pelvic irradiation now presents with acute oliguric renal failure. On physical examination, she has normal jugular venous pressure, is normotensive without orthostasis, and has a benign abdominal examination. Her urinalysis shows a specific gravity of 1.010, with no cells or casts on microscopy. Urinary FE_{Na} is 2%, and the Na level is 35 mEq/L. Which of the following is the best next step?
   A. Bolus of intravenous fluids
   B. Renal ultrasound
   C. Computed tomographic (CT) scan of the abdomen with intravenous contrast
   D. Administration of furosemide to increase her urine output

17.2   A 49-year-old man with a long-standing history of chronic renal fail-
        ure as a consequence of diabetic nephropathy is brought to the emergency
        room for nausea, lethargy, and confusion. His physical examination is
        significant for an elevated jugular venous pressure, clear lung fields, and
        harsh systolic and diastolic sounds heard over the precordium. Serum
        chemistries reveal K 5.1 mEq/L, CO_2 17 mEq/L, BUN 145 mg/dL, and
        creatinine 9.8 mg/dL. Which of the following is the most appropriate
        therapy?
        A. Administer IV insulin and glucose.
        B. Administer IV sodium bicarbonate.
        C. Administer IV furosemide.
        D. Urgent hemodialysis.

17.3   A 62-year-old diabetic man underwent an abdominal aortic aneurysm
        repair 2 days ago. He is being treated with gentamicin for a urinary
        tract infection. His urine output has fallen to 300 mL over 24 hours,
        and his serum creatinine has risen from 1.1 mg/dL on admission to
        1.9 mg/dL. Which of the following laboratory values would be most
        consistent with a prerenal etiology of his renal insufficiency?
        A. FE_{Na} of 3%
        B. Urinary sodium level of 10 mEq/L
        C. Central venous pressure reading of 10 mm Hg
        D. Gentamicin trough level of 4 μg/mL

ANSWERS

17.1   **B.** Renal ultrasound is the next appropriate step to assess for
        hydronephrosis and to evaluate for bilateral ureteral obstructions,
        which are common sites of metastases of cervical cancer. Her physical
        examination and urine studies (showing a FE > 1%) are inconsistent
        with hypovolemia, so intravenous infusion is unlikely to improve her
        renal function. Use of loop diuretics may increase her urine output
        somewhat but does not help to diagnose the cause of her renal fail-
        ure or to improve her outcome. Further imaging may be necessary
        after the ultrasound, but use of intravenous contrast at this point may
        actually worsen her renal failure.

17.2   **D.** The patient has uremia, hyperkalemia, and (likely) uremic peri-
        carditis, which may progress to life-threatening cardiac tamponade
        unless the underlying renal failure is treated with dialysis. As for the
        other treatments, insulin plus glucose would treat hyperkalemia, and
        bicarbonate would help with both metabolic acidosis and hyper-
        kalemia, but in this patient, his potassium and bicarbonate levels are
        only mildly abnormal and are not immediately life-threatening.
        Furosemide will not help because he does not have pulmonary edema.

17.3   **B.** Prerenal insufficiency connotes insufficient blood volume, typically with FE_{Na} less than 1% and urinary sodium less than 20 mEq/L. Supporting information would be a low central venous pressure reading (normal central venous pressure is 4-8 mm Hg). The gentamicin level of 4 µg/mL is elevated (normal <2 µg/mL) and may predispose to kidney damage.

Clinical Pearls

➤ The two main causes of renal failure in hospitalized patients are prerenal azotemia and acute tubular necrosis.

➤ In the anuric patient, one must quickly determine if the kidneys are obstructed or if the vascular supply is interrupted.

➤ Treatment of prerenal renal failure is volume replacement; treatment of postrenal failure is relief of the obstruction.

➤ The main causes of postrenal failure are obstruction caused by prostatic hypertrophy in men and bilateral ureteral obstruction caused by abdominal or pelvic malignancy in either gender.

➤ Uremic pericarditis is an indication for urgent hemodialysis. Other indications include hyperkalemia, metabolic acidosis, severe hyperphosphatemia, and volume overload when refractory to medical management.

➤ Treatment of hyperkalemia: C BIG K (calcium, bicarbonate/beta-agonist, insulin, glucose, Kayexalate).

➤ Hyperkalemia is treated initially with calcium to stabilize cardiac membranes; insulin and beta-agonists to redistribute potassium intracellularly (sodium bicarbonate if there is a severe metabolic acidosis); and then loop diuretics, a potassium exchange resin, or hemodialysis to remove excess potassium from the body.

➤ Indications for dialysis: AEIOU (acidosis, electrolyte disturbances, ingestions, overload, uremia).

REFERENCES

Lameire N, Van Biesen W, Vanholder R. Acute renal failure. *Lancet.* 2005;365:417-430.

Liu KD, Chertow GM. Acute renal failure. In: Kasper DL, Braunwald E, Fauci AS, et al. eds. *Harrison's Principles of Internal Medicine*. 17th ed. New York, NY: McGraw-Hill; 2008:1752-1761.

Rose BD, Post TW. Hyperkalemia. In: *Clinical Physiology of Acid-Base and Electrolyte Disorders*. 5th ed. New York, NY: McGraw-Hill; 2001:913-919.

Case 18

A 27-year-old woman presents to the emergency room complaining of retrosternal chest pain for the past 2 days. The pain is constant, not associated with exertion, worsens when she takes a deep breath, and is relieved by sitting up and leaning forward. She denies any shortness of breath, nausea, or diaphoresis.

On examination, her temperature is 99.4°F, heart rate 104 bpm, and blood pressure 118/72 mm Hg. She is sitting forward on the stretcher, with shallow respirations. Her conjunctivae are clear and her oral mucosa is pink, with two aphthous ulcers. Her neck veins are not distended; her chest is clear to auscultation and is mildly tender to palpation. Her heart rhythm is regular, with a harsh leathery sound over the apex heard during systole and diastole. Her abdominal examination is benign, and her extremities show warmth and swelling of the proximal interphalangeal (PIP) joints of both hands.

Laboratory studies are significant for a white blood cell (WBC) count of 2100/mm³, hemoglobin concentration 10.4 g/dL with mean corpuscular volume (MCV) 94 fL, and platelet count 78,000/mm³. Her blood urea nitrogen (BUN) and creatinine levels are normal. Urinalysis shows 10 to 20 WBCs and 5 to 10 red blood cells (RBCs) per high-powered field (hpf). A urine drug screen is negative.

Chest X-ray is read as normal, with a normal cardiac silhouette and no pulmonary infiltrates or effusions. The electrocardiogram (ECG) is shown in Figure 18–1.

➤ What is the most likely diagnosis?

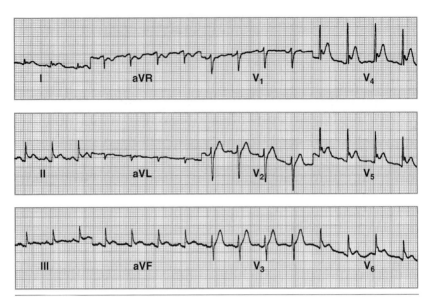

Figure 18–1. Electrocardiogram. *Reproduced, with permission, from Stead LG, Stead SM, Kaufman MS.* First Aid for the Medicine Clerkship. *2nd ed. New York, NY: McGraw-Hill;* 2006:33.

ANSWER TO CASE 18:

Acute Pericarditis Caused by Systemic Lupus Erythematosus

Summary: A 27-year-old woman presents with nonexertional pleuritic chest pain that is relieved with sitting forward. In addition, she has a pericardial friction rub and ECG changes consistent with acute pericarditis. She has no radiographic evidence of a large pericardial effusion and no clinical signs of cardiac tamponade. Regarding the etiology of her pericarditis, she has pancytopenia and an active urinary sediment, which could be caused by infection but may also represent a connective tissue disease such as systemic lupus erythematosus (SLE).

➤ **Most likely diagnosis:** Acute pericarditis as a consequence of SLE.

ANALYSIS

Objectives

1. Know the clinical and ECG features of pericarditis and be able to recognize a pericardial friction rub.
2. Know the causes of pericarditis and its treatment.

3. Know the diagnostic criteria for SLE.
4. Know the major complications of SLE and its treatment.

Considerations

In patients with chest pain, one of the primary diagnostic considerations is always myocardial ischemia or infarction. This is particularly true when the ECG is abnormal with changes that may represent myocardial injury, such as ST-segment elevation. However, other conditions may produce ST-segment elevation, such as acute pericarditis. ECG findings can help distinguish between these two diagnoses.

APPROACH TO
Acute Pericarditis

DEFINITIONS

ACUTE PERICARDITIS: An inflammation of the pericardial sac surrounding the heart.

PERICARDIAL FRICTION RUB: Harsh, high-pitched, scratchy sound, with variable intensity, usually best heard at the left sternal border by auscultation, due to pericarditis.

CLINICAL APPROACH

Acute pericarditis can result from a multitude of disease processes, but the most common causes are listed in Table 18–1.

There is a wide spectrum of clinical presentations, from subclinical or inapparent inflammation, to the classic presentation of acute pericarditis with

Table 18–1 COMMON CAUSES OF ACUTE PERICARDITIS

Idiopathic pericarditis: specific diagnosis unidentified, presumably either viral or autoimmune and requires no specific management

Infectious: viral, bacterial, tuberculous, parasitic

Vasculitis: autoimmune diseases, postradiation therapy

Hypersensitivity/immunologic reactions, eg. Dressler syndrome

Diseases of contiguous structures, eg, during transmural myocardial infarction

Metabolic disease, eg, uremia, Gaucher disease

Trauma: penetrating or nonpenetrating chest injury

Neoplasms: usually thoracic malignancies such as breast, lung, or lymphoma

Data from Spodick DH. Acute pericarditis: current concepts and practice. JAMA. 2003;289:1150-1153.

chest pain, to subacute or chronic inflammation, persisting for weeks to months. Most patients with acute pericarditis seek medical attention because of **chest pain**. The classic description is a sudden onset of substernal chest pain, which worsens on inspiration and with recumbency, that often radiates to the trapezius ridge and is improved by sitting and leaning forward. Other clinical features vary according to the cause of the pericarditis, but most patients are thought to have viral infection and often present with low-grade fever, malaise, or upper respiratory illness symptoms.

A **pericardial friction rub** is pathognomonic and virtually 100% specific for acute pericarditis. The sensitivity of this sign varies, though, because friction rubs tend to come and go over hours. Classically, a rub is harsh, high-pitched, scratchy sound, with variable intensity, usually best heard at the left sternal border. It can have one, two, or three components: presystolic (correlating with atrial systole), systolic, and diastolic. The large majority of rubs are triphasic (all three components) or biphasic, having a systolic and either an early or late diastolic component. In these cases, it usually is easy to diagnose the pericardial friction rub and acute pericarditis. When the rub is monophasic (just a systolic component), it often is difficult to distinguish a pericardial friction rub from a harsh murmur, making bedside diagnosis difficult and uncertain. In these cases, one should look for ECG evidence of pericarditis (Table 18–2) and perform serial examinations because the rub may vary with time.

The classic ECG findings in **acute pericarditis** as seen in this patient include **diffuse ST-segment elevation** in association with PR-segment depression. The opposite findings (PR-segment elevation and ST-segment depression) are often seen in leads aVR and V_1. Because of the presentation with chest pain and ST-segment elevation on ECG, acute pericarditis may be confused with acute myocardial infarction (MI). This is potentially a serious problem because if the patient is treated with **thrombolytics** for infarction, the patient may develop **pericardial hemorrhage and cardiac tamponade**. Several clinical features

Table 18–2 PERICARDITIS VERSUS MYOCARDIAL INFARCTION

ECG	ACUTE PERICARDITIS	ACUTE MI
ST-segment elevation	Diffuse: in limb leads as well as V_2-V_6	Regional (vascular territory), eg, inferior, anterior, or lateral
PR-segment depression	Present	Usually absent
Reciprocal ST-segment depression	Absent	Typical, eg, ST-segment depression inferiorly with anterior ischemia (ST-segment elevation)
QRS complex changes	Absent	Loss of R-wave amplitude and development of Q waves

can help to differentiate the two conditions: acute ischemia is more likely to have a gradual onset of pain with crescendo pattern; it usually is described as a heavy pressure or squeezing sensation rather than the sharp pain of pericarditis; it typically does not vary with respiration; and it is relieved with nitrates, whereas the pain of pericarditis is not. In addition, several ECG features can help to make the distinction (Table 18–2). Also, if the ECG reveals arrhythmias or conduction abnormalities, the condition is much more likely to represent ischemia rather than pericarditis.

Most patients with acute viral or idiopathic pericarditis have excellent prognoses. Treatment is mainly symptomatic, with aspirin or another nonsteroidal anti-inflammatory drug (NSAID), such as indomethacin, for relief of chest pain. Some physicians favor ibuprofen with colchicine, and use of corticosteroids for refractory symptoms. In most patients, symptoms typically resolve within days to 2 to 3 weeks. Any form of pericarditis can cause pericardial effusion and bleeding; however, the most serious consequence would be cardiac tamponade. It is a common misconception that a pericardial friction rub cannot coexist with an effusion (both are very common in uremic pericarditis). Therefore, it is important to monitor these patients for signs of developing hemodynamic compromises, such as cardiac tamponade.

Our patient is very young and has no significant previous medical history. The presence of symmetric arthritis as well as laboratory findings suggest a systemic disease, such as SLE, as the cause of her pericarditis. SLE is a systemic inflammatory disease that mainly affects women. It is characterized by autoimmune multiorgan involvement, such as pericarditis, nephritis, pleuritis, arthritis, and skin disorders. To diagnose SLE, the patient must meet 4 of the 11 criteria listed in Table 18–3 (96% sensitive and 96% specific).

Table 18–3 DIAGNOSTIC CRITERIA FOR SLE

Malar rash: fixed erythema, flat or raised over the malar area, that tends to spare nasolabial folds

Discoid rash: erythematous raised patches with adherent keratotic scaling and follicular plugging

Photosensitivity: skin rash as a result of exposure to sunlight

Oral or vaginal ulcers: usually painless

Arthritis: nonerosive, involving two or more peripheral joints with tenderness, swelling, and effusion

Serositis: usually pleuritis or pericarditis

Renal involvement: persistent proteinuria or cellular casts

Neurologic disorder: seizure or psychosis

Hematologic disorder: hemolytic anemia or leukopenia (<4000/mm^3) on two or more occasions, or lymphopenia <1500/mm^3) on two or more occasions, or thrombocytopenia (<100,000/mm^3)

Immunologic disorder: positive LE (lupus erythematosus) cell preparation or positive anti-dsDNA (anti–double-stranded DNA) or positive anti-Sm (anti-Smith antibody)

Antinuclear antibody (ANA): positive ANA

Our patient has serositis (pericarditis), oral ulcers, hematologic disorders (leukopenia, lymphopenia, thrombocytopenia), arthritis, and renal involvement (hematuria)—she clearly meets the criteria for SLE. Although the patient in the scenario, like most lupus patients, sought medical attention because of the pain of arthritis or serositis, both these problems are generally manageable or self-limited. The arthritis is generally nonerosive and nondeforming, and the serositis usually resolves spontaneously without sequelae. The major complication of SLE usually is related to renal involvement, which can cause hypertension, chronic renal failure, nephrotic syndrome, or end-stage renal disease. In the past, renal disease was the most common cause of death of SLE patients, but now it can be treated with powerful immunosuppressants, such as high-dose corticosteroids or cyclophosphamide. Other serious complications of lupus include central nervous system (CNS) disorders, which are highly variable and unpredictable and can include seizures, psychosis, stroke syndromes, and cranial neuropathies. In addition to renal failure and CNS involvement, the most common causes of death in SLE patients are infection (often related to the immunosuppression used to treat the disease) and vascular disease, for example, myocardial infarction.

Comprehension Questions

18.1   A 68-year-old man with a history of end-stage renal disease is admitted to the hospital for chest pain. On examination, a pericardial friction rub is noted. His ECG shows diffuse ST-segment elevation. Which of the following is the best definitive treatment?

A. NSAIDs
B. Dialysis
C. Steroids
D. Kayexalate (sodium polystyrene sulfonate)

18.2   The patient described in question 18.1 is hospitalized, but there is a delay in initiating treatment. You are called to the bedside because he has become hypotensive with systolic blood pressure of 85/68 mm Hg, a heart rate of 122 bpm, and you note pulsus paradoxus. A repeat ECG is unchanged from admission. Which of the following is the most appropriate immediate intervention?

A. Draw blood cultures and initiate broad spectrum antibiotics for suspected sepsis.
B. Intravenous furosemide for fluid overload.
C. Echocardiographic-guided pericardiocentesis.
D. Percutaneous coronary intervention for acute myocardial infarction.

18.3 A 25-year-old woman complains of pain in her PIP and metacar-pophalangeal (MCP) joints and reports a recent positive ANA laboratory test. Which of the following clinical features would not be consistent with a diagnosis of SLE?

A. Pleural effusion
B. Malar rash
C. Sclerodactyly
D. Urinary sediment with RBC casts

ANSWERS

18.1 **B.** Uremic pericarditis is considered a medical emergency and an indication for urgent dialysis.

18.2 **C.** The clinical picture suggests the patient has developed pericardial tamponade, which may be life-threatening and often requires urgent pericardiocentesis.

18.3 **C.** Sclerodactyly, which is thickened and tight skin of the fingers and toes, is a classic feature of patients with scleroderma (who may also have a positive ANA test), but is not seen in SLE. The other findings (malar rash, serositis, glomerulonephritis) are typical of SLE, but not seen in scleroderma.

Clinical Pearls

➤ Acute pericarditis is characterized by pleuritic chest pain, a pericardial friction rub, and ECG findings of diffuse ST-segment elevation and PR-segment depression.

➤ Pericardial friction rub does not exclude a pericardial effusion; patients with acute pericarditis should be monitored for development of effusion and tamponade.

➤ Treatment of pericarditis is directed at the underlying cause; for example, for uremic pericarditis, urgent dialysis is necessary. For viral or inflammatory causes, treatment is nonsteroidal anti-inflammatory drugs or corticosteroids for refractory cases.

➤ Systemic lupus erythematosus can be diagnosed if a patient has four of the following features: malar rash, discoid rash, photosensitivity, oral ulcers, arthritis, serositis, renal disease, neurologic manifestations, hematologic cytopenias, immunologic abnormalities (eg, false-positive Venereal Disease Research Laboratory [VDRL] test), and positive antinuclear antibody.

➤ The major morbidity and mortality of systemic lupus erythematosus are consequences of renal disease, central nervous system involvement, or infection.

REFERENCES

Hahn BH. Systemic lupus erythematosus. In: Kasper DL, Braunwald E, Fauci AS, et al. eds. *Harrison's Principles of Internal Medicine*. 17th ed. New York, NY: McGraw-Hill; 2008:2075-2083.

Lange RA, Hillis LD. Acute pericarditis. *N Engl J Med*. 2004;351:2195-2202.

Spodick DH. Acute pericarditis: current concepts and practice. *JAMA*. 2003;289: 1150-1153.

Case 19

A 27-year-old man presents to the outpatient clinic complaining of 2 days of facial and hand swelling. He first noticed swelling around his eyes 2 days ago, along with difficulty putting on his wedding ring because of swollen fingers. Additionally, he noticed that his urine appears reddish-brown and that he has had less urine output over the last several days. He has no significant medical history. His only medication is ibuprofen that he took 2 weeks ago for fever and a sore throat, which have since resolved. On examination, he is afebrile, with heart rate 85 bpm and blood pressure 172/110 mm Hg. He has periorbital edema; his funduscopic examination is normal without arteriovenous nicking or papilledema. His chest is clear to auscultation, his heart rhythm is regular with a nondisplaced point of maximal impulse (PMI), and he has no abdominal masses or bruits. He does have edema of his feet, hands, and face. A dipstick urinalysis in the clinic shows specific gravity of 1.025 with 3+ blood and 2+ protein, but it is otherwise negative.

➤ What is the most likely diagnosis?

➤ What is your next diagnostic step?

ANSWERS TO CASE 19:

Acute Glomerulonephritis, Poststreptococcal Infection

Summary: A 27-year-old man complains of several days of facial and hand swelling, decreased urine output, and reddish-brown urine. He took ibuprofen for fever and a sore throat 2 weeks ago. He is afebrile, hypertensive with a blood pressure of 172/110 mm Hg, and has periorbital edema but a normal funduscopic examination. His cardiac, pulmonary, and abdominal examinations are normal, but he does have edema of his feet, hands, and face. A dipstick urinalysis in the clinic shows specific gravity of 1.025 with 3+ blood and 2+ protein.

➤ **Most likely diagnosis:** Acute glomerulonephritis (GN).

➤ **Next diagnostic step:** Examine a fresh spun urine specimen to look for red blood cell (RBC) casts or dysmorphic red blood cells.

ANALYSIS

Objectives

1. Be able to differentiate glomerular from nonglomerular bleeding.
2. Understand the clinical features of GN.
3. Know how to evaluate and treat a patient with GN.
4. Be familiar with the evaluation of a patient with nonglomerular hematuria.

Considerations

A young man without a significant medical history now presents with new onset of hypertension, edema, and hematuria following an upper respiratory tract infection. He has no history of renal disease, does not have manifestations of chronic hypertension, and has not received any nephrotoxins. He does not have symptoms of systemic diseases such as systemic lupus erythematosus. The presentation of acute renal failure, hypertension, edema, and hematuria in a young man with no significant medical history is highly suggestive of glomerular injury (GN). He likely has acute GN, either postinfectious (streptococcal) or immunoglobulin (Ig)A nephropathy. The reddish-brown appearance of the urine could represent hematuria, which was later suggested by dipstick urinalysis (3+ blood); hence, microscopic examination of the urine for RBCs is very important. Together, the history and the examination suggest that the patient likely has acute GN, either primary GN of unknown etiology (no concomitant systemic disease is mentioned) or secondary GN as a result of recent upper respiratory infection (postinfectious GN). The next logical step in diagnosing GN should be to examine the precipitate of a freshly spun urine sample for

Table 19–1 SEROLOGIC MARKERS OF GLOMERULONEPHRITIS

Complement levels (C3, C4): low in complement-mediated GN (SLE, MPGN, infective endocarditis, poststreptococcal/postinfectious GN, cryoglobulin-induced GN)
Antineutrophil cytoplasmic antibody levels (p-ANCA and c-ANCA): positive in Wegener, microscopic polyangiitis, Churg-Strauss
ANA: positive in SLE (anti-dsDNA, anti-Smith)
Antiglomerular basement membrane (anti-GBM) antibody levels : positive in anti-GBM GN and Goodpasture
ASO titers: elevated in poststreptococcal GN (postinfectious GN)
Blood cultures: positive in infective endocarditis
Cryoglobulin titers: positive in cryoglobulin-induced GN
Hepatitis serologies: hepatitis C and hepatitis B associated with cryoinduced GN

active sediment (cellular components, red cell cast, dysmorphic red cells). If present, these are signs of inflammation and establish the diagnosis of acute GN. Although likely to be present, these markers do not distinguish among the distinct immune-mediated causes of GN; they merely allow us to make the diagnosis of acute GN (primary or secondary). Further evaluation with serologic markers, such as complement levels and antistreptolysin-O (ASO) titers (Table 19–1), may help to further classify the GN.

APPROACH TO
Suspected Glomerulonephritis

DEFINITIONS

HEMATURIA: Presence of blood in the urine
GROSS HEMATURIA: Blood in the urine visible to the eye
MICROSCOPIC HEMATURIA: Red blood cells in the urine that require microscopy for diagnosis

CLINICAL APPROACH

The term *hematuria* describes the presence of blood in the urine. Although direct visualization of a urine sample (gross hematuria) or dipstick examination (positive blood) can be helpful, the **diagnosis of hematuria is made by microscopic confirmation of the presence of red blood cells** (microscopic hematuria). The first step in evaluating a patient who complains of red-dark urine is to differentiate between true hematuria (presence of RBCs in urine) and pigmented urine (red-dark urine). The breakdown products of muscle cells and red blood cells (myoglobin and hemoglobin, respectively) are heme-containing compounds capable of turning the color of urine dark red or brown in the absence of true hematuria (red blood cells). A dipstick urinalysis positive for blood without the presence of RBCs (negative microscopic cellular sediment) is suggestive of hemoglobinuria or myoglobinuria.

After confirmation, the etiology of the hematuria should be determined. **Hematuria** can be classified into two broad categories: **intrarenal and extrarenal** (Table 19–2). The history and physical examination are very helpful in the evaluation (age, fever, pain, family history). Laboratory analysis and imaging studies often are necessary, and considering the potential clinical implications, the etiology of hematuria should be pursued in all cases of hematuria. First, examination of the cellular urine sediment can help to differentiate glomerular from nonglomerular hematuria. The presence of **dysmorphic/fragmented RBCs or red cell casts** is indicative of **glomerular origin** (GN); renal biopsy may offer further confirmation if indicated. Second, the urine Gram stain and culture can aid in the diagnosis of infectious hematuria. Third, the urine sample should be sent for cytologic evaluation when the diagnosis of malignancy is suspected. Finally, renal imaging via ultrasound or intravenous pyelogram (IVP) can help in the visualization of the renal parenchyma and vascular structures. Cystoscopy can be used to assess the bladder; and abdominal CT (computed tomography) or MRI (magnetic resonance imaging) can be performed to assess mass effect and surrounding structures.

However, a complete workup for hematuria is rarely needed because the initial evaluation of the patient and urinalysis often lead to the appropriate diagnosis.

Table 19–2 COMMON CAUSES OF HEMATURIA

Intrarenal hematuria
- Kidney trauma
- Renal stones and crystals
- Glomerulonephritis
- Infection (pyelonephritis)
- Neoplasia (renal cell carcinoma)
- Vascular injury (vasculitis, renal thrombosis)

Extrarenal hematuria
- Trauma (eg, Foley placement)
- Infections (urethritis, prostatitis, cystitis)
- Nephrolithiasis (ureteral stones)
- Neoplasia (prostate, bladder)

Glomerular Disease

Rarely do patients with glomerular disease present according to the description in textbooks. In clinical medicine, glomerulopathies are encountered mainly in the form of two distinct syndromes: nephritic or nephrotic (or, more often, as an overlap of the two syndromes). **Nephritis** (nephritic syndrome) is defined as an **inflammatory** renal syndrome that presents as hematuria, edema, hypertension, and a low degree of proteinuria (<3.5 g over 24 hours). **Nephrosis** (or the nephrotic syndrome) is a **noninflammatory** (no active sediment in the urine) glomerulopathy. Glomerular injury may result from a variety of insults and presents either as the sole clinical finding in a patient (primary renal disease) or as part of a complex syndrome of a systemic disorder (secondary glomerular disease). Although all glomerular disorders are often given the all encompassing name of *glomerulonephritis,* this term specifically describes an inflammatory intraglomerular process associated with cellular proliferation that results in hematuria and renal failure (*nephritis* or nephritic syndrome) and excludes the nonproliferative, noninflammatory glomerulopathies (ie, *nephrosis* or nephrotic syndrome). For the purpose of this discussion, *glomerulonephritis* (GN) includes only the inflammatory glomerulopathies.

Nephritic Syndrome

The presentation of acute renal failure with associated hypertension, hematuria, and edema is consistent with acute GN. Acute renal failure, as manifested by a decrease in urine output and azotemia, results from impaired urine production and ineffective filtration of nitrogenous waste by the glomerulus, respectively. The glomerular apparatus (endothelial and epithelial components) is responsible for the ultrafiltration of blood in the kidney and the initial formation of what will later become the urine. Glomerular injury leads to impaired/ineffective filtration of sodium, glucose, nitrogenous products, and amino acids/proteins and its consequent clinical manifestations. Common signs suggesting an inflammatory glomerular cause of renal failure (ie, acute GN) include hematuria (caused by ruptured capillaries in the glomerulus), proteinuria (caused by altered permeability of the capillary walls), edema (caused by salt and water retention), and hypertension (caused by fluid retention and disturbed renal homeostasis of blood pressure). The presence of this constellation of signs in a patient makes the diagnosis of glomerulonephritis very likely. However, it is important to note that often patients present with an overlap syndrome, sharing signs of both nephritis and nephrosis. Moreover, the presence of hematuria in itself is not pathognomonic for GN because there are multiple causes of hematuria of nonglomerular origin. Therefore, confirmation of the presumptive diagnosis of acute glomerulonephritis requires microscopic examination of a urine sample from the suspected patient. The presence of red cell casts (inflammatory cast) or dysmorphic RBCs (caused by filtration through damaged glomeruli) in a sample of spun urine establishes the diagnosis of GN.

Acute GN is a condition characterized by an inflammatory attack of the glomerular apparatus. The different types of GN have a variety of causes, outcomes, and responses to treatment. Once the presumptive diagnosis of acute GN is made, they can be broadly classified as either *primary* (present clinically as a renal disorder) or *secondary* (renal injury caused by a systemic disease). In the case of primary glomerular disorders, the inciting cause is rarely known (no associated systemic disease), and the pathophysiology is often poorly understood (eg, IgA nephropathy or membranoproliferative glomerulonephritis [MPGN]). In general, primary GN is named by the histopathologic appearance and clinical manifestation of the injured kidney (mesangioproliferative GN, MPGN, fibrillary GN, crescentic GN, rapidly progressive GN; Table 19–3). In the case of secondary GN, the inflammatory systemic disorder causes glomerular injury and presents with the clinical manifestations of acute GN (eg, SLE, hepatitis C, HIV, and a variety of vasculitis; Table 19–3). Secondary GN may be classified further by their histopathologic appearance. Because the etiology of inflammation and the degree of cellular proliferation vary widely among the different GNs, alternatively GN can be classified by the mechanism of immune-mediated injury to the glomeruli. In this classification, the injury patterns of all GNs generally fall under three categories: (1) complement-mediated GN, (2) antibody-mediated GN, or (3) non-antibody and complement-mediated (ANCA-mediated) GN, also known as pauci-immune GN. Glomerular injury occurs via circulating immune complexes (antibody and complement-mediated) that precipitate on the glomeruli or by direct attack on the glomerular

Table 19–3 CLASSIFICATION OF GLOMERULONEPHRITIS

Primary renal disorders (based on histopathology)

Membranoproliferative glomerulonephritis (MPGN, types I and II) Mesangioproliferative glomerulonephritis (MSGN)
Crescentic glomerulonephritis
  • Immune deposit (anti-GBM)
  • Pauci-immune (ANCA)
Fibrillary glomerulonephritis
Proliferative glomerulonephritis (IgA nephropathy)

Secondary renal disorders (based on clinical presentation)

Lupus nephritis
Postinfectious glomerulonephritis (poststreptococcal GN)
Hepatitis C/hepatitis B-related glomerulonephritis (cryo-GN)
Vasculitis-related glomerulonephritis (Wegener, Churg-Strauss, polyarteritis nodosa, microscopic polyangiitis, Henoch-Schönlein purpura)
Infective endocarditis-related glomerulonephritis

membranes (antibody-, complement-, and ANCA-mediated). This injury pattern can be visualized via immunofluorescence for specific staining patterns (IgG, IgA) and under electron microscopy of the injured glomeruli for characteristic deposit patterns (linear, granular, pauci-immune, etc).

Therefore, it is easy to see that although the diagnosis of primary versus secondary GN can be made simply by obtaining a detailed medical history, physical examination, and routine laboratory tests, the classification of a specific GN into a given immune-mediated category requires further microscopic analysis, blood tests, and sometimes a kidney biopsy.

Diagnostic Approach to Glomerulonephritis

The approach to the patient with glomerular disease should be systematic and undertaken in a stepwise fashion. The history should be approached meticulously, looking for evidence of preexisting renal disease, systemic disease, and exposure to nephrotoxins. Likewise, the physical examination should assess for blood pressure, evidence of hypertension, presence of edema, renal and vascular bruits, and evidence of systemic disease. The urine should be analyzed for hematuria and sediment. Proteinuria should be categorized as nephrotic (>3.5 g over 24 hours) versus nephritic range (<3.5 g over 24 hours). When erythrocyte casts or dysmorphic red cells are seen in the urine, a diagnosis of GN can be made. Although likely to be present, these markers do not distinguish among the distinct immune-mediated causes of GN; they merely allow us to make the diagnosis of acute GN (primary or secondary). Serologic markers of systemic diseases should be obtained, if indicated (Figure 19–1) in order to further classify the GN. The serologic workup of GN should be guided by the history and physical examination and the clinical suspicion for an individual entity to exist.

Once the appropriate serologic tests have been reviewed, a kidney biopsy may be required. A biopsy sample can be examined under the light microscope in order to determine the primary histopathologic injury to the nephron (MPGN, crescentic GN, etc). Further examination of an immunofluorescent stained sample for immune recognition (IgG, IgA, IgM, C3, C4, or pauci-immune staining) of the affected glomerular membrane (capillary, epithelial, etc.) and under electron microscopy for characteristic patterns of immune deposition (granular, linear GN) may provide a definitive diagnosis of the immune-mediated injury to the glomeruli. Figure 19–1 shows an algorithmic approach to the patient with acute GN.

Treatment of Glomerulonephritis

It is difficult to predict the prognosis and outcome of most GNs. Whereas some are self-limiting and largely asymptomatic (eg, IgA-associated), others may progress to end-stage renal failure (ANCA-mediated GN) without treatment. Unfortunately, as is the case with a number of immune-mediated

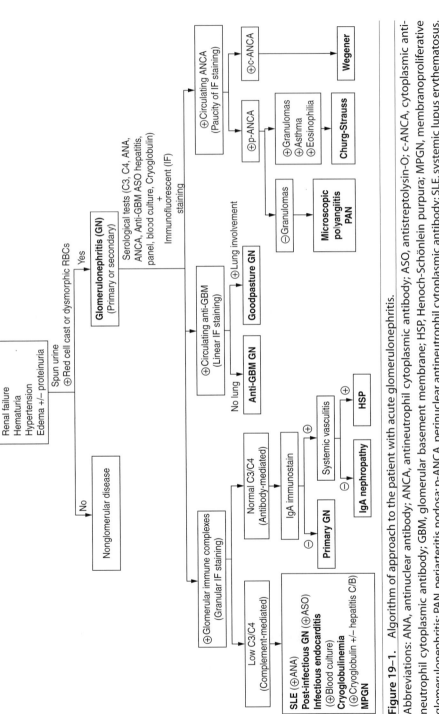

Figure 19-1. Algorithm of approach to the patient with acute glomerulonephritis.

Abbreviations: ANA, antinuclear antibody; ANCA, antineutrophil cytoplasmic antibody; ASO, antistreptolysin-O; c-ANCA, cytoplasmic antineutrophil cytoplasmic antibody; GBM, glomerular basement membrane; HSP, Henoch-Schönlein purpura; MPGN, membranoproliferative glomerulonephritis; PAN, periarteritis nodosa; p-ANCA, perinuclear antineutrophil cytoplasmic antibody; SLE, systemic lupus erythematosus.

disorders, treatment currently is limited to supportive therapy (hemodialysis for renal failure, antihypertensive medications and diuretics for edema) with or without immunosuppressive drugs. When appropriate, the underlying disease should be treated (infective endocarditis, hepatitis, SLE, or vasculitis). The use of steroids and cyclophosphamide has been advocated in the treatment of ANCA-induced GN, while other antibody-mediated GNs might require plasmapheresis in order to eliminate the inciting antibody–immune complex. Although the diagnosis of acute GN may be straightforward, the ensuing therapy often is frustrating and ineffective and leaves the clinician at the mercy of supportive measures.

Comprehension Questions

19.1 An 18-year-old marathon runner has been training during the summer. He is brought to the emergency room disoriented after collapsing on the track. His temperature is 102°F. A Foley catheter is placed and reveals reddish urine with 3+ blood on dipstick and no cells seen microscopically. Which of the following is the most likely explanation for his urine?

A. Underlying renal disease
B. Prerenal azotemia
C. Myoglobinuria
D. Glomerulonephritis

19.2 Which of the following laboratory findings is most consistent with poststreptococcal glomerulonephritis?

A. Elevated serum complement levels
B. Positive antinuclear antibody titers
C. Elevated ASO titers
D. Positive blood cultures
E. Positive cryoglobulin titers

19.3 A 22-year-old man complains of acute hemoptysis over the past week. He denies smoking or pulmonary disease. His blood pressure is 130/70 mm Hg, and his physical examination is normal. His urinalysis also shows microscopic hematuria and red blood cell casts. Which of the following is the most likely etiology?

A. Metastatic renal cell carcinoma to the lungs
B. Acute tuberculosis of the kidneys and lungs
C. Systemic lupus erythematosus
D. Goodpasture disease (antiglomerular basement membrane)

ANSWERS

19.1   **C.** This individual is suffering from heat exhaustion, which can lead to rhabdomyolysis and release of myoglobin. Myoglobinuria leads to a reddish appearance and positive urine dipstick reaction for blood, but microscopic analysis of the urine likely will demonstrate no red cells.

19.2   **C.** The antistreptolysin-O titers typically are elevated and serum complement levels are decreased in poststreptococcal GN.

19.3   **D.** Goodpasture (antiglomerular basement membrane) disease typically affects young males, who present with hemoptysis and hematuria. Antibody against type IV collagen, expressed in the pulmonary alveolar and glomerular basement membrane, leads to the pulmonary and renal manifestations. Hypertension typically is absent. After the initial clinical signs, renal insufficiency usually progresses rapidly. Anti-GBM antibodies almost always are present; the gold standard for diagnosis is renal biopsy.

Clinical Pearls

➤ Finding red blood cell casts or dysmorphic red blood cells on urinalysis differentiates glomerular bleeding (eg, glomerulonephritis) from nonglomerular bleeding (eg, kidney stones).

➤ Glomerulonephritis is characterized by hematuria, edema, and hypertension caused by volume retention.

➤ Gross hematuria following an upper respiratory illness suggests either immunoglobulin A nephropathy or poststreptococcal glomerulonephritis.

➤ Patients with nonglomerular hematuria and no evidence of infection should undergo investigation with imaging (ultrasound or intravenous pyelogram) or cystoscopy to evaluate for stones or malignancy.

REFERENCES

Hricik DE, Chung-Park M, Sedor JR, et al. Glomerulonephritis. *N Engl J Med.* 1998; 339:888-899.

Johnson RJ, Freehally J, eds. *Comprehensive Clinical Nephrology.* St. Louis, MO: CV Mosby; 2000.

Lewis JB, Neilson EG. Glomerular diseases. In: Kasper DL, Braunwald E, Fauci AS, et al. eds. *Harrison's Principles of Internal Medicine.* 17th ed. New York, NY: McGraw-Hill; 2008:1782-1797.

Case 20

A 48-year-old Hispanic woman presents to your office complaining of persistent swelling of her feet and ankles, so much so that she cannot put on her shoes. She first noted mild ankle swelling approximately 2 to 3 months ago. She borrowed a few diuretic pills from a friend; the pills seemed to help, but now she has run out. She also reports that she has gained 20 to 25 lb over the last few months, despite regular exercise and trying to adhere to a healthy diet. Her medical history is significant for type 2 diabetes, for which she takes a sulfonylurea agent. She neither sees a doctor regularly nor monitors her blood glucose at home. She denies dysuria, urinary frequency, or urgency, but she does report that her urine has appeared foamy. She had no fevers, joint pain, skin rashes, or gastrointestinal (GI) symptoms.

Her physical examination is significant for mild periorbital edema, multiple hard exudates, and dot hemorrhages on funduscopic examination, and pitting edema of her hands, feet, and legs. Her chest is clear, her heart rhythm is regular without murmurs, and her abdominal examination is benign. She has diminished sensation to light touch in her feet and legs to mid-calf. A urine dipstick performed in the office shows 2+ glucose, 3+ protein, and negative leukocyte esterase, nitrates, and blood.

➤ What is the most likely diagnosis?

➤ What is the best intervention to slow disease progression?

ANSWERS TO CASE 20:

Nephrotic Syndrome, Diabetic Nephropathy

Summary: A 48-year-old woman with long-standing diabetes now presents with edema and significant proteinuria on a urine dipstick. She has diabetic retinopathy, some peripheral neuropathy, and no other findings suggestive of any other systemic disease.

➤ **Most likely diagnosis:** Nephrotic syndrome as a consequence of diabetic nephropathy.

➤ **Best intervention:** Angiotensin-converting enzyme (ACE) inhibitors.

ANALYSIS

Objectives

1. Recognize the clinical features and complications of nephrotic syndrome.
2. Know the most common causes of nephrotic syndrome.
3. Understand the natural history of diabetic renal disease and how to diagnose and manage it.
4. Learn the principles of treatment of nephrotic syndrome.

Considerations

Patients develop significant proteinuria as a result of glomerular damage, which can result from many systemic diseases. It is important to screen for diseases such as human immunodeficiency virus (HIV), autoimmune diseases, and malignancy by history, physical examination, and sometimes laboratory investigation to determine the underlying cause and appropriate treatment of the renal manifestations.

APPROACH TO

Nephrotic Syndrome

DEFINITION

NEPHROTIC SYNDROME: Urine protein excretion more than 3.5 g over 24 hours, serum hypoalbuminemia (<3 g/dL), and edema.

CLINICAL APPROACH

Normally, the kidneys do not excrete appreciable amounts of protein (<150 mg/d) because serum proteins are excluded from the urine by the glomerular filter both by their large size and their net negative charge. Thus, the appearance of significant proteinuria heralds glomerular disease, with disruption of its normal barrier function. Proteinuria in excess of 3 to 3.5 g of protein per 1.73 m^2 body surface area (normal adult male body surface area) per day is considered to be in the nephrotic range. The key feature of nephrotic syndrome is the heavy proteinuria, which leads to loss of albumin and other serum proteins. The hypoalbuminemia and hypoproteinemia result in decreased intravascular oncotic pressure, leading to tissue edema that usually starts in dependent areas such as the feet but may progress to involve the face, hands, and ultimately the whole body (anasarca). The decreased oncotic pressure also triggers the liver to start lipoprotein synthesis, thus leading to hyperlipidemia.

Patients typically present to the doctor complaining of the edema and have the laboratory features described earlier. Urinalysis usually shows few or no cellular elements and may show waxy casts and oval fat bodies (which look similar to maltese crosses under polarized light) if hyperlipidemia is present.

In adults, one-third of patients with nephrotic syndrome have a systemic disease that involves the kidneys, such as diabetes or lupus; the rest have a primary renal disease, with one of four pathologic lesions: minimal change disease, membranous nephropathy, focal segmental glomerulosclerosis (FSGS), or membranoproliferative glomerulonephritis (MPGN). Thus, a new diagnosis of nephrotic syndrome warrants further investigation into an underlying systemic disease. Common tests include serum glucose and glycosylated hemoglobin levels to evaluate for diabetes, antinuclear antibody (ANA) to screen for systemic lupus erythematosus, serum and urine protein electrophoresis to look for multiple myeloma or amyloidosis, and viral serologies, because HIV and viral hepatitis can cause nephrosis. Less common causes include various cancers, medications such as nonsteroidal anti-inflammatory drugs (NSAIDs), heavy metals such as mercury, and hereditary renal conditions. Of these causes, diabetes mellitus is by far the most common, as in the patient presented in this scenario.

Adults with nephrotic syndrome usually undergo renal biopsy, especially if the underlying diagnosis is unclear, or if there is a possibility of a treatable or reversible condition. Patients with advanced diabetes who have heavy proteinuria and microvascular disease, such as retinopathy, but no active (cellular components) on a urinary sediment are generally presumed to have diabetic nephropathy. These patients typically do not undergo renal biopsy because the nephrotic proteinuria represents irreversible glomerular damage.

Treatment of nephrotic syndrome consists of treatment of the underlying disease, if present, as well as management of the edema and attempts to limit the progression of the renal disease. For edema, all patients require strict **salt restriction**, but most patients will also need **diuretics**. Because both thiazide and loop diuretics are highly protein bound, there is reduced delivery to the kidney, and often very large doses are required to manage the edema. Counterintuitively for a patient with hypoproteinemia, dietary protein restriction usually is recommended. It is thought that high-protein intake only causes heavier proteinuria, which can have an adverse effect on renal function. Additionally, use of **angiotensin-converting enzyme (ACE) inhibitors** or angiotensin receptor blockers (ARBs) reduces proteinuria and slows the progression of renal disease in diabetics with proteinuria.

Besides the edema, patients with nephrotic syndrome have other consequences of renal protein wasting. They have **decreased levels of antithrombin III and proteins C and S**, and often are **hypercoagulable**, with formation of venous thromboembolism, including renal vein thrombosis. Patients with evidence of thrombus formation require anticoagulation, often for life. Other complications include hypogammaglobulinemia with **increased infection risk** (especially pneumococcal infection), iron deficiency anemia caused by hypotransferrinemia, and vitamin D deficiency because of loss of vitamin D–binding protein.

In the progression of diabetic nephropathy, initially the glomerular filtration rate (GFR) is elevated and then declines over time. Prior to the decline in GFR, the earliest stages of diabetic nephropathy can be detected as **microalbuminuria**. This is defined as a urine albumin excretion between 30 and 300 mg/d. It is possible to measure this in a random urine sample rather than a timed collection, because a ratio of albumin (in milligrams) to creatinine (in grams) of 30 to 300 usually correlates with the total excretion described. When albuminuria exceeds 300 mg/d, it is detectable on ordinary urine dipsticks, and the patient is said to have **overt nephropathy**.

After the development of microalbuminuria, most patients will remain asymptomatic, but the glomerulopathy will continue to progress over the subsequent 5 to 10 years until overt nephropathy develops. At this point, many patients have some edema, and nearly all patients have developed hypertension. The presence of hypertension will markedly accelerate the decline of renal function. If left untreated, patients then progress to **end-stage renal disease (ESRD)**, requiring dialysis or transplant, within a 5- to 15-year period.

The development of nephropathy and proteinuria is very significant because they are associated with a much higher risk for cardiovascular disease, which is the leading cause of death in patients with diabetes. By the time patients with diabetes develop ESRD and require dialysis, the average life expectancy is less than 2 years.

Thus, the development of microalbuminuria in diabetic patients is extremely important because of the progressive disease it heralds and because it is potentially reversible, or at least its progression to overt proteinuria can be slowed via medications. The **ACE inhibitors slow the progression of renal disease** and should be initiated even when patients are normotensive. Tight **glycemic control** with a goal hemoglobin A_{1c} less than 6.5 to 7.0 has also been shown to slow or prevent the progression of microvascular complications of diabetes, such as retinopathy and nephropathy. If overt nephropathy and hypertension have developed, **blood pressure control** with a goal less than 130/80 mm Hg (or <125/75 mm Hg if heavy proteinuria >1 g/d) is essential to slow progression.

In addition, because cardiovascular disease is the major killer of patients with diabetes, aggressive risk factor reduction should be attempted, including smoking cessation and reduction of hypercholesterolemia. In the newest recommendations regarding management of cholesterol, patients with diabetes now are regarded as the highest risk category, along with patients who already have established coronary artery or other atherosclerotic vascular disease; they should be treated with diet and statins with a goal of low-density lipoprotein (LDL) cholesterol less than 100 mg/dL.

Comprehension Questions

20.1   A 49-year-old woman with type 2 diabetes presents to your office for new onset swelling in her legs and face. She has no other medical problems and says that at her last ophthalmologic appointment she was told that the diabetes had started to affect her eyes. She takes glyburide daily for her diabetes. Physical examination is normal except for pitting edema of bilateral upper and lower extremities, hard exudates and dot hemorrhages on funduscopic examination, and diminished sensation to the mid-shin bilaterally. Urine analysis shows 3+ protein and 2+ glucose (otherwise negative). Which of the following is the best treatment for this patient?

   A. Have the patient return in 6 weeks and check a repeat urine analysis at that time.
   B. Start metoprolol.
   C. Change the glyburide to glipizide and have the patient return for follow-up in 6 weeks.
   D. Start lisinopril.
   E. Refer the patient to a cardiologist.

20.2. A 19-year-old man was seen at the university student health clinic a week ago complaining of pharyngitis, and now returns because he has noted discoloration of his urine. He is noted to have elevated blood pressure (178/110 mm Hg) and urinalysis reveals RBC casts, dysmorphic RBCs, and 1+ proteinuria. Which of the following is the most likely diagnosis?

   A. Systemic lupus erythematosus (SLE)
   B. Amyloidosis
   C. Post-streptococcal glomerulonephritis
   D. HIV nephropathy
   E. Diabetic nephropathy

20.3   Which of the following is the best screening test for early diabetic nephropathy?

   A. Urine microalbuminuria
   B. Dipstick urinalysis
   C. Renal biopsy
   D. Fasting blood glucose
   E. 24-Hour urine collection for creatinine clearance

20.4   A 58-year-old man with type 2 diabetes is normotensive but has a persistent urine albumin/creatinine ratio of 100, but no proteinuria on urine dipstick. Which of the following is the best management for this patient?

   A. Start ACE inhibitor.
   B. Start high-protein diet.
   C. Switch from oral agent to insulin.
   D. Refer to ophthalmologist for examination.

ANSWERS

20.1   **D.** Beta-blockers are a good first-choice agent for a patient with hypertension and no comorbidities. However, for the patient with diabetes and nephropathy described in the clinical vignette, the benefit of an ACE inhibitor for decreasing proteinuria makes this the best choice for initial treatment. Changing from one sulfonylurea to another is of no benefit because all are equally efficacious. There is no indication for referral to a cardiologist based on the information provided in the vignette.

20.2   **C.** The patient has hypertension, and a urinary sediment consistent with a nephritic rather than nephrotic syndrome (RBC casts, mild degree of proteinuria). Given his recent episode of pharyngitis, the most likely cause would be post-infectious, probably due to streptococcal infection. SLE can produce a variety of renal diseases, including both nephritic and nephrotic manifestions, but it would be unlikely in a male patient, especially without other clinical manifestations of lupus such as arthritis. Amyloidosis, diabetes, and HIV all cause renal disease, but usually produce the nephrotic syndrome (heavy proteinuria >3gm/day, edema, hypoalbuminemia).

20.3   **A.** Although a 24-hour urine collection for creatinine may be useful in assessing declining GFR, it is not the best screening test for the diagnosis of early diabetic nephropathy. In the outpatient setting, a dipstick urinalysis is readily available but will detect only patients with overt nephropathy (proteinuria >300 mg/d). Thus, a random urinary albumin/creatinine ratio of 30/300 is the best test to screen for early diabetic nephropathy. A fasting blood glucose may aid in the diagnosis of diabetes but not nephropathy. Finally, although most patients with nephrotic syndrome require a renal biopsy for diagnosis, a patient with worsening renal function who has had long-standing diabetes is assumed to have renal disease secondary to diabetic nephropathy, and the majority of these patients do not undergo a renal biopsy.

20.4   **A.** The albumin/creatinine ratio of 100 is indicative of microalbuminuria. Screening for microalbuminuria is very important because it is the one aspect of the disease that is reversible and to which physicians can target therapy to blunt the progression to overt renal failure. Disease progression is slowed with ACE inhibitors, blood pressure control, limited dietary protein intake, weight loss, and improved glycemic control.

Clinical Pearls

➤ Nephrotic syndrome is characterized by more than 3.5 g proteinuria over 24 hours, hypoalbuminemia, and edema. Often, hypercoagulability and hyperlipidemia are present.

➤ Nephrotic syndrome can be a result of a primary renal disease but is often a manifestation of a systemic disease such as diabetes, HIV infection, an autoimmune disease, or a malignancy.

➤ Patients with diabetes should be screened for microalbuminuria (albumin excretion 30-300 mg/d); if present, treatment should be initiated with an angiotensin-converting enzyme inhibitor, even if the patient is normotensive.

➤ Patients with diabetic nephropathy and proteinuria are at very high risk for cardiovascular disease, so aggressive risk factor reduction, such as use of statins, is important.

REFERENCES

Gross JL, de Azevedo MJ, Silveiro SP, et al. Diabetic nephropathy: diagnosis, prevention, and treatment. *Diabetes Care*. 2005;28:164-176.

Lewis JB, Neilson EG. Glomerular diseases. In: Kasper DL, Braunwald E, Fauci AS, et al. eds. *Harrison's Principles of Internal Medicine*. 17th ed. New York, NY: McGraw-Hill; 2008:1782-1797.

Powers AC. Diabetes mellitus. In: Fauci AS, Braunwald E, Kasper DL. *Harrison's Principles of Internal Medicine*. 17th ed. New York, NY: McGraw-Hill; 2008: 2275-2304.

Case 21

A 48-year-old man comes to your office complaining of severe right knee pain for 8 hours. He states that the pain, which started abruptly at 2 AM and woke him from sleep, was quite severe, so painful that even the weight of the bed sheets on his knee was unbearable. By the morning, the knee had become warm, swollen, and tender. He explains that he prefers to keep his knee bent, and extending his leg to straighten the knee causes the pain to worsen. He has never had pain, surgery, or injury to his knees. A year ago, he did have some pain and swelling at the base of his great toe on the left foot, which was not as severe as this episode, and resolved in 2 or 3 days after taking ibuprofen. His only medical history is hypertension, which is controlled with hydrochlorothiazide. He works as a financial analyst; he is married and does not smoke, but he does consume one or two drinks after work one to two times per week.

On examination, his temperature is 100.6°F, heart rate 104 bpm, and blood pressure 136/78 mm Hg. His head and neck examinations are unremarkable, his chest is clear, and his heart is tachycardic but regular, with no gallops or murmurs. His right knee is swollen, with a moderate effusion, and appears erythematous, warm, and very tender to palpation. He is unable to fully extend the knee because of pain. He has no other joint swelling, pain, or deformity, and no skin rashes.

➤ What is the most likely diagnosis?

➤ What is your next step?

➤ What is the best initial treatment?

ANSWERS TO CASE 21:
Acute Monoarticular Arthritis—Gout

Summary: A 48-year-old hypertensive man complains of acute onset of severe right knee pain of 8-hour duration. He denies previous pain, surgery, or injury to his knees. One year ago, he had great toe pain and swelling for several days that resolved with ibuprofen. He takes hydrochlorothiazide and occasionally drinks alcohol. On examination, his temperature is 100.6°F, heart rate 104 bpm, and blood pressure 136/78 mm Hg. His right knee is swollen, with a moderate effusion, and appears erythematous, warm, and very tender to palpation. He is unable to fully extend the knee because of pain. He has no other joint swelling, pain, or deformity, and no skin rashes.

➤ **Most likely diagnosis:** Acute monoarticular arthritis, likely crystalline or infectious, most likely gout because of history.

➤ **Next step:** Aspiration of the knee joint to send fluid for cell count, culture, and crystal analysis.

➤ **Best initial treatment:** If the joint fluid analysis is consistent with infection, he needs drainage of the infected fluid by aspiration and administration of antibiotics. If analysis is suggestive of crystal-induced arthritis, he can be treated with colchicine, nonsteroidal anti-inflammatory drugs (NSAIDs), or corticosteroids.

ANALYSIS

Objectives

1. Be familiar with the use of synovial fluid analysis to determine the etiology of arthritis.
2. Know the stages of gout and the appropriate treatment for each stage.
3. Know about the similarities and differences between gout and pseudogout.

Considerations

A middle-aged man presents with an acute attack of monoarticular arthritis, as evidenced by knee effusion, limited range of motion, and signs of inflammation (low-grade fever, erythema, warmth, tenderness). The two most likely causes are infection (eg, *Staphylococcus aureus*) and crystalline arthritis (eg, gout or pseudogout). If the patient is at risk, gonococcal arthritis is also a possibility. The previous less severe episode involving his first metatarsophalangeal (MTP) joint sounds like **podagra**, the most common presentation of gout.

The previous attack of arthritis in the first MTP joint and the very rapid onset of severe symptoms during the current attack are consistent with acute gouty arthritis. In this patient, the attack could have been precipitated by the use of alcohol, which increases uric acid production, and his use of thiazide diuretics, which decrease renal excretion of uric acid.

Although the first attack was typical of gout, which makes this episode very likely to also be acute gouty arthritis, the current presentation is also entirely consistent with bacterial infection. Untreated septic arthritis could lead to rapid destruction of the joint, so joint aspiration and empiric antibiotic therapy are appropriate until his cultures and crystal analysis are available.

APPROACH TO
Monoarticular Arthritis

DEFINITIONS

MONOARTHRITIS: Inflammation of a single joint.

GOUT: A disturbance of uric-acid metabolism occurring mainly in men, characterized by painful inflammation of the joints, especially of the feet and hands, and arthritic attacks resulting from elevated levels of uric acid in the blood and the deposition of urate crystals around the joints.

CLINICAL APPROACH

Almost any joint disorder may begin as monoarthritis, or inflammation of a single joint; however, the primary concern is always **infectious arthritis**, because it may lead to **joint destruction and resultant severe morbidity**. For that reason, **acute monoarthritis should be considered a medical emergency** and investigated and treated aggressively.

Monoarthritis may be a result of infection (eg, bacterial, fungal, Lyme disease, tuberculosis) or crystal-induced arthritis (eg, pseudogout and gout); less often, it may be the presentation of a systemic disease typically associated with polyarticular disease, such as rheumatoid arthritis or systemic lupus erythematosus. It may also be a result of noninflammatory causes such as trauma or osteoarthritis.

Accurate diagnosis starts with a good history and physical examination supplemented by additional diagnostic testing, such as **synovial fluid analysis, radiography**, and occasionally **synovial biopsy**. A history of episodes of arthritis suggests crystalline disease or other noninfectious arthropathies. Patients with crystal-induced arthritis may give a history of recurrent, self-limited episodes. Precipitation of an attack by surgery or some other stress can occur with both crystalline disorders, but **gout is far more common than is pseudogout**. The clinical course can provide some clues to the etiology: septic arthritis usually worsens unless treated; osteoarthritis worsens with physical activity.

The location of joint involvement may be helpful. **Gout** most commonly involves the **first MTP joint (podagra), ankle, mid-foot, or knee.** Pseudogout most commonly affects the large joints, such as the knee; it may also affect the wrist or the first MTP joint (hence, the name pseudogout). In **gonococcal** arthritis, there are often **migratory arthralgias and tenosynovitis,** often involving the wrist and hands, associated with **pustular skin lesions,** before progressing to a purulent monoarthritis or oligoarthritis. Nongonococcal causes of septic arthritis often involve large weight-bearing joints, such as the knee and hip.

The basic approach in physical examination is to differentiate arthritis from inflammatory conditions adjacent to the joint, such as cellulitis or bursitis. **True arthritis** is characterized by **swelling and redness around the joint, and painful limitation of motion in all planes,** during **active and passive motion. Joint movement that is not limited by passive motion** suggests **a soft tissue disorder such as bursitis** rather than arthritis.

Diagnostic arthrocentesis usually is necessary when evaluating an acute monoarthritis and is always essential when infection is suspected. Synovial fluid analysis helps to differentiate between inflammatory and noninflammatory causes of arthritis. Fluid analysis typically includes gross examination, cell count and differential, Gram stain and culture, and crystal analysis. Table 21–1 gives the typical results that can help one distinguish between noninflammatory conditions such as osteoarthritis, inflammatory arthritis such as crystalline disease, and septic arthritis, which most often is a bacterial infection.

Normal joints contain a small amount of fluid that is essentially acellular. Noninflammatory effusions should have a white blood cell count less than 1000 to 2000/mm^3 with less than 25% to 50% polymorphonuclear (PMN) cells. **If the fluid is inflammatory, the joint should be considered infected until proven otherwise,** especially if the patient is febrile.

Crystal analysis requires the use of a polarizing light microscope. Monosodium urate crystals, the cause of **gout,** are **needle-shaped,** typically **intracellular** within a PMN cell, and are **negatively birefringent, appearing yellow** under the polarizing microscope. Calcium pyrophosphate dehydrate (CPPD) crystals, the cause of **pseudogout,** are **short and rhomboid,** and are **weakly positively birefringent,** appearing blue under polarized light. **Even if crystals are seen, infection must be excluded when the synovial fluid is inflammatory!** Crystals and infection may coexist in the same joint, and chronic arthritis or previous joint damage, such as occurs in gout, may predispose that joint to hematogenous infection.

In septic arthritis, Gram stain and culture of the synovial fluid is positive in 60% to 80% of cases. False-negative results may be related to prior antibiotic use or fastidious microorganisms. For example, in **gonococcal arthritis, joint fluid cultures typically are negative, whereas cultures of blood or the pustular skin lesions may be positive.** Sometimes, the diagnosis rests upon demonstration of gonococcal infection in another site, such as urethritis, with the typical arthritis-dermatitis syndrome. **Synovial biopsy** may be required

Table 21–1 JOINT ASPIRATE CHARACTERISTICS

GROSS EXAMINATION	NORMAL	NONINFLAMMATORY	INFLAMMATORY	SEPTIC
Volume (knee)	<1 mL	Often >1 mL	Often >1 mL	Often >1 mL
Viscosity	High	High	Low	Variable
Color	Colorless to straw	Straw to yellow	Yellow	Variable
Clarity	Transparent	Transparent	Translucent	Opaque
Leukocytes/mm^3	<200	50-1000	2000-75,000	Often >100,000
Polymorphonuclear cells	<25%	<25%	Often >50%	>85%
Culture results	Negative	Negative	Negative	Often positive
Glucose	Nearly equal to blood	Nearly equal to blood	<50 mg/dL lower than blood	<50 mg/dL lower than blood

Data from: Koch AE. Approach to the patient with pain in one or a few joints. In: H. David Humes ed. Kelly's Textbook of Internal Medicine. New York, NY: Lippincott Williams and Wilkins; 2000:1322.

when the cause of monoarthritis remains unclear, and is usually **necessary to diagnose arthritis caused by tuberculosis or hemochromatosis.**

Plain radiographs usually are unremarkable in cases of inflammatory arthritis; the typical finding is soft tissue swelling. **Chondrocalcinosis** or linear calcium deposition in joint cartilage suggests pseudogout. They are often found when evaluating for fracture in patients with a history of trauma.

Generally, patients require initiation of treatment before all test results are available. When septic arthritis is suspected, the clinician should culture the joint fluid and start antibiotic therapy; the antibiotic choice should be initially based on the Gram stain and, when available, the culture results. If the Gram stain is negative, the clinical picture should dictate antimicrobial selection. For example, if the patient has the typical presentation of **gonococcal arthritis, intravenous ceftriaxone** is the usual initial therapy, usually with rapid improvement in symptoms. Nongonococcal septic arthritis usually is caused by gram-positive organisms, most often *S aureus,* so treatment would involve an **antistaphylococcal penicillin such as nafcillin,** or vancomycin when methicillin resistance is suspected. **It is essential to drain the purulent joint fluid, usually by repeated percutaneous aspiration.** Open surgical drainage or arthroscopy is required when joint fluid is loculated, or when shoulders, hips, or sacroiliac joints are involved.

Gout classically progresses through four stages.

Stage 1 is **asymptomatic hyperuricemia**. Patients have elevated uric acid levels without arthritis or kidney stones. The majority of patients with hyperuricemia never develop any symptoms, but higher the uric acid level and the longer the duration of hyperuricemia, the greater the likelihood of the patient developing gouty arthritis.

Stage 2 is **acute gouty arthritis,** which most often involves the acute onset of severe **monoarticular pain,** often occurring at night, in the first MTP joint, ankle, or knee, with rapid development of joint swelling and erythema and sometimes associated with systemic symptoms such as fever and chills. This usually follows decades of asymptomatic hyperuricemia. Attacks may last hours or up to 2 weeks.

Stage 3 is **intercritical gout,** or the period between acute attacks. Patients are generally completely asymptomatic. The vast majority of patients will have another acute attack within 1 to 2 years. The presence of these completely asymptomatic periods between monoarthritic attacks is so uncommon, except in crystalline arthritis, that it is often used as a diagnostic criterion for gout.

Stage 4 is **chronic tophaceous gout,** which usually occurs after 10 or more years of acute intermittent gout. In this stage, the intercritical periods are no longer asymptomatic; the involved joints now have chronic swelling and discomfort, which worsens over time. Patients also develop subcutaneous tophaceous deposits of monosodium urate.

In general, **asymptomatic hyperuricemia requires no specific treatment**. Lowering the urate level does not necessarily prevent the development of gout, and most of these patients will never develop any symptoms. Acute gouty arthritis is treated with therapies to reduce the inflammatory reaction to the presence of the crystals, all of which are most effective if started early in the attack. **Potent NSAIDs, such as indomethacin, are the mainstay of therapy.** Alternatively, oral colchicine can be taken every hour until the joint symptoms abate, but dosing is limited by gastrointestinal side effects such as nausea and diarrhea. Individuals affected by acute joint pain with **renal insufficiency,** for which **NSAIDs or colchicine** is relatively **contraindicated,** usually benefit **from intraarticular glucocorticoid injection or oral steroid therapy.** Steroids should be used only if infection has been excluded. Treatment to lower uric acid levels is inappropriate during an acute episode because any sudden increase or decrease in urate levels may precipitate further attacks.

During intercritical gout, the focus shifts to preventing further attacks by lowering uric acid levels. Dietary restriction is mainly aimed at avoiding organ-rich foods, such as liver, and avoiding alcohol. Patients taking thiazide diuretics should be switched to another antihypertensive if possible. Urate lowering can be accomplished by therapy to increase uric acid excretion by the kidney, such as with probenecid. Uricosuric agents such as this are ineffective in patients with renal failure, however, and are contraindicated in patients with a history of uric acid kidney stones. In these patients, allopurinol can be used to diminish uric acid production. In either case, urate lowering can precipitate acute attacks, so initial prophylaxis with daily low-dose colchicine usually is necessary.

Patients with tophaceous gout are managed as previously described during acute attacks and treated with allopurinol to help tophaceous deposits resolve. Surgery may be indicated if the mass effect of tophi causes nerve compression, joint deformity, or chronic skin ulceration with resultant infection.

Patients with pseudogout are treated similarly for acute attacks (NSAIDs, colchicine, systemic or intraarticular steroids). Prophylaxis with colchicine may be helpful in patients with chronic recurrent attacks, but there is no effective therapy for preventing CPPD crystal formation or deposition.

Comprehension Questions

21.1   A previously healthy 18-year-old college freshman presents to the student health clinic complaining of pain on the dorsum of her left wrist and in her right ankle, fever, and a pustular rash on the extensor surfaces of both her forearms. She has mild swelling and erythema of her ankle, and pain on passive flexion of her wrist. Less than 1 mL of joint fluid is aspirated from her ankle, which shows 8000 polymorphonuclear (PMN) cells per high-power field (hpf) but no organisms on Gram stain. Which of the following is the best initial treatment?

   A. Indomethacin orally
   B. Intravenous ampicillin
   C. Colchicine orally
   D. Intraarticular prednisone
   E. Intravenous ceftriaxone

21.2   Which of the following diagnostic tests is most likely to give the diagnosis for the case in Question 21.1?
        A. Crystal analysis of the joint fluid
        B. Culture of joint fluid
        C. Blood culture
        D. Cervical culture

21.3   A 30-year-old man is noted to have an acutely swollen and red knee. Joint aspirate reveals numerous leukocytes and polymorphonuclear leukocytes, but no organisms on Gram stain. Analysis shows few negatively birefringent crystals. Which of the following is the best initial treatment?
        A. Oral corticosteroids
        B. Intraarticular corticosteroids
        C. Intravenous antibiotic therapy
        D. Oral colchicine

ANSWERS

21.1   **E.** The patient described best fits the picture of disseminated gonococcal infection. She has the rash, which typically is located on extensor surfaces of distal extremities. Pain on passive flexion of her wrist indicates likely tenosynovitis of that area. The fluid is inflammatory, but gonococci are typically not seen on Gram stain. Ceftriaxone is the usual treatment of choice for gonococcal infection. Nafcillin would be useful for staphylococcal arthritis and would be the more likely choice if she were older, had some chronic joint disease such as rheumatoid arthritis, or were immunocompromised. Gonococcal arthritis is the most common cause of infectious arthritis in patients younger than 40 years. Indomethacin or colchicine would be useful if she had a crystalline arthritis, but that is unlikely in this clinical picture. Intraarticular prednisone is contraindicated while infectious arthritis is a possibility.

21.2   **D.** Synovial fluid cultures usually are sterile in gonococcal arthritis (in fact, the arthritis is more likely caused by immune complex deposition than by actual joint infection), and blood cultures are positive less than 50% of the time. Diagnosis is more often made by finding gonococcal infection in a more typical site, such as urethra, cervix, or pharynx.

21.3   **C.** Corticosteroids should not be used until infection is ruled out. The inflammatory arthritis as shown by Gram stain of the joint aspirate is suspicious for infection, even with no organisms seen on Gram stain. Also, the presence of a few crystals does not eliminate an infection.

Clinical Pearls

➤ In the absence of trauma, acute monoarthritis is most likely to be caused by septic or crystalline arthritis.

➤ In a febrile patient with a joint effusion, diagnostic arthrocentesis is mandatory. Inflammatory fluid, that is, a white blood cell count more than 2000/mm^3, should be considered infected until proven otherwise.

➤ Gonococcal arthritis usually presents as a migratory tenosynovitis, often involving the wrists and hands, with few vesiculopustular skin lesions. Nongonococcal septic arthritis is most often caused by *Staphylococcus aureus* and most often affects large weight–bearing joints.

➤ Monosodium urate crystals in gout are needle-shaped and negatively birefringent (yellow) under the polarizing microscope. Calcium pyrophosphate dihydrate crystals in pseudogout are rhomboid and positively birefringent (blue).

➤ Treatment of gout depends on the stage: nonsteroidal anti-inflammatory drugs, colchicine, or steroids for an acute gouty arthritis, and urate lowering with probenecid or allopurinol during the intercritical period.

REFERENCES

Campion EW, Glynn RJ, DeLabray LO. Asymptomatic hyperuricemia: risk and consequences in the Normative Aging Study. *Am J Med.* 1987;82:421-426.

Klippel JH, Crofford L, eds. *Primer on the Rheumatic Diseases.* 12th ed. Atlanta, GA: Arthritis Foundation; 2001:Chapters 12, 13, 15.

Madoff LC. Infectious arthritis. In: Fauci AS, Braunwald E, Kasper DL, eds. *Harrison's Principles of Internal Medicine.* 17th ed. New York, NY: McGraw-Hill; 2008:2169-2175.

Schumacher HR, Chen LX. Gout and other crystal-associated arthropathies. In: Fauci AS, Braunwald E, Kasper DL, eds. *Harrison's Principles of Internal Medicine.* 17th ed. New York, NY: McGraw-Hill; 2008:2165-2169.

Terkeltaub RA. Gout. *N Engl J Med.* 2003;349:1647-1655.

Case 22

A 32-year-old nurse presents to your office with a complaint of intermittent episodes of pain, stiffness, and swelling in both hands and wrists for approximately 1 year. The episodes last for several weeks and then resolve. More recently, she noticed similar symptoms in her knees and ankles. Joint pain and stiffness are making it harder for her to get out of bed in the morning and are interfering with her ability to perform her duties at work. The joint stiffness usually lasts for several hours before improving. She also reports malaise and easy fatigability for the past few months, but she denies having fever, chills, skin rashes, and weight loss. Physical examination reveals a well-developed woman, with blood pressure 120/70 mm Hg, heart rate 82 bpm, and respiratory rate 14 breaths per minute. Her skin does not reveal any rashes. Head, neck, cardiovascular, chest, and abdominal examinations are normal. There is no hepatosplenomegaly. The joint examination reveals the presence of bilateral swelling, redness and tenderness of most proximal interphalangeal (PIP) joints, metacarpophalangeal (MCP) joints, the wrists, and the knees. Laboratory studies show a mild anemia with hemoglobin 11.2 g/dL, hematocrit 32.5%, mean corpuscular volume (MCV) 85.7 fL, white blood cell (WBC) count 7.9/mm³ with a normal differential, and platelet count 300,000/mm³. The urinalysis is clear with no protein and no red blood cells (RBCs). The erythrocyte sedimentation rate (ESR) is 75 mm/h, and the kidney and liver function tests are normal.

➤ What is your most likely diagnosis?

➤ What is your next diagnostic step?

ANSWERS TO CASE 22:
Rheumatoid Arthritis

Summary: This is a 32-year-old woman with a 1-year history of symmetric polyarticular arthritis and morning stiffness. Joint examination reveals the presence of bilateral swelling, redness and tenderness of her PIP joints, MCP joints, wrists, and knees. She has a mild normocytic anemia with an otherwise normal complete blood count (CBC). Urinalysis, renal, and liver function tests are normal. The ESR is elevated, suggesting an inflammatory cause of her arthritis.

➤ **Most likely diagnosis:** Rheumatoid arthritis (RA).

➤ **Next diagnostic step:** Rheumatoid factor and antinuclear antibody titer.

ANALYSIS

Objectives

1. Discern between the clinical presentation of RA and other symmetric polyarthritis syndromes.
2. Learn about the clinical course and treatment of RA.

Considerations

This patient's history, including the symmetric peripheral polyarthritis and duration of symptoms, is suggestive of RA. Rheumatoid arthritis is a systemic autoimmune disorder of unknown etiology. Its major distinctive feature is a chronic symmetric and erosive synovitis of peripheral joints, which, if untreated, leads to deformity and destruction of joints due to erosion of cartilage and bone. The diagnosis of RA is a clinical one, based on the presence of a combination of clinical findings, laboratory abnormalities, and radiographic erosions.

APPROACH TO
Polyarticular Arthritis

CLINICAL APPROACH

The first and most important step in evaluating a patient with polyarticular joint pain is determining whether or not **synovitis/arthritis** is present, producing soft tissue swelling, joint effusion, tenderness, warmth of the joint, and limitation of both active and passive range of motion. If the only finding is pain without inflammatory changes, then the diagnostic considerations include noninflammatory diseases such as osteoarthritis (OA), fibromyalgia, hypothyroidism, neuropathic pain, and depression. The presence of soft tissue swelling and tenderness with limited active range of motion but normal passive range of motion suggests the problem is extraarticular soft tissue inflammation, such as bursitis or tendonitis.

If there is active synovitis/arthritis, it is clinically useful to distinguish between monoarticular/oligoarticular arthritis (see Chapter 21) and polyarticular arthritis. In polyarticular disease, the next diagnostic clue is the duration of symptoms. If symptoms are relatively acute (<6 weeks), the major considerations are arthritis due to **viral infection** (such as hepatitis B or C, rubella, or parvovirus B19) or the earliest manifestation of a true rheumatic disease. Viral serologies and compatible clinical history of exposure often can make the diagnosis at this point and obviate need for further rheumatologic evaluation. Treatment of a viral arthritis usually is limited to symptom relief with nonsteroidal anti-inflammatory drugs (NSAIDs) because the conditions are generally self-limited.

Symmetric peripheral polyarthritis is the most characteristic feature of RA. Other autoimmune rheumatic diseases, such as systemic lupus erythematosus (SLE) and psoriatic arthritis are often asymmetric. **Lupus,** which may present with a symmetric polyarthritis, usually is characterized by the presence of other symptoms, such as malar rash, serositis (pleuritis and pericarditis), renal disease with proteinuria or hematuria, central nervous system (CNS) manifestations, as well as hematologic disorders, such as hemolytic anemia, leucopenia, lymphopenia, or thrombocytopenia. **Rheumatic fever,** which can cause symmetric polyarthritis, is an acute febrile illness lasting only 6 to 8 weeks. In **psoriatic arthritis** the pattern of joint involvement varies widely. The vast majority of patients have peripheral joint involvement of more than five joints. Others have a pauciarticular asymmetric arthritis or exclusive distal interphalangeal (DIP) involvement. Inflammation is not limited to the joints but also occurs at the periosteum, along tendons, and at the insertion points into the bone, resulting in the development of "sausage digits," which are typical of psoriatic arthritis (and Reiter syndrome). Although the arthritis can precede the development of a skin rash, the definite diagnosis of psoriatic arthritis cannot be made without the evidence of skin or nail changes typical of psoriasis. Reactive arthritis as an asymmetric inflammatory arthritis which follows infection of the gastrointestinal (GI) or genitourinary (GU) tract with bacteria such as *Salmonella, Shigella, Campylobacter, Yersinia,* or *Chlamydia.* **Reiter syndrome** is a form of reactive arthritis with the **triad of arthritis, uveitis, and urethritis.**

The peripheral polyarthritis of **RA** most typically involves the wrists and the MCP or **PIP joints** of both hands; the DIP joints usually are spared. It is useful to contrast the typical pattern of joint involvement of RA from those of degenerative OA. Degenerative joint disease may affect multiple joints, but it occurs in older age groups, usually is not associated with inflammation or constitutional symptoms, and tends not to be episodic. Also, in **OA** the hand joints most commonly involved are the **DIP joints,** where the formation of **Heberden nodes** can be noted (Figure 22–1). **Ulnar deviation of the MCP joints** is often associated with **radial deviation of the wrists; swan-neck**

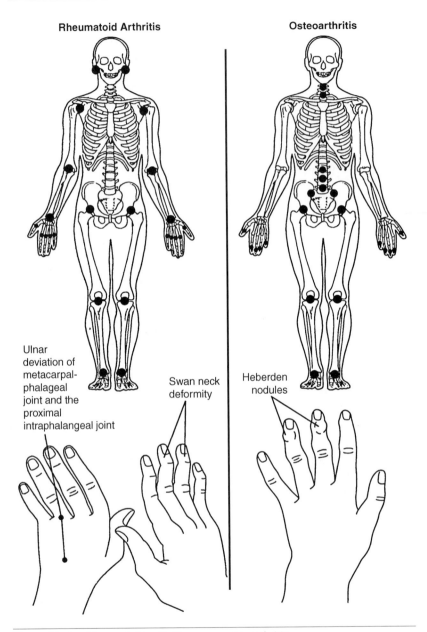

Figure 22–1.   Rheumatoid arthritis versus osteoarthritis.

deformities can develop as well as the **boutonnière deformity (Figure 22–2).**
Swan-neck deformity results from contracture of the interosseous and flexor
muscles and tendons, which causes a flexion contracture of the MCP joint,
hypertension of the PIP joint, and flexion of the DIP joint. In the boutonnière

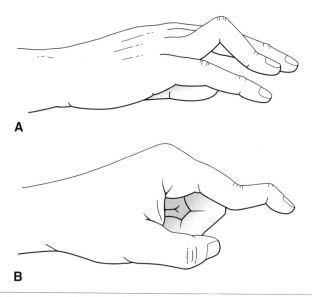

Figure 22–2.   Boutonnière (A) and swan-neck (B) deformities.

deformity, there is a flexion of the PIP and hyperextension of the DIP joints. These findings are typical of advanced RA.

Morning stiffness or stiffness after any prolonged inactivity is a common feature of many arthritic disorders. However, stiffness that lasts more than 1 hour is seen only in inflammatory conditions such as RA and reflects the severity of joint inflammation. See Table 22-1 for diagnostic criteria.

Rheumatoid nodules are subcutaneous nodules typically found over extensor surfaces of the proximal ulna or other pressure points. They only occur in 20% to 30% of patients with RA but are believed to have a high diagnostic specificity for RA.

Rheumatoid factors (RFs) are **immunoglobulins** that react to the F_C **portion of immunoglobulin (Ig)G molecules.** The usual serologic tests used in clinical laboratories detect IgM RFs, which are found in 80% to 85% of patients with RA. Rheumatoid factor is not specific for RA, as it is found in 5% of healthy patients, but it can support the diagnosis when clinical features are suggestive. High RF titers have a prognostic utility for more severe systemic and progressive disease.

Radiologic findings in RA, such as erosion of periarticular bone and cartilage destruction with loss of joint space, may help the diagnosis. On X-rays, the typical findings are joint space narrowing, subchondral polysclerosis, marginal osteophyte formation, and cyst formation. Usually, though, the typical X-ray findings do not develop until later in the disease process after a diagnosis

Table 22–1 1987 CRITERIA FOR THE CLASSIFICATION OF ACUTE RHEUMATOID ARTHRITIS*

CRITERION	DEFINITION
1. Morning stiffness	Morning stiffness in and around the joints, lasting at least 1 h before maximal improvement.
2. Arthritis of 3 or more joint areas	3 or more of the following joints noted to have soft tissue swelling or fluid: PIP, MCP, wrist, elbow, knee, ankle, or MTP.
3. Arthritis of hand joints	At least one wrist, MCP, or PIP joint with soft tissue swelling or fluid.
4. Symmetric arthritis	Simultaneous involvement of the same joint areas (as defined in criterion 2) on both sides of the body (bilateral involvement of PIPs, MCPs, or MTPs is acceptable without absolute symmetry).
5. Rheumatoid nodules	Subcutaneous nodules, over bony prominences, or extensor surfaces, or in juxtaarticular regions, observed by a physician.
6. Serum rheumatoid factor	Demonstration of abnormal amounts of serum rheumatoid factor by any method for which the result has been positive in <5% of normal control subjects.
7. Radiographic changes	Radiographic changes typical of rheumatoid arthritis on posteroanterior hand and wrist radiographs, which must include erosions or unequivocal bony decalcification localized in or most marked adjacent to the involved joints (osteoarthritis changes alone do not qualify).

*Rheumatoid arthritis is strongly suspected when 4 of 7 criteria are met.

has been made based on clinical findings. Joint deformities in RA occur from several different mechanisms, all related to synovitis and pannus formation with resulting cartilage destruction and erosion of periarticular bone. The structural damage to the joint is irreversible and worsens with disease progression. Multiple different joints may be affected, such as hand, foot, ankle, hip, shoulders, elbow, and cervical spine.

There are several **extraarticular manifestations in RA**, including vasculitic lesions with the development of ischemic ulcers, which implies systemic involvement; ocular manifestations with symptoms of **keratoconjunctivitis sicca** (Sjögren syndrome); respiratory manifestations caused by **interstitial lung disease;** cardiac manifestations; and several neurologic manifestations, such as myelopathy, related to cervical spine instability. Although not common, the continuous bone erosion may result in an atlantoaxial subluxation with cervical dislocation and spinal cord compression. Entrapment neuropathy may develop, such as carpal tunnel syndrome. Hematologic manifestations include anemia, typically anemia of chronic disease. The combination of **RA, splenomegaly, leucopenia, lymphadenopathy**, and **thrombocytopenia** is called **Felty syndrome.** Felty syndrome is most common with severe nodule-forming RA.

At this stage in the disease process, our patient is presenting with joint complaints, fatigue, and malaise. No other extraarticular manifestations have developed yet. At the very onset of RA, the characteristic symmetric inflammation of the joints and the typical serologic findings may not be evident. Therefore, initially distinguishing RA from other conditions, such as lupus, may be difficult. Usually, the development of extraarticular phenomenon allows the physician to make a more specific diagnosis.

Treatment

Several drugs currently are used for treatment of RA. **Nonsteroidal antiinflammatory drugs** (NSAIDs) or cyclooxygenase-2 (COX-2) inhibitors such as celecoxib may control local inflammatory symptoms. **Corticosteroids** have an immediate and dramatic effect on joint symptoms, but were historically thought not alter the natural progression of the disease. Recent evidence suggests that low-dose corticosteroids may retard the progression of bone erosions.

Disease-modifying antirheumatic drugs (DMARDs) may have a favorable impact on the natural course of the disease, reducing joint inflammation and disease activity, and improving functional status in patients with RA. The DMARDs include methotrexate, hydroxychloroquine, sulfasalazine, oral and parenteral gold, and penicillamine. There is controversy regarding which DMARD is the most effective, but **methotrexate** is often used as the first drug of choice because of its rapid onset of action and higher tolerability and patient compliance. Toxicity of the various DMARDs is often the most important determinant of which drug is used, and if the patient fails to respond or develops unacceptable side effects, they may be tried on a different agent.

More recently, the biologic agents **tumor necrosis factor (TNF) antagonists** (etanercept, infliximab, and adalimumab) have been found to reduce disease activity within weeks, unlike other DMARDs, which may take several months to act, and may also control signs and symptoms in patients who have failed DMARD therapy. Side effects of TNF blockers may include increased risk of infection, such as reactivation tuberculosis.

Immunosuppressive agents such as azathioprine, leflunomide, cyclosporine, and cyclophosphamide are as effective as DMARDs in controlling symptoms, but are considerably more toxic, so are generally reserved for patients who have failed DMARDs and biologics.

Comprehension Questions

22.1   A 72-year-old man develops severe pain and swelling in both knees, shortly after undergoing an abdominal hernia repair surgery. Physical examination shows warmth and swelling of both knees with large effusions. Arthrocentesis of the right knee reveals the presence of intracellular and extracellular *weakly positive birefringent crystals* in the synovial fluid. Gram stain is negative. Which of the following is the most likely diagnosis?
   A. Gout
   B. Septic arthritis
   C. Calcium oxalate deposition disease
   D. Reactive arthritis
   E. Pseudogout

22.2   A 65-year-old man with a history of chronic hypertension, diabetes mellitus, and degenerative joint disease presents with acute onset of severe pain of the metatarsophalangeal (MTP) joint and swelling of the left first toe. Physical examination shows exquisite tenderness of the joint, with swelling, warmth, and erythema. The patient has no history of trauma or other significant medical problems. Synovial fluid analysis and aspiration is most likely to show which of the following?
   A. Hemorrhagic fluid
   B. Needle-shaped, negatively birefringent crystals
   C. Gram-negative organisms
   D. Noninflammatory fluid
   E. Rhomboidal, positively birefringent crystals

22.3   A 17-year-old sexually active adolescent male presents with a 5-day history of fever, chills, and persistent left ankle pain and swelling. On physical examination, maculopapular and pustular skin lesions are noted on the trunk and extremities. He denies any symptoms of genitourinary tract infection. Synovial fluid analysis is most likely to show which of the following?
   A. WBCs 75,000/mm^3 with 95% polymorphonuclear leukocytes
   B. RBCs 100,000/mm^3, WBCs 1000/mm^3
   C. WBCs 48,000/mm^3 with 80% lymphocytes
   D. WBCs 500/mm^3 with 25% polymorphonuclear leukocytes

22.4 A 22-year-old man presents with complaints of low back pain for 3 to 4 months and stiffness of the lumbar area, which worsen with inactivity. He reports difficulty in getting out of bed in the morning and may have to roll out sideways, trying not to flex or rotate the spine to minimize pain. A lumbosacral (LS) spine X-ray film would most likely show which of the following?

A. Degenerative joint disease with spur formation
B. Sacroiliitis with increased sclerosis around the sacroiliac joints
C. Vertebral body destruction with wedge fractures
D. Osteoporosis with compression fractures of L3-L5
E. Diffuse osteonecrosis of the LS spine

22.5 A 36-year-old woman was seen by her physician due to pain in her hands, wrists, and knees. She is diagnosed with rheumatoid arthritis. Which of the following treatments will reduce joint inflammation and slow progression of the disease?

A. NSAIDs
B. Joint aspiration
C. Methotrexate
D. Systemic corticosteroids

ANSWERS

22.1 **E.** Pseudogout is diagnosed by positive birefringent crystals.

22.2 **B.** The involvement of the great toe is most likely gout, and the synovial fluid is likely to show **needle-shaped, negatively birefringent crystals**.

22.3 **A.** This history is suggestive of gonococcal arthritis, and the rash is suggestive of disseminated gonococcal disease. The synovial fluid would most likely show an acute inflammatory exudate, WBCs 72,000/mm^3 with 75% polymorphonuclear cells.

22.4 **B.** A young man is not likely to have osteoporosis, osteoarthritis, or compression fractures. His morning stiffness, which worsens with rest, suggests an inflammatory arthritis, such as ankylosing spondylitis, which would include sacroiliitis with increased sclerosis around the sacroiliac joints.

22.5 **C.** Although NSAIDs and corticosteroids may help to relieve symptoms, they typically do not alter the disease course significantly. Disease-modifying mediations include methotrexate, hydroxychloroquine, sulfasalazine, oral and parenteral gold, and penicillamine. Of these agents, methotrexate is thought to be the first line.

Clinical Pearls

> ➤ Rheumatoid arthritis is a chronic systemic inflammatory disorder characterized by the insidious onset of symmetric polyarthritis and extraarticular symptoms.
> ➤ Rheumatoid factor is found in the serum of 85% of patients with rheumatoid arthritis.
> ➤ In nearly all patients with rheumatoid arthritis, the wrist, metacarpophalangeal joints, and proximal interphalangeal joints are affected, whereas the distal interphalangeal joints are spared.
> ➤ Distal interphalangeal joints and large weight–bearing joints are most commonly involved in osteoarthritis.
> ➤ The typical X-ray finding in rheumatoid arthritis—periarticular bone erosion (loss of joint space)—may not develop until later in the disease process, when the diagnosis has already been made based on clinical findings.

REFERENCES

American College of Rheumatology Subcommittee on Rheumatoid Arthritis Guidelines. Guidelines for management of rheumatoid arthritis: 2002 update. *Arthritis Rheum*. 2002;46:328-346.

Lee DM, Weinblatt ME. Rheumatoid arthritis. *Lancet*. 2001;358:903-911.

Lipski PE. Rheumatoid arthritis. In: Kasper DL, Braunwald E, Fauci AS, et al., eds. *Harrison's Principles of Internal Medicine*. 17th ed. New York, NY: McGraw-Hill; 2008:2083-2092.

Case 23

A 36-year-old man comes to the office complaining of 7 to 10 days of low-grade fevers with fatigue, myalgias, and headaches, which he attributes to the "flu." When he awoke this morning, he noticed that he had weakness of the right side of his face. He denies cough, congestion, sore throat, abdominal pain, diarrhea, or any urinary symptoms. He has had a mildly pruritic rash near his waist for the last several days, which he thought was "jock itch." He works as a Wall Street commodities broker, is married, and is monogamous. He recently accompanied his son on a weekend Boy Scout camping trip in New Jersey, but he does not recall any bites or injury.

On physical examination, his temperature is 100.8°F, heart rate 94 bpm, and blood pressure 128/79 mm Hg. He is alert and talkative, and he appears comfortable. He has drooping of the right corner of his mouth and inability to elevate his eyebrow on the right. His conjunctivae are clear, and he has no oral lesions. His neck is somewhat stiff when passively flexed. His chest is clear, and his heart rhythm is regular without murmurs. His abdominal examination is benign, without liver or splenic enlargement. He has a 10 × 6-cm raised erythematous annular plaque with partial central clearing at his waistline (Figure 23–1). He has no joint swelling or erythema, and except for the facial weakness, he has no focal neurologic deficits.

➤ What is the most likely diagnosis?

➤ What is the most appropriate next step?

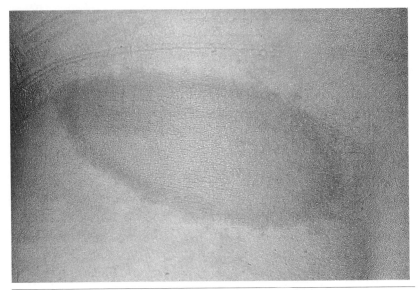

Figure 23-1. Skin rash. *Reproduced, with permission, from Fitzpatrick TB, Johnson RA, Wolff K, et al.* Color Atlas and Synopsis of Clinical Dermatology. *3rd ed. New York, NY: McGraw-Hill; 1997:679.*

ANSWERS TO CASE 23:

Lyme Disease

Summary: A 36-year-old man presents with a peripheral facial nerve palsy occurring in the setting of a febrile illness associated with arthralgias, myalgias, neck stiffness, and an erythematous annular plaque at his waistline. He recently went on a camping trip, but he shows no specific tick or other arthropod exposure. The rash is consistent with erythema migrans, the distinctive lesion of early Lyme disease, and all of the clinical features are consistent with that disease.

➤ **Most likely diagnosis:** Lyme disease, probably early disseminated stage.

➤ **Most appropriate next step:** Lumbar puncture to evaluate for meningitis and look for antibody production against *Borrelia burgdorferi*.

ANALYSIS

Objectives

1. Understand the distinctive features of common diseases that present with fever and a rash.
2. Know the clinical features and phases of Lyme disease.
3. Learn the appropriate treatment for Lyme disease based on the stage of disease.

Considerations

This patient has fever, headache, stiff neck, and an acute neurologic deficit. It is essential to exclude serious central nervous system (CNS) pathology, such as meningitis or Guillain-Barré syndrome, which necessitates a lumbar puncture. The **diagnosis of Lyme disease is made on clinical grounds**, and serologic testing is performed for confirmation. Treatment is primarily undertaken to prevent late chronic cardiac and neurologic sequelae.

APPROACH TO
Suspected Lyme Disease

DEFINITIONS

ERYTHEMA MIGRANS: An annular rash of usually 5-7 cm in diameter with a "bull's eye" appearance that often is seen with Lyme disease.
BORRELIA BURGDOFERI: A spirochete of the genus Borrelia that is the agent of Lyme disease, transmitted by the tick bite.

CLINICAL APPROACH

The evaluation of the patient who presents with fever and a rash is a very common problem that often frustrates and confuses beginning clinicians, partly because of their unfamiliarity with many typical rash patterns, and partly because the rash may be an incidental nonspecific finding (as in miliaria or heat rash), may be a sign of serious, even fatal illness (as in the purpuric rash of meningococcemia), or may be the pathognomonic finding that yields the diagnosis, as in the case of the **erythema migrans rash of Lyme disease.** Table 23–1 lists some important clinical features of systemic febrile syndromes associated with rash.

Lyme disease is diagnosed by the clinical presentation of the patient and can be verified by serologic tests at the earliest 6 weeks after the initial infection; thus, the patient's history is the key to the diagnosis. Lyme disease can present in three different stages; early localized (stage 1), early disseminated (stage 2), and late disease (stage 3). The **early localized stage** occurs **within the first month of the tick bite.** It presents with the **classic erythema migrans,** an expanding lesion that may or may not have a central clearing. It occurs most commonly around the belt line or the axilla because the ticks favor these areas. The erythema migrans is most often asymptomatic and therefore can be overlooked by the patient, although it sometimes is associated with burning, itching, or pain. In the first stage of the illness, the patient may complain of a viral-like syndrome with fatigue, headaches, myalgias, and

Table 23–1 DIFFERENTIAL DIAGNOSIS OF RASH AND FEVER

	LYME DISEASE	RHEUMATIC FEVER	ROCKY MOUNTAIN SPOTTED FEVER	TOXIC SHOCK SYNDROME	MEASLES
Organism	*Borrelia burgdorferi*	Group A *Streptococcus*	*Rickettsia rickettsii*	*Staphylococcus aureus*	Paramyxovirus
Characteristic rash	Erythema migrans: papule that expands to an *annular lesion with central clearing,* aka "bull's-eye" Usually occurs at the belt line or the axilla	Erythema marginatum: nonpruritic, erythematous papules occurring in polycyclic waves over the trunk, *sparing the face*	Rash begins on *wrists and ankles* and spreads centripetally Appears on palms and soles later	Diffuse *erythema involving the palms followed by desquamation after 7-10 d*	Discrete lesions that become confluent as the *rash proceeds from the hairline down, but spares the palms and the soles*
Clinical features	• Initially viral-like syndrome • Cardiac and neurologic manifestations if no initial treatment • Migratory oligoarticular (knee) or polyarticular arthritis weeks to months later	• Streptococcal pharyngitis • Migratory polyarthritis • Carditis: cardiac valvular and muscle damage • Rheumatic heart disease (10-20 y after original attack) Chorea: abrupt, purposeless nonrhythmic, involuntary movements Subcutaneous nodules	• Headache, myalgias, abdominal pain • 40% mortality if not treated	• Fever >102°F, hypotension, multiorgan dysfunction • Menstruating woman with tampon placed for a long period of time • Wound or skin infections	• Cough, conjunctivitis, coryza, severe prostration • Koplik spots: 1- to 2-mm bluish lesions with an erythematous halo on buccal mucosa pathognomonic for measles
Treatment	• Doxycycline (first line) • Amoxicillin	• Anti-inflammatory agents, usually aspirin • Corticosteroids if carditis present • Penicillin for pharyngitis	• Doxycycline (first line) • Tetracycline	• Penicillin or oxacillin plus clindamycin	• Supportive therapy • Antibiotics for otitis and pneumonia

arthralgias. Physical examination during this stage may or may not show the skin lesion, as well as generalized lymphadenopathy or organomegaly.

The **early disseminated (second stage)** disease occurs **days to months after the initial tick bite**, and there may be additional skin lesions similar to the primary skin lesion. There may be systemic symptoms of headache, mild neck stiffness, malaise, fatigue, fever, and chills. Commonly, there is also **migratory musculoskeletal pain without joint inflammation** that can last from hours to days and can affect one or two locations at a time. This stage may also include cardiac or neurologic manifestations. **Cardiac manifestations** of the disease may include conduction disturbances, myocarditis, or pericarditis. This problem usually resolves within weeks without any antibiotics; however, in some instances, it can progress to cardiomyopathy (this most often occurs in Europe) or permanent heart block. Neurologic manifestations can occur in 10% of untreated patients after several weeks to months. They can present as cranial nerve palsies, most commonly facial nerve palsy that may be bilateral. **Meningitis** with a lymphocytic pleocytosis and elevated protein level in the cerebrospinal fluid (CSF) or a mild encephalitis are possible. There may also be a sensory radiculoneuropathy. In Asia and Europe, the first characteristic neurologic sign is radicular pain, followed by the development of cerebrospinal fluid (CSF) pleocytosis, which is known as Bannwarth syndrome.

The third stage of the disease represents late or persistent infection. This occurs months to years after initial infection, usually when the initial presentation of the disease was not recognized or was not treated with medications. The common presentation is that of generalized musculoskeletal pain and a migratory polyarthritis that may mimic juvenile rheumatoid arthritis in 50% of the cases. There are also intermittent attacks of oligoarthritis most often involving the knees; the episodes can last from weeks to months within the involved joint. Aspiration of joint fluid shows white blood cells approximately $25,000/mm^3$ with a predominance of polymorphonuclear leukocytes. This may develop into a chronic inflammatory joint disease lasting 5 to 8 years, especially if no treatment is given. Late neurologic manifestations or tertiary borreliosis in the form of subtle encephalitis, neurocognitive dysfunction, or peripheral neuropathy occur in this stage.

Treatment of Lyme disease consists of antibiotics. It is important to recognize the illness in the early phase to prevent progression to the later and more chronic stages. Most patients with Lyme disease, including those with skin or joint manifestations, can be treated with oral antibiotics, preferably **doxycycline** 100 mg twice daily. Other choices include **amoxicillin** 500 mg three times daily, **cefuroxime** 500 mg twice daily, or **erythromycin** 250 mg four times daily. In more severe manifestations of the disease, such as **third-degree heart block or neurologic** manifestations, **intravenous** delivery of antibiotics is preferred, usually ceftriaxone 2 g daily, cefotaxime 2 g every 8 hours, or penicillin G 5 million units every 6 hours. The duration of therapy depends on the stage and severity of disease: 14 days for localized skin infection, 21 days for early disseminated infection, and 1 month for patients with arthritis, neurologic, or cardiac involvement.

Comprehension Questions

23.1   A 45-year-old woman complains of near syncope. Her heart rate is 50 bpm.
       On ECG, third-degree heart block is noted. She had been in good
       health, but she spent time camping in the woods of New Hampshire
       and had numerous tick bites 6 months previously. Which of the following
       is the best treatment for this condition?
       A. Oral doxycycline
       B. Intravenous lidocaine
       C. Oral amoxicillin
       D. Intravenous ceftriaxone

For the following questions (23.2 to 23.4), choose the Lyme disease stage
(A–D) that matches the clinical manifestations.
       A. First stage (localized infection)
       B. Second stage (disseminated infection)
       C. Third stage (persistent infection)
       D. Not consistent with Lyme disease

23.2   A 35-year-old woman with heart rate of 54 bpm, slightly irregular, with
       second-degree atrioventricular block on electrocardiogram (ECG)

23.3   A 22-year-old man who has facial weakness on the right, headache,
       and fever

23.4   A 28-year-old man who complains of 2 weeks of headache, fatigue,
       myalgias, and a rash along the belt line

ANSWERS

23.1   **D.** Intravenous antibiotics are indicated with severe disease such as
       neurologic or severe cardiac disease.

23.2   **B.** Heart block occurs in approximately 8% of patients in the second
       stage (early disseminated) of Lyme borreliosis.

23.3   **B.** Fluctuating symptoms of meningitis with facial nerve palsy are
       often seen in the early disseminated stage. Facial weakness and car-
       diac heart block both are within the second (early disseminated)
       stage of the disease.

23.4   **A.** The first stage of Lyme disease consists of the acute symptoms of
       headache, fatigue, low-grade fever, myalgias, and the typical erythema
       migrans rash along the axilla or belt line.

Clinical Pearls

➤ The diagnosis of Lyme disease is made on clinical grounds; serologic testing is only confirmatory, that is, a positive serologic test in an asymptomatic patient is not meaningful.

➤ Erythema migrans, particularly with the classic "bull's-eye" lesion, is the only pathognomonic feature of Lyme disease.

➤ The treatment of Lyme disease is oral doxycycline or amoxicillin for early localized disease.

➤ Intravenous cephalosporins are used to treat early disseminated or late disease.

REFERENCES

Kaye ET, Kaye KM. Fever and a rash. In: Kasper DL, Braunwald E, Fauci AS, et al. eds. *Harrison's Principles of Internal Medicine*. 17th ed. New York, NY: McGraw-Hill; 2008:121-130.

Steere AC. Lyme disease. *N Engl J Med*. 2001;345:115.

Steere AC. Lyme borreliosis. In: Fauci AS, Braunwald E, Kasper DL, eds. *Harrison's Principles of Internal Medicine*. 17th ed. New York, NY: McGraw-Hill; 2008:1055-1059.

Treatment of Lyme disease. *Med Letter Drugs Ther*. 2005;47:41-43.

Case 24

An obese 35-year-old housekeeper presents with low back pain and requests an X-ray. She has had this pain off and on for several years; however, for the past 2 days it is worse than it has ever been. It started after she vigorously vacuumed a rug, is primarily on the right lower side, radiates down her posterior right thigh to her knee, but is not associated with any numbness or tingling. It is relieved by laying flat on her back with her legs slightly elevated and lessened somewhat when she takes ibuprofen 400 mg. Except for moderate obesity and difficulty maneuvering onto the examination table because of pain, her examination is fairly normal. The only abnormalities you note are a positive straight leg raise test, with raising the right leg eliciting more pain than the left. Her strength, sensation, and deep tendon reflexes in all extremities are normal.

➤ What is your diagnosis?

➤ What is your next step?

ANSWERS TO CASE 24:

Low Back Pain

Summary: An obese 35-year-old woman with acute worsening of chronic low back pain complains of shooting pain down her right leg. Her physical examination is normal.

➤ **Most likely diagnosis:** Musculoskeletal low back pain, possible sciatica without neurologic deficits.

➤ **Next step:** Encourage continuation of usual activity, avoiding twisting motions or heavy lifting. Use nonsteroidal anti-inflammatory drugs (NSAIDs) on a scheduled basis; you can also recommend muscle relaxants, although these drugs may cause sleepiness. Massage might be helpful. Follow-up in 4 weeks. Long-term advice includes weight loss and back-strengthening exercises.

ANALYSIS

Objectives

1. Learn the history and physical examination findings that help to distinguish benign musculoskeletal low back pain from more serious causes of low back pain.
2. Understand the variety of treatment options and their effectiveness in low back pain.
3. Learn the judicious use of laboratory and imaging tests in evaluating low back pain.

Considerations

This young patient with chronic back pain has an acute exacerbation with pain radiating down her leg, which may indicate possible sciatic nerve compression. She has no other neurologic abnormalities, such as sensory deficits, motor weakness, or "red flag" symptoms of more serious etiologies of back pain, which if present would demand a more urgent evaluation. Thus, this individual has a good prognosis for recovery with conservative therapy, perhaps time being the most important factor. If she does not improve after 6 weeks, then imaging studies can be considered.

APPROACH TO
Low Back Pain

DEFINITIONS

CAUDA EQUINA SYNDROME: Lower back pain, saddle anesthesia, and bowel or bladder dysfunction with possible lower extremity weakness and loss of reflexes caused by compression of multiple sacral nerve roots. Cauda equine syndrome is a surgical emergency.

SCIATICA: Pain in the distribution of the lumbar or sacral nerve roots, with or without motor or sensory deficits.

SPONDYLOLISTHESIS: Anterior displacement of an upper vertebral body on the lower body, which can cause symptoms and signs of spinal stenosis. This condition can result from spondylolysis or from degenerative disk disease in the elderly.

SPONDYLOLYSIS: Defect in the pars interarticularis, either congenital or secondary to a stress fracture.

CLINICAL APPROACH

Low back pain is experienced by two-thirds of all adults at some point in their lives. Approximately 2% of adults miss work each year because of low back pain. This complaint is most common in adults in their working years, usually affecting patients between 30 and 60 years of age. Although it is common in workers required to perform lifting and twisting, it is also a common complaint in those who sit or stand for prolonged periods. Low back pain is a recurrent disease that tends to be mild in younger patients, often resolving by 2 weeks, but can be more severe and prolonged as the patient ages. It is one of the most common reasons for young adults to seek medical care, second only to upper respiratory infections, and millions of health-care dollars are expended on this problem each year. In evaluating patients with low back pain, the clinician needs to exclude potentially serious conditions, such as **malignancy, infection,** and dangerous neurologic processes, such as **spinal cord compression or cauda equina syndrome.** Individuals without these conditions are initially managed with conservative therapy. Nearly all patients recover spontaneously within 4 to 6 weeks; only 3% to 5% remain disabled for more than 3 months. If patients do not improve within 4 weeks with conservative management, they should undergo further evaluation to rule out systemic or rheumatic disease and to clarify the anatomic cause, especially patients with localized pain, nocturnal pain, or sciatica.

Table 24–1 ETIOLOGIES OF LOW BACK PAIN	
CAUSES OF LOW BACK PAIN	INCIDENCE
Musculoskeletal low back or leg pain	97%
• Lumbar sprain or strain	70%
• Degenerative disk disease	10%
• Herniated disk	4%
• Spinal stenosis	3%
• Trauma	1%
• Congenital disease, eg, kyphoscoliosis	<1%
Referred or visceral pain	2%
• Pelvic disease	
• Renal disease	
• Aortic aneurysm	
• Gastrointestinal disease	
Nonmechanical low back pain	1%
• Neoplasia	
• Infection	
• Inflammatory arthritis	
• Paget disease	

Data from Deyo RA. Low back pain. N Engl J Med. 2001;344:365.

The potential causes of back pain are numerous (Table 24–1). Pain can emanate from the bones, ligaments, muscles, or nerves. Rarely, it can be a result of referred pain from a visceral organ or other structure. Back pain with **radiation down the back of the leg** suggests **sciatic nerve root compression**, generally caused by a herniated intervertebral disk at the **L4-L5** or **L5-S1** level. Patients typically report aching pain in the buttock and paresthesias radiating into the posterior thigh and calf or lateral foreleg. When pain radiates below the knee, it is more likely to indicate a true radiculopathy than radiation only to the posterior thigh. A history of persistent leg numbness or weakness further increases the likelihood of neurologic involvement.

Most cases are idiopathic, and this group, in general, is referred to as musculoskeletal low back pain. **Imaging studies and other diagnostic tests are generally not helpful in managing these cases.** Studies show that the history and physical examination can help separate the majority of patients with simple and self-limited musculoskeletal back pain from the minority with more serious underlying causes. Finding "red-flag" symptoms can help the physician use diagnostic tests in a more judicious manner (Table 24–2). **Malignancy** should be considered in patients with **systemic symptoms and who have pain at night or pain that is not relieved by lying** in a supine position. **Primary cancers** which commonly metastasize to the spine include **lung, breast, prostate,**

Table 24–2 "RED FLAG" SIGNS AND SYMPTOMS OF LOW BACK PAIN
New onset of pain in a patient older than 50 y or younger than 20 y
Fever
Unintentional weight loss
Severe nighttime pain or pain that is worse in the supine position
Bowel or bladder incontinence
History of cancer
Immunosuppression (chemotherapy or HIV)
Saddle anesthesia
Major motor weakness

lymphoma, and gastrointestinal (GI) tumors and melanoma. **Multiple myeloma** is a plasma cell neoplasm which can present with **bone pain, renal failure, and anemia.** When the patient has worrisome symptoms or signs, in most cases, the most effective initial evaluation is plain anteroposterior and lateral radiographs of the involved area of the spine, a sedimentation rate, and a complete blood count. More expensive tests, such as magnetic resonance imaging (MRI), should be reserved for those patients for whom surgery is being considered, because it is not required to make most diagnoses.

It is rare that the patient can recall a precipitating event. Patients often have a history of recurrent episodes of low back pain. Psychological causes have not been consistently related to low back pain; however, there does seem to be an association with job satisfaction. During the physical examination, palpable point tenderness over the spinous processes may indicate a destructive lesion of the spine itself; however, those with musculoskeletal back pain most often have tenderness in the muscular paraspinal area. Strength, sensation, and reflexes should be assessed, especially in those with complaints of radicular or radiating pain. **Straight leg raise testing,** in which the examiner holds the patient's ankle and passively elevates the patient's leg to 45°, is helpful if it elicits pain in the lower back. However, it is **not a very sensitive or specific test.** The Patrick maneuver, in which the patient externally rotates the hip, flexes the knee, and crosses the knee of the other leg with the ankle (like a number 4) while the examiner simultaneously presses down on the flexed knee and the opposite side of the pelvis, can help distinguish pain emanating from the sacroiliac joint.

In treating idiopathic low back pain, various modalities have been shown to be equally effective in the long run. Randomized, controlled trials have shown that encouraging the patient to continue his or her **usual activity is superior to recommendations for bedrest.** Patients without disability and without evidence of nerve root compression probably can maintain judicious activity rather than undergoing bedrest. Bedrest probably is appropriate only for individuals with severe pain or neurologic deficits. The patient should be instructed to position himself or herself so as to minimize pain; this usually consists of lying supine with the upper body slightly elevated and a pillow under the knees. Nonsteroidal anti-inflammatory medications (on a scheduled rather than on an as-needed basis), nonaspirin analgesics, and muscle relaxants may help in the acute phase. Because most cases of disk herniation with radiculopathy resolve spontaneously within 4 to 6 weeks without surgery, this is the initial regimen recommended for these patients as well. Narcotic analgesics are also an option in cases of severe pain; however, because idiopathic low back pain is often a chronic problem, their prolonged use beyond the initial phase is discouraged. Chiropractic, physical therapy, massage therapy, and acupuncture have been studied (in trials of varying quality), with results comparable to traditional approaches. **Referral** to a surgeon may be considered for those patients with radicular pain with or without neuropathy that **does not resolve with 4 to 6 weeks of conservative management.**

Comprehension Questions

24.1   A 35-year-old obese hotel housekeeper presents with 1 week of lower back pain. Her history and examination are without "red flag" symptoms and completely normal, except for her weight. Which of the following is the best next step?
   A. Regular doses of a nonnarcotic analgesic
   B. Six weeks of bedrest
   C. MRI of the lumbar spine
   D. Plain film X-ray of lumbosacral spine

24.2   A 32-year-old woman from Nigeria presents with a 12-week history of persistent lower lumbar back pain, associated with a low-grade fever and night sweats. She denies any extremity weakness or HIV (human immunodeficiency virus) risk factors. Her examination is normal except for point tenderness over the spinous processes of L4-5. Which of the following is the most likely diagnosis?
   A. *Staphylococcus aureus* osteomyelitis
   B. Tuberculous osteomyelitis
   C. Given her age, idiopathic low back pain
   D. Metastatic breast cancer
   E. Multiple myeloma

24.3 A 70-year-old woman presents with a 4-week history of low back pain, generalized weakness, and a 15-lb weight loss over the last 2 months. Her medical history is unremarkable, and her examination is normal except that she is generally weak. Initial laboratory tests reveal an elevated sedimentation rate, mild anemia, creatinine level 1.8 mg/dL, and calcium level 11.2 mg/dL. Which of the following is the most likely diagnosis?

    A. Osteoporosis with compression fractures
    B. Renal failure with osteodystrophy
    C. Multiple myeloma
    D. Lumbar strain
    E. Osteomyelitis

24.4 A 45-year-old man complains of decreased sensation in his buttocks and inability to achieve an erection. On examination he has decreased anal sphincter tone and decreased ankle reflexes bilaterally. Which of the following is the best next step in management?

    A. Bedrest and follow-up in 4 to 6 weeks
    B. Plain film X-ray of lumbosacral spine
    C. Sedimentation rate and complete blood count
    D. Immediate referral for surgical decompression

ANSWERS

24.1 **A.** Bedrest has not been shown to improve outcome in idiopathic low back pain compared to encouraging usual activities that do not exacerbate the pain. Imaging is not necessary with uncomplicated back pain.

24.2 **B.** The patient's country of origin, the chronic and slowly progressive nature of the pain in association with fever, and night sweats are highly suggestive of tuberculous osteomyelitis of the spine, or Pott disease. Bacterial osteomyelitis presents more acutely, often with high, spiking fevers. Metastatic breast cancer and multiple myeloma are extremely rare in this age group. The fevers, night sweats, and persistent and progressive nature of her back pain make a musculoskeletal cause unlikely.

24.3 **C.** This patient has many "red flag" symptoms in her presentation: her age, new onset pain, and history of weight loss. The elevated calcium level and mild renal failure are classic for multiple myeloma. Plain radiographs of the spine and, more likely, of the skull may illustrate the punched out lytic bone lesions often seen in this disease. Bence Jones proteins in the urine is also a finding in multiple myeloma.

24.4   **D.** This individual has cauda equine syndrome, and requires imme-
         diate surgical decompression to avoid long-term nerve denervation
         and incontinence/lower extremity weakness. The decreased anal
         sphincter tone and decreased ankle reflexes indicate a peripheral
         neuropathy. Bedrest with follow-up is indicated when no "red flag"
         symptoms and signs are present. The plain film X-ray is often normal
         in patients with cauda equine syndrome.

Clinical Pearls

➤ In 90% of patients, acute low back pain, even with sciatic nerve involvement, resolves within 4 to 6 weeks.

➤ Analgesics, such as nonsteroidal anti-inflammatory drugs or narcotics, muscle relaxants, and attempts at maintaining some level of activity are helpful in managing acute low back pain; bedrest does not help.

➤ Pain that interferes with sleep, significant unintentional weight loss, or fever suggests an infectious or neoplastic cause of back pain.

➤ Imaging studies, such as magnetic resonance imaging, are useful only if surgery is being considered (persistent pain and neurologic symptoms after 4 to 6 weeks of conservative care in patients with herniated disks) or if a neoplastic or inflammatory cause of back pain is being considered.

REFERENCES

Deyo RA, Weinstein JN. Low back pain. *N Engl J Med.* 2001;344:363-370.

Engstrom JW. Back and neck pain. In: Fauci AS, Braunwald E, Kasper DL, eds. *Harrison's Principles of Internal Medicine.* 17th ed. New York, NY: McGraw-Hill; 2008:107-117.

Jarvik JG, Deyo RA. Diagnostic evaluation of low back pain with emphasis on imaging. *Ann Intern Med.* 2002;137:586-597.

Staal JB, Hlobil H, Twisk, JW, et al. Graded activity for low back pain in occupational health care: a randomized, controlled trial. *Ann Intern Med.* 2004;140:77-84.

Case 25

A healthy 52-year-old man presents to the doctor's office complaining of increasing fatigue for the past 4 to 5 months. He exercises every day, but lately he has noticed becoming short of breath while jogging. He denies orthopnea, paroxysmal nocturnal dyspnea (PND), or swelling in his ankles. The patient reports occasional joint pain, for which he uses over-the-counter ibuprofen. He denies bowel changes, melena, or bright red blood per rectum, but he reports vague left-side abdominal pain for a few months off and on, not related to food intake. The patient denies fever, chills, nausea, or vomiting. He has lost a few pounds intentionally with diet and exercise.

On examination, he weighs 205 lb, and he is afebrile. There is slight pallor of the conjunctiva, skin, and palms. No lymphadenopathy is noted. Chest is clear to auscultation bilaterally. Examination of the cardiovascular system reveals a regular rate and rhythm, with no rub or gallop. There is a systolic ejection murmur. His abdomen is soft, nontender, and without hepatosplenomegaly. Bowel sounds are present. He has no extremity edema, cyanosis, or clubbing. His peripheral pulses are palpable and symmetric. Hemoglobin level is 8.2 g/dL.

➤ What is the most likely diagnosis?

➤ What is your next diagnostic step?

ANSWERS TO CASE 25:
Iron-Deficiency Anemia

Summary: A healthy 52-year-old man complains of a 4- to 5-month history of increasing exercise intolerance, but he denies orthopnea, PND, edema, or other signs of heart failure. The patient uses a nonsteroidal anti-inflammatory drug (NSAID) regularly. He has not had any overt gastrointestinal (GI) blood loss. On examination, he weighs 205 lb, and he has slight pallor of the conjunctiva, skin, and palms. He is anemic, with a hemoglobin level of 8.2 g/dL.

> ➤ **Most likely diagnosis:** Iron-deficiency anemia as a result of chronic blood loss.

> ➤ **Next diagnostic step:** Analyze the complete blood count (CBC), particularly the mean corpuscular volume (MCV), to determine if the anemia is microcytic, normocytic, or macrocytic; assess the leukocyte count and platelet count.

ANALYSIS

Objectives

1. Understand that iron-deficiency anemia is the most common cause of anemia.
2. Know the diagnostic approach to anemia.
3. Be familiar with the treatment of iron-deficiency anemia.

Considerations

This 52-year-old man presents to the doctor's office with complaints of fatigue and dyspnea on exertion for the few months prior to the office visit. His physical examination is significant only for pallor. The serum hemoglobin level confirms anemia. The next step would be to characterize the anemia as microcytic, which would be consistent with iron deficiency, and confirmed with further testing for total iron-binding capacity (TIBC) and ferritin. The most likely source of blood loss in male patients is the GI tract; therefore, finding iron-deficiency anemia should suggest the presence of a possible GI source of bleeding, with colon cancer the most serious possibility. This patient is using ibuprofen, which may predispose to erosive gastritis. Once iron-deficiency anemia is confirmed, a thorough evaluation of the GI tract, including upper and lower endoscopy, is needed.

APPROACH TO
Suspected Iron-Deficiency Anemia

DEFINITIONS

ANEMIA: Decreased red blood cell (RBC) mass, leading to less oxygen-carrying capacity. Hemoglobin levels less than 13 g/dL in men and less than 12 g/dL in women are generally used.

IRON STUDIES: Ferritin is a marker of iron stores, but it also is an acute-phase reactant, which is decreased in iron deficiency but increased with chronic disease. The TIBC is an indirect measure of transferrin saturation levels and is increased in iron deficiency.

MEAN CORPUSCULAR VOLUME (MCV): Average RBC volume. This offers a method of categorizing anemias as microcytic (MCV <80 fL), normocytic (MCV 80-100 fL), and macrocytic (MCV >100 fL).

RETICULOCYTE: New RBC that usually is 1 to 1.5 days old.

RETICULOCYTE COUNT: Fraction of RBCs consisting of reticulocytes that indirectly indicates the bone marrow activity of the erythrocyte line. It usually is expressed as a percentage and normally is 1%. Corrected reticulocyte count accounts for anemia.

CLINICAL APPROACH

Iron Deficiency

Although anemia may be caused by disorders of bone marrow production, red cell maturation, or increased destruction, iron deficiency is the most common cause of anemia in the United States, affecting all ages and both genders. Iron is essential to the synthesis of hemoglobin. The normal daily intake of elemental iron is approximately 15 mg, of which only 1 to 2 mg is absorbed. The daily iron losses are about the same, but menstruation adds approximately 30 mg of iron lost each month. The primary etiology for iron-deficiency anemia is blood loss (Table 25–1). **In men, the most frequent cause is chronic GI tract occult bleeding.** In women, menstrual loss may be the main mechanism, but other sites must be considered. Supplemental iron is needed during pregnancy because of iron transfer from the mother to the developing fetus. Iron deficiency may also be a result of increased iron requirements, diminished iron absorption, or both. Iron deficiency can develop during the first 2 years of life if dietary iron is inadequate for the demands of rapid growth. Adolescent girls may become iron deficient from inadequate diet plus the added loss from menstruation. The growth spurt in adolescent boys may also produce a significant increase in demand for iron. Other possible causes of anemia are decreased

Table 25–1 COMMON CAUSES OF IRON-DEFICIENCY ANEMIA

Blood loss

Gastrointestinal blood loss
- Esophageal varices
- Peptic ulcer disease
- Gastritis, eg, NSAID induced
- Small-bowel polyp or carcinoma
- Colonic angiodysplasia
- Colon cancer
- Inflammatory bowel disease, eg, ulcerative colitis
- Hookworm infestation

Uterine blood loss
- Menstruation/menorrhagia
- Uterine fibroids

Other blood loss
- Chronic hemodialysis
- Surgical blood loss
- Repeated blood donation or phlebotomy
- Paroxysmal nocturnal hemoglobinuria

Malabsorption

- Gastrectomy
- Celiac disease
- Inflammatory bowel disease, eg, Crohn disease

Inadequate dietary intake/increased physiologic demands

- Infancy/adolescence
- Pregnancy
- Vegetarian diet

iron absorption after gastrectomy and upper-bowel malabsorption syndrome, but such mechanisms are rare when compared to blood loss.

When iron loss exceeds intake, iron deposits are progressively depleted. Hemoglobin and serum iron levels may remain normal in the initial stages, but the **serum ferritin** level (iron stores) will start to fall. As serum iron levels fall, the percent of transferrin saturation falls and the **TIBC will increase**, leading to a progressive decrease in iron available for RBC formation. At this point, anemia will develop initially with normal-appearing RBCs. As the iron deficiency becomes more severe, microcytosis and hypochromia will develop. Later in the disease process, iron deficiency will affect other tissues, resulting in a variety of symptoms and signs.

Typical symptoms of anemia include fatigue, shortness of breath, dizziness, headache, palpitations, and impaired concentration. Additionally, patients with chronic severe iron deficiency may develop **cravings for dirt, paint (pica),** or ice (pagophagia). Glossitis, cheilosis, or koilonychia may develop and, in rare advanced cases, dysphagia, associated with a postcricoid esophageal web (Plummer-Vinson syndrome). When the anemia develops over a long period, the typical symptoms of fatigue and shortness of breath may not be evident. Many patients with iron-deficiency anemia may be asymptomatic. The lack of symptoms reflects the very slow development of iron deficiency and the ability of the body to adapt to lower iron reserves and anemia.

Evaluation of Anemia

Once anemia is discovered, a CBC with differential, platelets, and RBC indices are helpful in narrowing the differential diagnosis. The first step is to look at the MCV to classify the common causes of anemia (Table 25–2). Iron deficiency usually leads to a microcytic anemia. The red blood cell distribution width (RDW) is a calculated index that quantitates the variation in the size of RBCs. RDW is a quantitative measure of anisocytosis that helps to distinguish uncomplicated iron deficiencies from uncomplicated thalassemia. An increased RDW associated with microcytic anemia is suggestive of iron-deficiency anemia, because the bone marrow produces erythrocytes of various sizes. A normal RDW in the presence of microcytic anemia may be more suggestive of chronic disease, thalassemia, or even iron deficiency associated with anemia of a chronic disease. A detailed history, physical examination, and further laboratory data may be necessary to achieve a final diagnosis.

The reticulocyte count is another important parameter to help in the differential diagnosis of anemia. A new RBC remains a reticulocyte for 1 to 1.5 days, after which the RBC circulates for approximately 120 days. The blood normally

Table 25–2 CLASSIFICATION OF ANEMIA BY MCV

Microcytic (low MCV)
- Iron deficiency
- Thalassemia
- Sideroblastic anemia
- Lead poisoning

Normocytic (normal MCV)
- Acute blood loss
- Hemolysis
- Anemia of chronic disease
- Anemia of renal failure
- Myelodysplastic syndromes

Macrocytic anemia (high MCV)
- Folate deficiency
- Vitamin B_{12} deficiency
- Drug toxicity, eg, zidovudine
- Alcoholism/chronic liver disease

contains about 1 reticulocyte per 100 RBCs. The reticulocyte count, usually reported as a percentage of reticulocytes per 100 RBCs, may be falsely elevated in the presence of anemia. Therefore, a corrected reticulocyte percentage is calculated by multiplying the reported reticulocyte count by the patient's hematocrit divided by 45 (normal hematocrit). The reticulocyte may also be converted to an absolute number by multiplying the reported reticulocyte count by the RBC count and dividing by 100. The absolute reticulocyte count is normally 50,000 to 70,000 reticulocytes/mm^3. If the **reticulocyte count is low,** causes of **hypoproliferative bone marrow** disorders should be suspected. A **high reticulocyte count** may reflect **acute blood losses, hemolysis,** or a response to therapy for anemia.

Iron studies are very helpful to confirm a diagnosis of iron deficiency anemia and to help in the differential diagnosis with other types of anemia, such as anemia of chronic disease and sideroblastic anemia (Table 25–3). **Serum ferritin concentration is a reliable indication of iron deficiency.** Serum **ferritin values are increased with chronic inflammatory disease,** malignancy, or liver injury; therefore, serum ferritin concentration may be above normal when iron deficiency exists with chronic diseases, such as rheumatoid arthritis, Hodgkin disease, or hepatitis, among many other disorders. Measurement of serum iron

Table 25–3 DIFFERENT ANEMIAS WITH CHARACTERISTICS AND LABORATORY STUDIES

TESTS	IRON DEFICIENCY	INFLAMMATION	THALASSEMIA	SIDEROBLASTIC ANEMIA
Smear	Microcytic/ hypochromic	Normal microcytic/ hypochromic	Microcytic/ hypochromic with targeting	Variable
Serum iron (μg/dL)	<30	<50	Normal to high	Normal to high
TIBC (μg/dL)	>360	<300	Normal	Normal
Percent saturation	<10	10-20	30-80	30-80
Ferritin (μg/L)	<15	30-200	50-300	50-300
Hemoglobin electrophoresis	Normal	Normal	Abnormal	Normal

Abbreviations: SI, serum iron; TIBC, total iron-binding capacity.
Reproduced, with permission, from Adamson JW. Iron deficiency and other hypoproliferative anemias. In: Braunwald E., Fauci AS, Kasper KL, et al., eds. Harrison's Principles of Internal Medicine. 17th ed. New York, NY: McGraw-Hill; 2008:632.

concentration, serum TIBC, and calculation of percent saturation of transferrin has been widely used for diagnosis of iron deficiency. **True iron deficiency** is strongly suspected on the basis of **low serum iron level** and **normal or high binding capacity,** which will result in a low calculated saturation. In anemia of **chronic disease, serum iron concentration is low, but usually the TIBC is also reduced;** therefore, percent transferrin saturation typically is normal in anemia of chronic disease. **Chronic disease typically causes elevation in serum ferritin concentration.** When chronic disease and iron-deficiency anemia coexist, serum ferritin concentration may be normal. Sideroblastic anemia is commonly microcytic and hypochromic. The iron studies in **sideroblastic anemia** include **increases in serum iron and serum ferritin concentration and saturation of transferrin.** An important clue to the presence of sideroblastic anemia is the presence of **stippled RBCs** in the peripheral blood smear. Iron stain in the bone marrow reveals pathognomonic feature of engorged mitochondria in the developing RBCs called **ringed sideroblasts.**

Evaluating the peripheral blood smear for specific abnormalities in RBC morphology may be very useful for determining the etiology of anemia. In iron-deficiency anemia, the peripheral blood smear shows RBCs smaller than normal (microcytes) and hypochromia.

Although the treatment of iron deficiency is straightforward, finding the underlying etiology is paramount. Treatment of iron-deficiency anemia consists of iron replacement therapy, typically with **oral ferrous sulfate 325 mg two or three times daily.** Correction of anemia usually occurs **within 6 weeks,** but therapy should continue for at least 6 months to replenish the iron stores. A number of patients may develop GI side effects, such as constipation, nausea, and abdominal cramping. Taking the iron with meals may help with tolerance but can reduce absorption. Parenteral iron therapy is indicated in rare instances, such as in patients with a poor absorption state or with excessive intolerance to oral therapy. Caution must be taken with parenteral iron because **anaphylaxis** may occur.

Comprehension Questions

25.1   A 25-year-old man with a history of a duodenal ulcer is noted to have a hemoglobin level of 10 g/dL. Which of the following most likely will be seen on laboratory investigation?
   A. Reticulocyte count of 4%
   B. Elevated total iron-binding capacity
   C. Normal serum ferritin
   D. Mean corpuscular volume of 105 fL

25.2   A 22-year-old woman is pregnant and at 14-week gestation. Her hemo-
        globin level is 9 g/dL. She asks why she could have iron deficiency
        when she is no longer menstruating. Which of the following is the best
        explanation?
        A. Occult gastrointestinal blood loss
        B. Expanded blood volume and transport to the fetus
        C. Hemolysis
        D. Iron losses as a result of relative alkalosis of pregnancy

25.3   A 35-year-old man has undertaken a self-imposed diet for 3 months.
        He previously had been healthy but now complains of fatigue. His
        hemoglobin level is 10 g/dL, and his MCV is 105 fL. Which of the fol-
        lowing is the most likely etiology of his anemia?
        A. Iron deficiency
        B. Folate deficiency
        C. Vitamin B$_{12}$ deficiency
        D. Thalassemia
        E. Sideroblastic anemia

For the following questions (25.4 to 25.6) choose the laboratory parameter
(A-E) that matches the clinical picture.

	MCV	Ferritin	TIBC	RDW
A.	Elevated	Decreased	Elevated	Decreased
B.	Decreased	Decreased	Elevated	Increased
C.	Normal	Elevated	Normal	Normal
D.	Decreased	Increased	Normal	Normal
E.	Elevated	Increased	Decreased	Increased

25.4   A 20-year-old woman with heavy menses

25.5   A 34-year-old man of Mediterranean descent with a family history of
        anemia

25.6   A 50-year-old man with severe rheumatoid arthritis

ANSWERS

25.1   **B.** Chronic gastrointestinal blood loss leads to low ferritin levels
        reflecting diminished iron stores, elevated TIBC, and low iron satu-
        ration. There is a microcytic anemia (low MCV) with a low reticu-
        locyte count.

25.2   **B.** Iron deficiency occurs in pregnancy as a result of the expanded
        blood volume and active transport of iron to the fetus.

25.3   **B.** Macrocytic anemia is usually a result of folate or vitamin B$_{12}$ defi-
        ciency. Because vitamin B$_{12}$ stores last for nearly 10 years, a diet of
        several months would more likely cause folate deficiency. Folate is
        found in green leafy vegetables.

25.4   **B.** This laboratory finding is diagnostic of iron-deficiency anemia (microcytic, low ferritin, high TIBC, high RDW).

25.5   **D.** Thalassemia usually leads to a microcytic anemia with uniform red cell size (normal RDW) and excess iron stores.

25.6   **C.** Chronic disease generally leads to a normocytic anemia with elevated ferritin level (acute-phase reactant).

Clinical Pearls

➤ Anemia is a clinical finding, not a diagnosis, and requires some investigation to determine the underlying etiology.

➤ Iron-deficiency anemia in men or postmenopausal women is primarily a result of gastrointestinal blood losses; therefore, finding iron-deficiency anemia in this patient population warrants a thorough gastrointestinal workup.

➤ Iron-deficiency anemia in women of reproductive age is most often caused by menstrual blood loss.

➤ Fecal occult blood testing is negative in approximately 50% of patients with gastrointestinal cancer. Therefore, a negative fecal occult blood test in the presence of iron-deficiency anemia should not discourage you from pursuing a thorough gastrointestinal workup.

➤ The mean corpuscular volume, red blood cell distribution width, and reticulocyte index are important parameters in the evaluation of anemia.

REFERENCES

Adamson JW. Iron deficiency and other hypoproliferative anemias. In: Kasper DL, Braunwald E, Fauci AS, et al., eds. *Harrison's Principles of Internal Medicine*. 17th ed. New York, NY: McGraw-Hill; 2008:628-634.

Cook JD, Skikne BS. Iron deficiency: definition and diagnosis. *J Intern Med*. 1989; 226:349-355.

Weiss G, Goodnough LT. Anemia of chronic disease. *N Engl J Med*. 2005;352:1011-1023.

Case 26

A 61-year-old man comes to the emergency room complaining of 3 days of worsening abdominal pain. The pain is localized to the left lower quadrant of his abdomen. It began as an intermittent crampy pain and now has become steady and moderately severe. He feels nauseated, but he has not vomited. He had a small loose stool at the beginning of this illness, but he has not had any bowel movements since. He has never had symptoms like this before, nor any gastrointestinal (GI) illnesses.

On examination, his temperature is 100.2°F, heart rate 98 bpm, and blood pressure 110/72 mm Hg. He has no pallor or jaundice. His chest is clear, and his heart rhythm is regular without murmurs. His abdomen is mildly distended with hypoactive bowel sounds and marked left lower quadrant tenderness with voluntary guarding. Rectal examination reveals tenderness, and his stool is negative for occult blood.

Laboratory studies are significant for a white blood cell (WBC) count of 11,800/mm^3 with 74% polymorphonuclear leukocytes, 22% lymphocytes, and a normal hemoglobin and hematocrit. A plain film of the abdomen shows no pneumoperitoneum and a nonspecific bowel gas pattern.

➤ What is the most likely diagnosis?

➤ What is the most appropriate next step?

ANSWERS TO CASE 26:
Acute Sigmoid Diverticulitis

Summary: A 61-year-old man has 3 days of new-onset, worsening, left lower quadrant abdominal pain. He feels nauseated, and he has not had any bowel movements since the illness began. His temperature is 100.2°F and he has no pallor or jaundice. His abdomen is mildly distended with hypoactive bowel sounds and marked left lower quadrant tenderness with voluntary guarding. Rectal examination reveals tenderness, and his stool is negative for occult blood. The WBC count is 11,800/mm^3 with 74% polymorphonuclear cells, 22% lymphocytes, and a normal hemoglobin and hematocrit. A plain film of the abdomen shows no acute changes.

➤ **Most likely diagnosis:** Acute sigmoid diverticulitis.

➤ **Most appropriate next step:** Admit to the hospital for intravenous antibiotics and monitoring. Computed tomographic (CT) scan of the abdomen will be very useful to confirm the diagnosis and to exclude pericolic abscess or other complications, such as fistula formation.

ANALYSIS

Objectives

1. Understand the complications of diverticular disease.
2. Understand the appropriate therapy of acute diverticulitis, which is dependent on the age of the patient and the severity of the disease presentation.
3. Learn the complications of diverticulitis and the indications for surgical intervention.

Considerations

This is an older patient with new-onset, progressively severe, lower abdominal pain. It is on the left side, suggesting diverticulitis as a diagnosis. The pattern of the pain suggests a bowel process because he has had nausea, no bowel movement, and pain that initially was crampy and intermittent but now is steady. The low-grade temperature is consistent with acute sigmoid diverticulitis, which is likely to improve with antibiotic therapy. Because the clinical presentation is similar, it is important to evaluate the patient for colon cancer with perforation, once all signs of inflammation have subsided. The abdominal film reveals no free air under the diaphragm. Ischemic colitis is another diagnostic consideration in an older patient, but it usually is associated with signs of bleeding, whereas diverticulitis is not.

APPROACH TO
Suspected Diverticulitis

DEFINITIONS

COLONIC DIVERTICULUM: Herniation of the mucosa and submucosa through a weakness of the muscle lining of the colon.

DIVERTICULITIS: Inflammation of the colonic diverticulum, typically on the left colon, such as the sigmoid.

DIVERTICULOSIS: Presence of diverticular disease in the colon with uninflamed diverticula.

CLINICAL APPROACH

Diverticulosis is extremely common, affecting 50% to 80% of people older than 80 years. Diverticula are, in fact, *pseudodiverticula* through a weakness in the muscle lining, typically at areas of vascular penetration to the smooth muscle. Therefore, their walls do not contain the muscle layers surrounding the colon. They are typically 5 to 10 mm in diameter and occur mainly in the distal colon in Western societies. The development of diverticula has been linked to insufficient dietary fiber leading to alteration in colonic transit time and increased resting colonic intraluminal pressure. The majority of patients will remain asymptomatic. However, some patients will have chronic symptoms resembling those of irritable bowel syndrome (nonspecific lower abdominal pain aggravated by eating with relief upon defecation, bloating, and constipation or diarrhea). They may even present with acute symptoms that could be confused with acute diverticulitis, but without evidence of inflammation upon further workup. This entity has been named "painful diverticular disease without diverticulitis." **Complications of diverticulosis** include **acute diverticulitis, hemorrhage, and obstruction.**

Diverticular hemorrhage, one of the most common causes of lower GI bleeding in patients older than 40 years, typically presents as **painless passage of bright red blood.** Generally, the hemorrhage is **abrupt in onset and abrupt in resolution.** The diagnosis may be established by finding diverticula on endoscopy without other pathology. Most diverticular hemorrhages are self-limited, and treatment is supportive, with intravenous fluid or blood replacement as needed. Treatment of diverticulosis consists of dietary measures with increased fiber. Avoidance of foods with small seeds (eg, strawberries) is traditionally advised, although data supporting this recommendation are scant. For patients with recurrent or chronic bleeding, resection of the affected colonic segment may be indicated.

Table 26–1 STAGES OF DIVERTICULITIS	
Stage I	Small, confined pericolic abscess
Stage II	Distant abscess (retroperitoneal or pelvic)
Stage III	Generalized suppurative peritonitis from rupture of abscess (noncommunicating with bowel lumen)
Stage IV	Fecal peritonitis caused by a free communicating perforation

Acute diverticulitis is the **most common complication of diverticulosis**, developing in approximately 20% of all patients with diverticula. Patients often present with acute abdominal pain and signs of peritoneal irritation localizing to the left lower quadrant and often throught of presenting like "left-sided appendicitis." Inspissated stool particles (fecaliths) appear to obstruct the diverticular neck, setting up for more inflammation and diminished venous outflow, as well as bacterial overgrowth, which ultimately leads to abrasion and perforation of the thin diverticular wall. It is classified into four stages according to the extent of the inflammation and perforation (Table 26–1).

Diagnosis

Patients usually present with visceral pain that localizes later to the **left lower quadrant** and is associated with fever, nausea, vomiting, or constipation. A right lower quadrant presentation would not exclude this diagnosis because ascending colon or cecal diverticulitis can occur. If a **colovesical fistula** is present, the patient may present with **pneumaturia** or **fecaluria** (a virtually pathognomic finding). On examination, the patient may have localized left lower quadrant tenderness or more diffuse abdominal tenderness with peritoneal irritation signs, such as guarding or rebound tenderness. The differential diagnosis includes painful diverticular disease without diverticulitis, acute appendicitis, Crohn disease, colon carcinoma, ischemic colitis, irritable bowel syndrome, and gynecologic disorders such as ruptured ovarian cyst, endometriosis, ectopic pregnancy, and pelvic inflammatory disease.

Plain film radiographs, including abdominal erect and supine films with a chest X-ray, are routinely performed but usually are not diagnostic. They help in identifying patients with pneumoperitoneum and assessing their cardiopulmonary status, especially in patients with other comorbid conditions. Contrast enemas are contraindicated for fear of perforation and spillage of contrast into the abdominal cavity, a catastrophic complication. Endoscopy is also relatively contraindicated in the acute phase and usually is reserved for use at least 6 weeks after resolution of the attack and then is performed primarily to exclude colonic neoplasia, which may have a similar findings on imagines studies, such as luminal narrowing or thickened colonic wall. **CT scan** typically is the **preferred modality of choice for diagnosing diverticulitis** if there is a high pretest probability from clinical suspicion. Findings consistent with diverticulitis include the presence of pericolic fat stranding, thickening of the bowel wall to more than 4 mm, or the finding of a peridiverticular abscess.

Therapy

Factors that advocate for **inpatient** therapy include the need for narcotics to control pain, presence of peritoneal signs, presence of comorbid illnesses, inability to tolerate oral liquids, or presence of any of the complications that may potentially require surgical intervention (abscess or peritonitis). Indications for **emergent surgical intervention** include **generalized peritonitis, uncontrolled sepsis, perforation, and clinical deterioration**. In the absence of acute complications, **elective resection** is undertaken later in cases of complications including fistula formation and when there are recurrent episodes of diverticulitis.

Individuals treated as outpatients should be placed on a broad-spectrum antibiotic regimen that covers abdominal gram-negative rods and anaerobes, such as trimethoprim/sulfamethoxazole, *or* ciprofloxacin with metronidazole *or* clindamycin with gentamicin. Patients should be placed on a clear liquid diet and undergo close follow-up.

The treatment priorities in hospitalized patients are intravenous hydration, correction of electrolyte imbalances, and bowel rest (nothing by mouth). Some recommended broad-spectrum intravenous antibiotic regimens include standard triple therapy (ampicillin, an aminoglycoside, and metronidazole) and beta-lactamase inhibitor combinations (ampicillin-sulbactam or ticarcillin-clavulanate), among others. More empiric agents, such as imipenem or meropenem, usually are reserved for more severe and complicated cases. Pain, fever, and leukocytosis are expected to diminish with appropriate management in the first few days of treatment, at which point the dietary intake can be advanced gradually. Further imaging may be indicated to identify complications (Table 26–2) such as abscess, stricture, or obstruction in the patient with persistent fever or pain.

Surgical management such as sigmoid resection may be indicated for patients who have suffered two or more documented episodes of diverticulitis requiring hospitalization. This is especially true for patients younger than 50 years of age, who may experience more aggressive disease.

Table 26-2 COMPLICATIONS OF DIVERTICULITIS

COMPLICATION	CHARACTERISTICS	TREATMENT
Abscess	Suspected in patients with a tender mass on examination, persistent fever and leukocytosis in spite of adequate therapy, or a suggestive finding on imaging studies.	Conservative management for small pericolic abscesses. A CT-guided percutaneous drainage or surgical drainage for other abscesses depending on the size, content, location, and peritoneal contamination.
Fistulas	Majority is colovesical with male predominance (because of bladder protection by the uterus in females). Others include colovaginal, coloenteric, colouterine, and coloureteral. Colocutaneous fistulas are extremely rare.	Single-stage surgery with fistula closure and primary anastomosis.
Obstruction	Either acutely or chronically. Ileus or pseudo-obstruction is more likely than complete mechanical obstruction. Small-bowel obstruction may occur if a small-bowel loop was incorporated in the inflamed mass.	Usually amenable to medical management. If not, prompt surgical intervention is required.
Strictures	Occur as a result of recurrent attacks of diverticulitis. Insidious-onset colonic obstruction is likely. Colonoscopy is important for an accurate diagnosis and to exclude a stenosing neoplasm as the cause of the stricture.	A trial of endoscopic therapy (bougienage, balloon, laser, electrocautery, or a blunt dilating endoscope) reasonably can be attempted. Surgery is indicated if neoplasm could not be excluded or if such trial has failed.

Comprehension Questions

26.1 A 48-year-old woman is admitted to the hospital with left lower quadrant abdominal pain, leukocytosis, and a CT showing sigmoid wall thickening consistent with diverticulitis. Her only significant medical history is a similar hospitalization with the same diagnosis less than a year previously. Which of the following is the most appropriate treatment?

A. Urgent surgical consultation for exploratory laparotomy and sigmoid resection.

B. Intravenous antibiotics with follow-up colonoscopy after hospital discharge, and surgical consultation for elective sigmoidectomy.

C. Intravenous antibiotics and barium enema to evaluate for possible colonic malignancy.

D. Intravenous antibiotics and recommendations for post discharge diet high in fiber with whole grains and nuts to minimize the risk of diverticular progression.

26.2 A 78-year-old is noted to have fever and chills, decreased mentation, tachycardia, and right lower quadrant abdominal tenderness and guarding. Which of the following is the most likely diagnosis?

A. Ruptured diverticulitis

B. Meningitis

C. Ruptured appendicitis

D. Ischemic bowel

E. Urosepsis

26.3 A 58-year-old man presents to the emergency room with a temperature of 102°F, abdominal pain localizing to the left lower quadrant, and mild rebound tenderness. Which of the following diagnostic tests is the best next step?

A. Barium enema

B. Lower endoscopy

C. CT imaging of the abdomen

D. Laparoscopic examination

ANSWERS

26.1 **B.** Patients with two or more episodes of diverticulitis should be considered for elective surgical management to try to prevent future complications such as fistulae, obstruction, or perforation. Colonoscopy is generally performed before surgical resection to exclude the possibility of malignancy, since the radiographic appearance of colonic wall inflammation and malignancy may be indistinguishable.

26.2   **C.** The most common cause of an acute abdomen at any age is appendicitis.

26.3   **C.** A CT imaging is the modality of choice in evaluating diverticulitis. Barium enema and endoscopy tend to increase intraluminal pressure and can worsen diverticulitis or lead to colonic rupture.

Clinical Pearls

➤ Acute diverticulitis usually presents with left lower quadrant pain, fever, leukocytosis, and constipation, and often with signs of peritoneal inflammation.

➤ A patient with mild diverticulitis can be treated as an outpatient with oral antibiotics; more severe cases require hospital admission for intravenous broad-spectrum antibiotics, bowel rest, and fluids.

➤ Diverticulitis can be complicated by perforation with peritonitis, pericolic abscess, fistula formation, often to the bladder, and strictures with colonic obstruction.

REFERENCES

Ferzoco LB, Raptopoulos V, Silen W. Acute diverticulitis. *N Engl J Med.* 1998; 338:1521-1526.

Gearhart SL. Diverticular disease and common anorectal disorders. In: Kasper DL, Braunwald E, Fauci AS, et al., eds. *Harrison's Principles of Internal Medicine.* 17th ed. New York, NY: McGraw-Hill; 2008:1903-1909.

Stollman N, Raskin J. Diverticular disease of the colon. *J Clin Gastroenterol.* 1999; 29:241-252.

Case 27

A 54-year-old man presents to the emergency room complaining of 24 hours of fevers with shaking chills. He is currently being treated for acute lymphoblastic leukemia (ALL). His most recent chemotherapy with hyperfractionated CVAD (cyclophosphamide, vincristine, doxorubicin, and dexamethasone) was 7 days ago. He denies any cough or dyspnea, headache, abdominal pain, or diarrhea. He has had no sick contacts or recent travel. On physical examination, he is febrile to 103°F, tachycardic with heart rate 122 bpm, blood pressure 118/65 mm Hg, and respiratory rate 22 breaths per minute. He is ill appearing; his skin is warm and moist but without any rashes. He has no oral lesions, his chest is clear to auscultation, his heart rhythm is tachycardic but regular with a soft systolic murmur at the left sternal border, and his abdominal examination is benign. The perirectal area is normal, digital rectal examination is deferred, but his stool is negative for occult blood. He has a tunneled vascular catheter at the right internal jugular vein with erythema overlying the subcutaneous tract, but no purulent discharge at the catheter exit site. Laboratory studies reveal a total white blood cell count of 1100 cells/mm^3, with a differential of 10% neutrophils, 16% band forms, 70% lymphocytes, and 4% monocytes (absolute neutrophil count 286). Chest radiograph and urinalysis are normal.

➤ What is the most likely diagnosis?

➤ What are your next therapeutic steps?

ANSWERS TO CASE 27:
Neutropenic Fever, Line Sepsis

Summary: A 54-year-old man with ALL is receiving immunosuppressive chemotherapy. He now presents with fever. He has no respiratory or abdominal symptoms, a clear chest X-ray, and an absolute neutrophil count of 286/mm³. He has redness and purulence along the tract of the vascular catheter.

➤ **Most likely diagnosis:** Neutropenic fever and infected vascular catheter.

➤ **Next therapeutic step:** After drawing blood cultures, the patient should undergo broad-spectrum intravenous antibiotic administration, including coverage for gram-positive organisms such as *Staphylococcus* spp. The vascular catheter should be removed, if possible.

ANALYSIS

Objectives

1. Be familiar with the possible sources of infection in a neutropenic patient.
2. Learn the management of a patient with neutropenic fever.
3. Be able to diagnose and treat a catheter-related infection.
4. Understand the techniques to prevent infection in immunosuppressed patients, including granulocyte colony-stimulating factor (G-CSF) and vaccination of household contacts.

Considerations

This patient is being treated for a hematologic malignancy with combination chemotherapy, which has a common side effect of leukopenia and, especially, neutropenia. Generally, the nadir of the white cell count occurs 7 to 14 days after the chemotherapy. This patient certainly has neutropenia, defined as an absolute neutrophil count less than 500 cells/mm³. Infection in this immunosuppressed condition is life-threatening, and immediate antibiotic coverage is paramount. Neutropenic patients are at risk for a variety of bacterial, fungal, or viral infections, but the most common sources of infection are gram-positive bacteria from the skin or oral cavity or gram-negative bacteria from the bowel. Infection of the indwelling catheter, as in this individual, is common. Rapid institution of empiric antibiotic therapy is critical while attempts to find a source of infection are in progress. Because the tract of the catheter is infected, the line usually must be removed.

APPROACH TO
Neutropenic Fever

DEFINITIONS

CVC: Central venous catheter.

FEVER: Single oral temperature measurement more than or equal to 101°F (38.3°C) or a temperature more than or equal to 100.4°F (38.0°C) for 1 hour or more.

MUCOSITIS: Breakdown of skin and mucosal barriers as a result of chemotherapy or radiation. Mucositis can result in bacteremia or fungemia.

NEUTROPENIA: Neutrophil count less than 500 cells/mm^3 or a count less than 1000 cells/mm^3 with a predicted decrease to less than 500 cells/mm^3.

CLINICAL APPROACH

Fever in a neutropenic patient with cancer should be considered a medical emergency. Approximately 5% to 10% of cancer patients will die of neutropenia-associated infection. Individuals with a hematologic malignancy (leukemias or lymphomas) are at even greater risk for sepsis as a result of lymphocyte or granulocyte dysfunction or because of abnormal immunoglobulin production. Chemotherapy often causes further bone marrow suppression and neutropenia. The incidence of an occult infection in a neutropenic patient increases with the **severity and duration of the neutropenia** (>7-10 days). Some neutropenic patients (eg, the elderly or those receiving corticosteroids) may not be able to mount a febrile response to infection; thus, **any neutropenic patient showing signs of clinical deterioration should be suspected of having sepsis.**

The typical signs and symptoms of infection noted in immunocompetent patients are the result of the host's inflammatory response and may be minimal or absent in neutropenic patients. Soft tissue infections may have diminished or absent induration, erythema, or purulence; pneumonia may not show a discernible infiltrate on a chest radiograph; meningitis may not reveal cerebrospinal fluid (CSF) pleocytosis; and urinary tract infection may be present without pyuria.

Empirical antibiotic therapy should be administered promptly to all neutropenic patients at the onset of fever. Historically, gram-negative bacilli, mainly enteric flora, were the most common pathogens in these patients. Because of their frequency and because of the high rate of mortality associated with gram-negative septicemia, empiric coverage for gram-negative bacteria, including *Pseudomonas aeruginosa*, is almost always indicated for neutropenic fever. Currently, as a consequence of frequent use of CVCs, gram-positive bacteria now account for 60% to 70% of microbiologically documented infections. Other clues that the infection is likely to be a gram-positive organism include the presence of obvious soft tissue infection, such as cellulitis or oral mucositis, which causes breaks in the mucosal barriers and allows oral flora to enter the bloodstream. If any of these factors are present, an appropriate agent, such as vancomycin, should be added to the regimen. If patients continue to be febrile despite antibacterial therapy, empiric antifungal therapy with either fluconazole or amphotericin B should be considered. Figure 27–1 shows a useful algorithm for patient management.

Central venous catheters are in widespread use and are a common site of infection in hospitalized patients and in those receiving outpatient infusion therapy. Infection may occur as a consequence of contamination by gram-positive skin flora or by hematogenous seeding, usually by enteric gram-negative organisms or *Candida* spp. Erythema, purulent drainage, and induration are evidence of infection. A variety of CVCs are frequently used, with different rates of infection.

The two main decisions impacting suspected catheter-related infection are (1) whether the catheter is really the source of infection and, if it is, (2) must the catheter be removed or can the infection be cleared with antibiotic therapy? **Most nontunneled or implanted catheters** should be **removed**. For the more

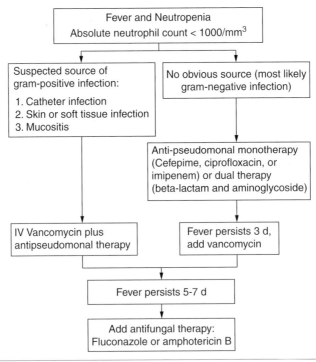

Figure 27–1. Algorithm of a suggested approach to neutropenic fever.

permanent catheters, the decision to remove the catheter depends on the patient's clinical state, identification of the organism, and the presence of complications such as endocarditis or septic venous thrombosis. Infected catheters may produce several manifestations, such as infections of the subcutaneous tunnel, infection at the exit site, or catheter-related bacteremia and sepsis. Generally, **erythema overlying the subcutaneous tract** of a tunneled catheter necessitates catheter removal. Leaving the catheter in place may result in severe cellulitis and soft tissue necrosis. If there is only erythema at the exit site, it may be possible to salvage the line using antibiotics, usually vancomycin through the CVC. Coagulase-negative staphylococci, such as *Staphylococcus epidermidis*, is the most common organism causing line infections.

In the absence of obvious tunnel or exit-site infection, authorities recommend obtaining two or more blood cultures to try to diagnose **catheter-related bacteremia**. Catheter-related infection is suspected when a patient has two or more positive blood cultures obtained from a peripheral vein, clinical manifestation of infection (eg, fever, chills, and/or hypotension), and no apparent source for bloodstream infection except for the catheter. In some institutions, quantitative blood cultures are obtained, that is, counting colony-forming units (CFUs), with the idea that heavier colony counts will be obtained from blood drawn through an infected catheter than from blood obtained from a peripheral vein. If the catheter is removed, the tip of the catheter may be cut off and rolled across a culture plate, again using a quantitative culture method.

Staphylococcus aureus and coagulase-negative *Staphylococcus* **are the most common causes of catheter-associated infections.** With coagulase-negative *Staphylococcus* bacteremia, response to **antibiotic therapy without catheter removal** is possible up to 80% of the time; that is, one may seek to "sterilize" the CVC if it is deemed necessary. However, this is usually not advisable in critically ill or hemodynamically unstable patients in whom immediate catheter removal and rapid administration of antibiotics are essential. Bacteremia as a consequence of *S aureus,* **gram-negative organisms, or fungemia caused by Candida spp respond poorly to antimicrobial therapy** alone, and **prompt removal of the catheter is recommended.**

Because of the serious complications associated with neutropenia, preventive measures are critical in cancer patients who are receiving chemotherapy. They should be **immunized against Pneumococcus and influenza,** but administration of live virus vaccines, such as measles-mumps-rubella or varicella-zoster, is contraindicated. **G-CSF,** which stimulates the bone marrow to produce neutrophils, is frequently used prophylactically in patients receiving chemotherapy to shorten the duration and depth of neutropenia, thereby reducing the risk of infection. It is sometimes used once a neutropenic patient develops a fever, but its use at that point is controversial. Prophylactic use of oral quinolones to prevent gram-negative infection or antifungal agents to prevent *Candida* infection may reduce certain types of infection but may select for resistant organisms and is not routinely used. In hospitalized patients with neutropenia, use of reverse isolation offers no benefit (the patient is most often infected with his or her own flora) and interferes with patient care.

Comprehension Questions

27.1   Which of the following infectious agents is the most likely etiology associated with an infected central venous catheter?
        A. *Staphylococcus aureus*
        B. *Pseudomonas aeruginosa*
        C. Coagulase-negative *Staphylococcus*
        D. *Klebsiella pneumoniae*
        E. *Candida albicans*

27.2   A 32-year-old man with acute myelogenous leukemia is undergoing chemotherapy. He was hospitalized 7 days ago for fever to 102°F with an absolute neutrophil count of 100 cells/mm^3, and he has been placed on intravenous imipenem and vancomycin. He continues to have fever to 103°F without an obvious source. Which of the following is the best next step?
        A. Lumbar puncture to assess cerebrospinal fluid.
        B. Continue present therapy.
        C. Stop all antibiotics because he likely has drug fever.
        D. Add an aminoglycoside antibiotic.
        E. Add an antifungal agent.

27.3   A 68-year-old woman is diagnosed with acute leukemia and is undergoing induction of chemotherapy. Last cycle, she developed neutropenia with an absolute neutrophil count of 350 cells/mm^3, which has now resolved. Which of the following is appropriate therapy?
        A. Immunization against varicella
        B. Immunization against mumps
        C. Use of recombinant erythropoietin before the next cycle of chemotherapy
        D. Use of G-CSF after the next cycle of chemotherapy

ANSWERS

27.1   **C.** Coagulase-negative staphylococci, such as *Staphylococcus epidermidis*, are the most common etiology of catheter-related infections.

27.2   **E.** Antifungal therapy should be added when the fever is persistent despite broad-spectrum antibacterial agents.

27.3   **D.** Granulocyte colony-stimulating factor given after chemotherapy can decrease the duration and severity of neutropenia and the subsequent risk of sepsis. Live vaccines, such as varicella and mumps, are contraindicated. Erythropoietin is not indicated because the patient is not anemic.

Clinical Pearls

➤ Fever in a neutropenic patient should be considered a medical emergency and is associated with a high mortality rate.

➤ The usual sources of bacterial infection in neutropenic patients are gram-positive skin or oral flora or gram-negative enteric flora, including *Pseudomonas*.

➤ Antifungal therapy should be started in neutropenic patients who have persistent fever despite broad-spectrum antibiotic therapy and who have no obvious source of infection.

➤ Vascular catheters with evidence of infection along a subcutaneous tract or purulent discharge at the exit site should be removed; replacement over a guidewire is insufficient.

➤ If a catheter is deemed necessary but it is infected with coagulase-negative staphylococci, antibiotic treatment may sterilize the catheter, allowing it to remain in place. For *Staphylococcus aureus,* gram-negative rods, or fungal catheter infections, the catheter usually requires removal.

REFERENCES

Finberg R. Infections in atients with cancer. In: Fauci AS, Braunwald E, Kasper DL, eds. *Harrison's Principles of Internal Medicine.* 17th ed. New York, NY: McGraw-Hill; 2008:533-541.

Hall K, et al. Diagnosis and management of long-term central venous catheter infections. *J Vasc Interv Radiol.* 2004;15:327.

Hughes WT, Armstrong D, Bodey GP, et al. Guidelines for the use of antimicrobial agents in neutropenia patients with cancer. *Clin Infect Dis.* 2002;34:730-751.

Pizzo PA. Fever in immunocompromised patients. *N Engl J Med.* 1999;341:893-900.

Case 28

A 25-year-old African American man is admitted to your service with the diagnosis of a sickle cell pain episode. He was admitted to the hospital six times last year with the same diagnosis, and he was last discharged 2 months ago. Again he presented to the emergency room complaining of abdominal and bilateral lower extremity pain, his usual sites of pain. When you examine him, you note he is febrile to 101°F, respiratory rate 25 breaths per minute, normal blood pressure, and slight tachycardia of 100 bpm. Lung examination reveals bronchial breath sounds and egophony in the right lung base. His oxygen saturation on 2 L/min nasal cannula is 92%. Besides the usual abdominal and leg pain, he is now complaining of chest pain, which is worse on inspiration. Although he is tender on palpation of his extremities, the remainder of his examination is normal. His laboratory examinations reveal elevated white blood cell and reticulocyte counts, and a hemoglobin and hematocrit that are slightly lower than baseline. Sickle and target cells are seen on the peripheral smear.

➤ What is the most likely diagnosis?

➤ What is your next step?

➤ What are the potential complications of this condition?

ANSWERS TO CASE 28:
Sickle Cell Crisis

Summary: A 25-year-old African American man with a history of numerous pain crises is admitted for abdominal and bilateral lower extremity pain. He is febrile to 101°F, respiratory rate 25 breaths per minute, and slight tachycardia of 100 bpm. Lung examination reveals bronchial breath sounds and egophony in the right lung base. His oxygen saturation on 2 L/min nasal cannula is 92%. He is now complaining of chest pain, which is worse on inspiration. He has a leukocytosis, an elevated reticulocyte count, and a hemoglobin and hematocrit that are slightly lower than baseline. Sickle and target cells are seen on the peripheral smear.

➤ **Most likely diagnosis:** Acute chest syndrome.

➤ **Next step:** Chest radiograph and empiric antibiotic therapy.

➤ **Potential complications:** Respiratory failure, possible death.

ANALYSIS

Objectives

1. Understand the pathophysiology of sickle cell anemia and acute painful episodes.
2. Learn the acute and chronic complications of sickle cell anemia.
3. Become familiar with treatment options available for the complications of sickle cell anemia.

APPROACH TO
Sickle Cell Anemia

DEFINITIONS

SICKLE CELL ANEMIA: A congenital defect in hemoglobin formation such that both genes code for hemoglobin S, leading to hemolysis and an abnormal shape of the red blood cell. Affected individuals have numerous complications including pain crises.

ACUTE CHEST SYNDROME: A condition found in individuals with sickle cell disease characterized by **fever, tachycardia, chest pain, leukocytosis, and pulmonary infiltrates.**

CLINICAL APPROACH

Pathophysiology

The molecular structure of a normal hemoglobin molecule consists of two alpha-globin chains and two beta-globin chains. Sickle cell anemia is an autosomal recessive disorder resulting from a substitution of valine for glutamine in the sixth amino acid position of the beta-globin chain. This substitution results in an alteration of the quaternary structure of the hemoglobin molecule. Individuals in whom only half of their beta chains are affected are heterozygous, a state referred to as *sickle cell trait*. When both beta chains are affected, the patient is homozygous and has sickle cell anemia. In patients with sickle cell disease, the altered quaternary structure of the hemoglobin molecule causes polymerization of the molecules under conditions of deoxygenation. These rigid polymers distort the red blood cell into a sickle shape, which is characteristic of the disease. **Sickling** is promoted by **hypoxia, acidosis, dehydration, or variations in body temperature.**

Epidemiology

Sickle cell anemia is the most common autosomal recessive disorder and the most common cause of hemolytic anemia in African Americans. Approximately 8% of African Americans carry the gene (ie, sickle cell trait), with one in 625 affected by the disease.

Complications of Sickle Cell Disease

Acute painful episodes, also known as *pain crisis*, are a consequence of microvascular occlusion of bones by sickled cells. The most common sites are the long bones of the arms, legs, vertebral column, and sternum. Acute painful episodes are precipitated by infection, cold exposure, dehydration, venous stasis, or acidosis. They usually last 2 to 7 days.

Infections are another complication. Patients with sickle cell disease are at greater risk for infections, especially with encapsulated bacterial organisms. **Autoinfarction of the spleen** occurs during early childhood secondary to microvascular obstruction by sickled red blood cells. The spleen gradually regresses in size and by age 4 years is no longer palpable. As a consequence of infarction and fibrosis, the immunologic capacity of the spleen is diminished. Patients with sickle cell disease are at greater risk for pneumonia, sepsis, and meningitis by encapsulated organisms such as *Streptococcus pneumonia* and *Haemophilus influenza*. For the same reason, patients with sickle cell disease are at greater risk for osteomyelitis with *Salmonella* spp.

Acute chest syndrome is a vasoocclusive crisis within the lungs and is associated with infection or pulmonary infarction. Patients with **acute chest syndrome** present with **hypoxia, dyspnea, fever, chest pain, and progressive pulmonary infiltrates** on radiography. These episodes may be precipitated by pneumonia causing sickling in the infected lung segments, or, in the absence of infection, intrapulmonary sickling can occur as a primary event. It is virtually impossible to clinically distinguish whether or not infection is present; thus, empiric antibiotic therapy is used.

Aplastic crisis occurs secondary to viral suppression of red blood cell precursors, most often by parvovirus B19. It occurs because of the very short half-life of sickled red blood cells and consequent need for brisk erythropoiesis. If red blood cell production is inhibited, even for a short time, profound anemia may result. The process is acute and usually reversible, with spontaneous recovery.

Other complications of sickle cell disease include hemorrhagic or ischemic stroke as a result of thrombosis, pigmented gallstones, papillary necrosis of the kidney, priapism, and congestive heart failure.

Treatment

The mainstay of treatment of pain crisis is hydration and pain control with nonsteroidal anti-inflammatory agents and narcotics. It is important to also provide adequate oxygenation to reduce sickling. One must search diligently for any underlying infection, and antibiotics are often used empirically when infection is suspected. **Acute chest syndrome** is treated with **oxygen, analgesia, and antibiotics.** Sometimes exchange transfusions are necessary. In general, blood transfusions may be required for aplastic crisis, for severe hypoxia in acute chest syndrome, or to decrease viscosity and cerebral thrombosis in patients with stroke. Transfusion does not shorten the duration of pain crisis. To protect against encapsulated organisms, all patients with sickle cell disease should receive **penicillin prophylaxis** and a **vaccination against pneumococcus.** **Hydroxyurea** is often used to reduce the occurrence of painful crisis by stimulating hemoglobin F production and thus decreasing hemoglobin S concentration, and should be considered in patients who have repeated episodes of acute chest syndrome, or frequent severe pain crises. The antineoplastic agent 5-deoxyazacytidine (**decitabine**) may also elevate levels of hemoglobin F without excessive side effects.

Comprehension Questions

28.1   Which of the following therapies would most likely decrease the number of sickle cell crises?
   A. Hydroxyurea
   B. Folate supplementation
   C. Prophylactic penicillin
   D. Pneumococcal vaccination

For the following questions (28.2 to 28.4) choose the finding (A-E) that best matches with the syndrome to which it is commonly associated in persons with sickle cell anemia.

A. *Salmonella* spp
B. *Streptococcus pneumonia*
C. Parvovirus B19
D. Fat embolus
E. Hematuria

28.2   Aplastic crisis

28.3   Osteomyelitis

28.4   Pneumonia

ANSWERS

28.1   **A.** Hydroxyurea and decitabine may decrease the incidence of sickle cell crises by increasing levels of hemoglobin F.

28.2   **C.** Parvovirus B19 is associated with aplastic crisis, especially in individuals with sickle cell disease.

28.3   **A.** Patients with sickle cell disease are at risk for *Salmonella* osteomyelitis.

28.4   **B.** *Streptococcus pneumoniae* is the most common causative agent for pneumonia.

Clinical Pearls

> Treatment of an acute painful episode in sickle cell disease includes hydration, narcotic analgesia, adequate oxygenation, and search for underlying infection.

> Acute chest syndrome is characterized by chest pain, cough, dyspnea, fever, and radiographic pulmonary infiltrate; it can be caused by pneumonia, vaso-occlusion, or pulmonary embolism.

> Blood transfusion may be required for aplastic crisis, for severe hypoxemia in acute chest syndrome, or to decrease viscosity and cerebral thrombosis in patients with stroke.

> Hydroxyurea and decitabine increase hemoglobin F production (decreasing hemoglobin S concentration) and thus reduce the frequency of pain crises and other complications.

REFERENCES

Benz, EJ. Disorders of hemoglobin. In: Fauci AS, Braunwald E, Kasper DL, eds. *Harrison's Principles of Internal Medicine*. 17th ed. New York, NY: McGraw-Hill; 2008:635-643.

Steinberg MH. Management of sickle cell disease. *N Engl J Med*. 1999;340:1021-1030.

Vichinsky E. New therapies in sickle cell disease. *Lancet*. 2002;360:629-631.

Vichinsky EP, Styles LA, Colangelo LH, et al. Acute chest syndrome in sickle cell disease: clinical presentation and course. Cooperative Study of Sickle Cell Disease. *Blood*. 1997;89:1787-1792.

Case 29

A 20-year-old college student is your next patient in the emergency room. When you walk into the room, he is lying on the examination table, on his side, with his arm covering his eyes. The light in the room is off. You look at his chart and see that the nurse recorded his temperature as 102.3°F, heart rate 110 bpm, and blood pressure 120/80 mm Hg. When you gently ask how he has been feeling, he says that for the past 3 days he has had fever, body aches, and a progressively worsening headache. The light hurts his eyes and he is nauseated, but he has not vomited. He has had some rhinorrhea, but no diarrhea, cough, or nasal congestion. He has no known ill contacts. On examination, he has no skin rash, but his pupils are difficult to assess because of photophobia. Ears and oropharynx are normal. Heart, lung, and abdomen examinations are normal. Neurologic examination reveals no focal neurologic deficits, but passive flexion of his neck worsens his headache, and he is unable to touch his chin to his chest.

➤ What condition are you concerned about?

➤ What diagnostic test would confirm the diagnosis?

ANSWERS TO CASE 29:

Bacterial Meningitis

Summary: A 20-year-old college student presents with a 3-day history of fever, headache, myalgias, and nausea. He has no respiratory or gastrointestinal symptoms, but now has developed photophobia. He is febrile to 102.3°F, tachycardic, and normotensive. His physical examination is generally unremarkable with a nonfocal neurologic examination but some neck stiffness, suggesting meningeal irritation. He has no skin lesions as might be seen in meningococcemia.

> **Most likely condition:** Meningitis.

> **Diagnostic test to confirm diagnosis:** Lumbar puncture (LP) for evaluation of the cerebrospinal fluid (CSF), possibly preceded by a computed tomographic (CT) scan of the head.

ANALYSIS

Objectives

1. Be familiar with the clinical presentations of viral and bacterial meningitis.
2. Know that LP is the diagnostic test of choice for meningitis.
3. Be familiar with the treatment for meningitis.

Considerations

This 20-year-old college student has headache, nausea, photophobia, fever, and neck pain and stiffness—all suggestive of meningitis, which could be bacterial or viral. Prompt LP and analysis of CSF are essential to establish the diagnosis. In a patient without focal neurologic signs and a normal level of consciousness, CT scan may be unnecessary prior to performing an LP. If he had a purpuric skin rash, one would be suspicious of *Neisseria* meningitis, and appropriate antibiotics should be administered immediately. Dosing of antibiotics in suspected meningococcal infection should not await the performance of any diagnostic test because progression of the disease is rapid, and mortality and morbidity are extremely high even when antibiotics are given in a timely manner.

APPROACH TO
Suspected Meningitis

DEFINITIONS

MENINGITIS: A serious inflammation of the meninges, the thin, membranous covering of the brain and the spinal cord, which can be caused by bacteria, viruses, fungi, or protozoa.

PAPILLEDEMA: Swelling of the optic nerve, caused by an increased intracranial pressure. On fundoscopic examination, the optic disc margin appears hazy.

CLINICAL APPROACH

Bacterial meningitis is the most common pus-forming intracranial infection, with an incidence of 2.5 per 10,000 persons. The microbiology of the disease has changed somewhat since the introduction of the *Haemophilus influenzae* type B vaccine in the 1980s. Now **Streptococcus pneumoniae is the most common bacterial isolate, with Neisseria meningitidis a close second. Group B streptococcus** or *Streptococcus agalactiae* occurs in approximately 10% of cases, more frequently in neonates or in patients older than 50 years or with chronic illnesses such as diabetes or liver disease. **Listeria monocytogenes** accounts for approximately 10% of cases and must be considered in pregnant women, the **elderly**, or patients with impaired cell-mediated immunity such as AIDS (acquired immunodeficiency syndrome) patients. *Haemophilus influenzae* is responsible for less than 10% of meningitis cases. Resistance to penicillin and some cephalosporins is now of great concern in the treatment of *S pneumoniae*.

Bacteria usually seed the meninges hematogenously after colonizing and invading the nasal or oropharyngeal mucosa. Occasionally, bacteria directly invade the intracranial space from a site of abscess formation in the middle ear or sinuses. The gravity and rapidity of progression of disease depend upon both host defense and organism virulence characteristics. For example, patients with defects in the complement cascade are more susceptible to invasive meningococcal disease. Patients with CSF rhinorrhea caused by trauma or postsurgical changes may also be more susceptible to bacterial invasion. **Staphylococcus aureus** and **Staphylococcus epidermidis** are common causes of meningitis in patients following **neurologic procedures** such as placement of **ventriculoperitoneal shunts**. The brisk host inflammatory response in the subarachnoid space may cause edema, vasculitis, and coagulation of vessels, leading to severe neurologic complications including seizures, increased intracranial pressure, and stroke. Acute bacterial meningitis can progress over hours to days. **Typical symptoms include fever, neck stiffness, and headache.** Patients may also complain of photophobia, nausea and vomiting, and more nonspecific constitutional symptoms. Approximately 75% of patients will experience some confusion or altered level of consciousness. Forty percent may experience seizures during the course of their illness.

Some physical examination findings may be useful in the evaluation of a patient with suspected meningitis. **Nuchal rigidity** is demonstrated when passive or active flexion of the neck results in an inability to touch the chin to the chest. Classic tests include Kernig and Brudzinski signs. **Kernig sign** can be elicited with the patient on his or her back. The hip and knees are flexed. The knee is then passively extended, and the test is positive if this maneuver elicits pain. **Brudzinski sign** is positive if the supine patient flexes the knees and hips when the neck is passively flexed. Neither sign is very sensitive for the presence of meningeal irritation, but, if present, both are highly specific. **Papilledema**, if present, would indicate **increased intracranial pressure**, and focal neurologic signs or altered level of consciousness or seizures may reflect ischemia of the cerebral vasculature or focal suppuration.

Differential Diagnosis

The differential diagnosis of bacterial meningitis is fairly limited and can be narrowed depending upon the patient's age, as discussed earlier, exposure history, and course of illness. Various viral infections may also cause meningitis. These include **enteroviruses**, which tend to be more common in the summer and fall, when patients may present with severe headache, accompanied by symptoms of gastroenteritis. The **CSF white blood cell (WBC) count will be elevated**, with a **predominance of lymphocytes**, and usually **glucose and protein levels are normal (Table 29–1)**. Either herpes simplex virus (HSV)-1 or HSV-2 can cause herpes simplex meningitis. The CSF of these patients will also have a normal glucose level, whereas protein and WBC counts will be elevated with a predominance of lymphocytes. Typically, these patients have a high CSF red blood cell count, which is not seen in bacterial meningitis in the absence of a traumatic spinal tap. In a patient with human immunodeficiency virus (HIV) infection, fungal meningitis, specifically caused by *Cryptococcus*, should be considered. Tuberculous meningitis presents subacutely and is more common in older, debilitated patients, or in patients with HIV. Rickettsial disease, specifically Rocky Mountain spotted fever, may also present with meningitis. Intracranial empyema, or brain or epidural abscess, should be considered, especially if the patient has focal neurologic findings. The one nonsuppurative diagnosis in the differential is **subarachnoid hemorrhage**. These patients present with sudden onset of the "worst headache of their lives" in the absence of other symptoms of infection. They may have photophobia, and the CSF will be grossly bloody; the supernatant will be xanthochromic, reflecting the breakdown of blood into bilirubin.

Table 29–1 CSF CHARACTERISTICS OF MENINGITIS

CAUSATIVE ORGANISM	OPENING PRESSURE	WHITE BLOOD CELL COUNT/TYPE	GLUCOSE	PROTEIN	RED BLOOD CELL COUNT	SPECIAL STAINS/ TESTS
Bacteria	High	Elevated, predominantly neutrophilic	Low, <40 mg/dL	Elevated	None	Gram stain
Viral	Normal	Elevated, predominantly lymphocytic	Normal	Normal	None	Cell culture or PCR
Herpes simplex	Normal to high	As in other viral meningitis	Normal	Normal to high	High	PCR
Tuberculosis	Normal to high	Elevated, monocytes may be elevated	Very low	Very high	None	PCR, AFB smear (usually negative), and culture

Abbreviations: AFB, acid fast bacillus; CSF, cerebrospinal fluid; PCR, polymerase chain reaction.

Blood cultures should be obtained in all patients with suspected meningitis. Critical to the diagnosis of meningitis is the LP and evaluation of the CSF. Table 29–1 lists typical findings in the CSF from various causes of meningitis.

The necessity of imaging of the head and brain prior to performing an LP is controversial. Studies show that in the patient with suspected meningitis who does not have papilledema, focal neurologic signs, or altered level of consciousness, an LP may be safely performed without preceding imaging. However, in instances in which performance of the LP may be delayed, antibiotics should be administered after blood cultures while awaiting the radiologic studies. Ideally, the CSF should be examined within 30 minutes of antibiotics, but it has been shown that if the LP is performed within 2 hours of antibiotic administration, it will not significantly alter the CSF protein, glucose, or WBC count, or Gram stain. If CSF is obtained, a culture and Gram stain should be sent. If enough fluid is available, it should also be sent for cell count and glucose and protein levels. Latex agglutination tests for S pneumoniae and H influenzae can be useful in patients pretreated with antibiotics, and, although not very sensitive, if positive they can rule in disease (high specificity). Polymerase chain reaction (PCR) testing is available for some bacteria; however, it may be more useful in the diagnosis of herpes simplex, enteroviral, or tuberculous meningitis. In all, no more than 3.5 to 4 mL of CSF is necessary. The most critical issue in a patient with suspected bacterial meningitis, however, is the initiation of antibiotics. The CSF examination and imaging studies can be deferred in this medical emergency.

During the course of treatment, most patients will undergo some cerebral imaging study. Computed tomographic (CT) scans are most useful in the initial presentation to exclude intracranial mass or bleeding, or to evaluate for other signs of increased intracranial pressure. However, magnetic resonance imaging (MRI) is most helpful for demonstrating any focal ischemia or infarction caused by the disease. When **HSV meningitis** is suspected, MRI should demonstrate **enhancement of the temporal lobes**. In tuberculous meningitis, enhancement of the basal region may be seen. An electroencephalogram (EEG) may be helpful in patients suspected of HSV meningitis. Within 2 to 15 days of the start of the illness, periodic sharp and slow wave complexes originating within the temporal lobes can be demonstrated at 2- to 3-second intervals. When the purpuric skin lesions are present, skin biopsy may demonstrate N meningitidis and can be helpful in the diagnosis. Age may give a clue regarding etiology of meningitis (Table 29–2).

Therapy

Treatment of meningitis often is empiric until specific culture data are available. Because of the growing incidence of resistant pneumococci as well as meningococci, the recommended empiric therapy in most areas is a **high-dose third-generation cephalosporin given concurrently with vancomycin**. In other areas, if the disease presentation is typical for meningococcus (with the

Table 29–2 ETIOLOGIES OF BACTERIAL MENINGITIS BY AGE

AGE OF PATIENT	BACTERIA	EMPIRIC TREATMENT	COMMENTS
Neonate	1. Gram-negative enteric bacteria (*Escherichia coli*) and group B streptococcus 2. *Listeria monocytogenes*	Ampicillin + cefotaxime	Vaginal organisms common
1-23 mo	1. *Streptococcus pneumoniae* 2. *Neisseria meningitides* 3. *Haemophilus influenzae* type b *(less since vaccine)*	Cefotaxime (or ceftriaxone) + vancomycin	Previous to vaccine, *H influenzae caused 70% of meningitis in children*
2-18 y	1. *N meningitides* 2. *S pneumoniae* 3. *H influenzae* type b (less common since vaccine)	Ampicillin + vancomycin ± ceftriaxone	
19-59 y	1. *S pneumoniae* 2. *N meningitides* 3. *H influenzae* type b	Ampicillin + vancomycin ± ceftriaxone	
60+ y	1. *S pneumoniae* 2. *Listeria monocytogenes* 3. Group B streptococcus	Ampicillin + vancomycin + ceftriaxone (or cefotaxime)	*Listeria* more common

Data from: Centers for Disease Control and Prevention, 2003.

typical rash) or the organism is identified quickly on Gram stain of the CSF, therapy with high-dose penicillin can be started if the meningococcus in that area is known to be sensitive. **Ampicillin is added when there is a suspicion of listeriosis. Acyclovir should be started for suspicion of HSV** or four-drug antituberculosis (TB) therapy started if the presentation is suspicious for tuberculous meningitis. The administration of **glucocorticoids** to reduce CNS (central nervous system) inflammation is controversial. One study in adults demonstrated decreased mortality in patients with S pneumoniae meningitis who were given glucocorticoids. There is stronger data for steroids for H influenzae and S pneumoniae meningitis in children. There is also some evidence for benefit of steroids in severe tuberculous meningitis.

Prevention of meningitis can be achieved through the administration of **vaccines and chemoprophylaxis** of close contacts. **Specific vaccinations are available for H influenzae type B and some strains of S pneumoniae** and are now routinely administered to **children. Meningococcal vaccination** is recommended for those living in dormitory situations, such as college students and military recruits, but not for the general population. **Rifampin given twice daily for 2 days** or a single dose of ciprofloxacin is recommended for **household and close contacts** of an index case of **meningococcemia or meningococcal meningitis.**

Comprehension Questions

29.1   An 18-year-old with a 1-week history of fever, headache, increasing confusion, and lethargy presents to the emergency room. His physical examination is normal, and he has no focal neurologic signs. The CT scan of his head is negative. An LP reveals a WBC count of 250/mm^3, with 78% lymphocytes and red blood cells (RBCs) 500/mm^3 in tube 1 and 630/mm^3 in tube 2, respectively. No organisms are seen on Gram stain. Which of the following is the best next step?

A. Intravenous ceftriaxone, acyclovir, and vancomycin
B. Intravenous fluconazole
C. Intravenous azithromycin
D. Careful observation with no antibiotics

29.2   A 55-year-old man with a long history of alcohol abuse presents with a 3-week history of progressive confusion and stupor. On examination he is afebrile, but he has a new right sixth cranial nerve palsy and tremulousness of all four extremities. His CSF has 250 WBCs/mm^3, with 68% lymphocytes. There are 300 RBCs/mm^3. Protein levels are high, and the ratio of CSF to serum glucose is very low. He is started on ceftriaxone, vancomycin, and acyclovir. A purified protein derivative (PPD) placed on admission is positive, and bacterial cultures are negative at 48 hours. Which of the following would help to confirm the diagnosis?

A. Gram stain of throat scrapings
B. CT of the head with contrast
C. MRI of the head
D. Repeat LP after 48 hours of therapy
E. Herpes simplex virus PCR

29.3   A 65-year-old man with colon cancer on chemotherapy presents with a fever and headache of 3-day duration. An LP is performed, and Gram stain reveals gram-positive rods. Which of the following therapies is most likely to treat the organism?

A. Vancomycin
B. Metronidazole
C. Ampicillin
D. Gentamicin
E. Ceftriaxone

ANSWERS

29.1   **A.** This young man most likely has a viral meningitis given the modest CSF pleocytosis count with predominant lymphocytes. Given the high RBC count, it may be HSV, so acyclovir should be instituted until more specific testing can be done. However, because bacterial meningitis cannot be excluded based on the CSF analysis alone, empiric antibacterials should be given until culture results are known, usually within 48 hours.

29.2   **D.** Tuberculous meningitis is extremely difficult to diagnose, and the index of suspicion should be high in susceptible individuals. Certain clinical findings, such as nerve palsies, and CSF findings, such as an extremely low glucose and high protein levels with a fairly low WBC count, are highly suggestive but not diagnostic. Mortality is high and related to the delay in instituting therapy. The only definitive test is acid fast bacillus (AFB) culture, but it can take 6 to 8 weeks to grow. PCR test for *Mycobacterium tuberculosis* is diagnostic if positive; however, the sensitivity is low, so a negative test does not rule out the disease. Findings such as a positive PPD, or CSF cell counts and protein levels that do not change with standard antimicrobial or antiviral therapies, can also suggest the diagnosis. Low CSF glucose is a hallmark of TB meningitis—if the glucose level falls at 48 hours, it is highly suggestive of TB. A CT scan and an MRI may demonstrate basilar meningitis in TB, but the finding is not specific.

29.3   **C.** *Listeria monocytogenes* is a gram-positive rod that causes approximately 10% of all cases of meningitis. It is more common in the elderly and in other patients with impaired cell-mediated immunity, such as patients on chemotherapy. It is also more common in neonates. It is not sensitive to cephalosporins, and specific therapy with ampicillin must be instituted if the suspicion for this disease is high.

Clinical Pearls

➤ In general, a lumbar puncture should not be delayed in a patient in whom meningitis is suspected. If lumbar puncture is contraindicated or impossible because of hemodynamic or other instability, empiric therapy should be started immediately after blood cultures are drawn.

➤ The most common cause of bacterial meningitis in adults is *Streptococcus pneumoniae*, followed by *Neisseria meningitides*. *Listeria monocytogenes* meningitis occurs in neonates and in immunocompromised or older patients.

➤ Patients who have undergone neurosurgical procedures or who have been subject to skull trauma are at risk for staphylococcal meningitis.

➤ Hemorrhagic cerebrospinal fluid with evidence of temporal lobe involvement by imaging or EEG suggests herpes simplex virus encephalitis; acyclovir is the treatment of choice.

REFERENCES

Hasbrun R, Abrahams J, Jekel J, et al. Computed tomography of the head before lumbar puncture in adults with suspected meningitis. *N Engl J Med*. 2001;345:1727-1733.

Roos KL, Tyler KL. Meningitis, encephalitis, brain abscess, and empyema. In: Fauci AS, Braunwald E, Kasper DL, eds. *Harrison's Principles of Internal Medicine*. 17th ed. New York, NY: McGraw-Hill; 2008: 2621-2641.

Thomas KE, Hasbrun R, Jekel J, et al. The diagnostic accuracy of Kernig's sign, Brudzinski's sign, and nuchal rigidity in adults with suspected meningitis. *Clin Infect Dis*. 2002;35:46-52.

Van de Beek D, de Gans J, Spanjaard L, et al. Clinical features and prognostic factors in adults with bacterial meningitis. *N Engl J Med*. 2004;351:1849-1859.

Wetzler LM. Meningococcal infections. In: Fauci AS, Braunwald E, Kasper DL, eds. *Harrison's Principles of Internal Medicine*. 17th ed. New York, NY: McGraw-Hill; 2008:908-914.

Case 30

A 28-year-old man comes to the emergency room complaining of 6 days of fevers with shaking chills. Over the past 2 days, he has also developed a productive cough with greenish sputum, which occasionally is blood streaked. He reports no dyspnea, but sometimes experiences chest pain on deep inspiration. He does not have headache, abdominal pain, urinary symptoms, vomiting, or diarrhea. He has no significant medical history. He smokes cigarettes and marijuana regularly, drinks several beers daily, but denies intravenous drug use.

On examination, his temperature is 102.5°F, heart rate 109 bpm, blood pressure 128/76 mm Hg, and respiratory rate 23 breaths per minute. He is alert and talkative. He has no oral lesions, and funduscopic examination reveals no abnormalities. His jugular veins show prominent V waves, and his heart rhythm is tachycardic but regular with a harsh holosystolic murmur at the left lower sternal border that increases with inspiration. Chest examination reveals inspiratory rales bilaterally. On both of his forearms, he has linear streaks of induration, hyperpigmentation, with some small nodules overlying the superficial veins, but no erythema, warmth, or tenderness.

Laboratory examination is significant for an elevated white blood cell (WBC) count at 17,500/mm^3, with 84% polymorphonuclear cells, 7% band forms, and 9% lymphocytes, a hemoglobin concentration of 14 g/dL, hematocrit 42%, and platelet count 189,000/mm^3. Liver function tests and urinalysis are normal. Chest radiograph shows multiple peripheral, ill-defined nodules, some with cavitation.

➤ What is the most likely diagnosis?

➤ What is your next step?

ANSWERS TO CASE 30:

Endocarditis (Tricuspid)/Septic Pulmonary Emboli

Summary: A 28-year-old man complains of shaking chills and fever. He also has a productive cough. He denies intravenous drug use. He has a temperature of 102.5°F, heart rate 109 bpm, and a new holosystolic murmur at the left lower sternal border, which increases with inspiration. He has linear streaks of induration on both forearms, and chest radiograph shows with multiple ill-defined nodules.

➤ **Most likely diagnosis:** Infective endocarditis involving the tricuspid valve, with probable septic pulmonary emboli.

➤ **Next step:** Obtain serial blood cultures and institute empiric broad-spectrum antibiotics.

ANALYSIS

Objectives

1. Understand the differences in clinical presentation between acute and sub-acute, and left-sided versus right-sided endocarditis.
2. Learn the most common organisms that cause endocarditis, including "culture-negative" endocarditis.
3. Know the diagnostic and therapeutic approach to infective endocarditis, including the indications for valve replacement.
4. Understand the complications of endocarditis.

Considerations

Although this patient denied parenteral drug use, his track marks on the fore-arms are very suspicious for intravenous drug abuse. He has fever, a new heart murmur very typical of tricuspid regurgitation, and a chest radiograph sugges-tive of septic pulmonary emboli. Serial blood cultures, ideally obtained before antibiotics are started, are essential to establish the diagnosis of infective endocarditis. The rapidity with which antibiotics are started depends on the clinical presentation of the patient: a septic, critically ill patient needs antibi-otics immediately; a patient with a subacute presentation can wait many hours while cultures are obtained.

APPROACH TO
Suspected Endocarditis

DEFINITIONS

INFECTIOUS ENDOCARDITIS: A microbial process of the endocardium, usually involving the heart valves.

JANEWAY LESIONS: Painless hemorrhagic macules on the palms and soles that are consistent with infectious endocarditis.

ROTH SPOTS: Hemorrhagic retinal lesions with white centers, due to infectious endocarditis.

CLINICAL APPROACH

The clinical presentation depends upon the valves involved (left-sided vs right-sided), as well as the virulence of the organism. Highly virulent species, such as *Staphylococcus aureus*, produce acute infection, and less virulent organisms, such as the viridans group of streptococci, tend to produce a more subacute illness, which may evolve over weeks. **Fever is present in 95% of all cases.** For **acute endocarditis**, patients often present with high fever, acute valvular regurgitation, and embolic phenomena (eg, to the extremities or to the brain, causing stroke). **Subacute endocarditis** more often is associated with constitutional symptoms such as anorexia, weight loss, night sweats, and findings attributable to immune-complex deposition and septic vasculitis; these include petechiae, splenomegaly, glomerulonephritis, **Osler nodes (tender nodules on the finger or toe pads), Janeway lesions (painless hemorrhagic macules** on the palms and soles), **Roth spots** (hemorrhagic retinal lesions with white centers), and **splinter hemorrhages**. These classic peripheral lesions, although frequently discussed, are actually seen in only 20% to 25% of cases.

Right-sided endocarditis usually involves the **tricuspid** valve, causing **pulmonary** emboli, rather than involving the systemic circulation. Accordingly, patients develop pleuritic chest pain, purulent sputum, or hemoptysis, and radiographs may show multiple peripheral nodular lesions, often with cavitation. The murmur of tricuspid regurgitation may not be present, especially early in the illness.

In all cases of endocarditis, the critical finding is bacteremia, which usually is sustained. The initiating event is a transient bacteremia, which may be a result of mucosal injury, as in dental extraction, or a complication of the use of intravascular catheters. Bacteria are then able to seed valvular endothelium. Previously damaged, abnormal, or prosthetic valves form vegetations, which are composed of platelets and fibrin, and are relatively avascular sites where bacteria may grow protected from immune attack.

Serial blood cultures are the most important step in the diagnosis of endocarditis. Acutely ill patients should have **three blood cultures** obtained over a **2- to 3-hour** period prior to initiating antibiotics. In **subacute** disease, **three blood cultures over a 24-hour** period maximize the diagnostic yield. Of course, if patients are critically ill or hemodynamically unstable, no delay in initiating therapy is appropriate, and cultures are obtained on presentation, even while broad-spectrum antibiotics are administered. Usually it is not difficult to isolate the infecting organism, because the hallmark of infective endocarditis is sustained bacteremia; thus, all blood cultures often are positive for the microorganism. Table 30–1 lists typical organisms, frequency of infection, and associated conditions.

Culture-negative endocarditis, an uncommon situation in which routine cultures fail to grow, is most likely a result of prior **antibiotic** treatment, **fungal** infection (fungi other than *Candida* spp. often require special culture media), or **fastidious** organisms. These organisms can include *Abiotrophia* spp, *Bartonella* spp, *Coxiella burnetii*, *Legionella* spp, *Chlamydia*, and the **HACEK organisms** (*Haemophilus aphrophilus/paraphrophilus*, *Actinobacillus actinomycetemcomitans*, *Cardiobacterium hominis*, *Eikenella corrodens*, *Kingella kingae*). The clinical features, blood cultures, and echocardiography are used to diagnose cases of infective endocarditis using the highly sensitive and specific **Duke criteria**. It should be noted that transesophageal echocardiography (TEE) rather than transthoracic

Table 30–1 ORGANISMS CAUSING ENDOCARDITIS

ORGANISM	FREQUENCY	ASSOCIATED CONDITIONS
Staphylococcus aureus	30%-40% of native valve infection	Intravascular catheter, intravenous drug use (tricuspid valve endocarditis)
Coagulase-negative staphylococci	30%-35% of early prosthetic valve infection	Neonates, prosthetic valves
Streptococcal viridans	40%-60% of native valve infection	Oral flora, after dental surgery
Enterococci	15%, usually in older patients	Previous genitourinary tract disease or instrumentation
Streptococcus bovis	5%-10%	Elderly patients, often with underlying GI mucosal lesion, eg, adenoma or malignancy
Candida spp	5%-10%	Intravascular catheters, intravenous drug use

echocardiography (TTE) is the method of choice in assessing these vegetations. Endocarditis is considered to definitely be present if the patient satisfies two major criteria; one major and three minor criteria; or five minor criteria (Table 30–2).

One life-threatening complication of endocarditis is **congestive heart failure,** usually as a consequence of **infection-induced valvular damage.** Other cardiac complications are intracardiac abscesses and conduction disturbances caused by septal involvement by infection. Systemic arterial embolization may lead to splenic or renal infarction or abscesses. Vegetations may embolize to the coronary circulation, causing a myocardial infarction, or to the brain, causing a cerebral infarction. A **stroke syndrome** in a **febrile** patient should always suggest the possibility of **endocarditis.** Infection of the vasa vasorum may weaken the wall of major arteries and produce mycotic aneurysms, which can occur anywhere but are most common in the cerebral circulation, sinuses of Valsalva, or abdominal aorta. These aneurysms may leak or rupture, producing sudden fatal intracranial or other hemorrhage.

Antibiotic treatment usually is begun in the hospital but because of the prolonged nature of therapy is often completed on an outpatient basis when the patient is clinically stable. **Treatment generally lasts 4 to 6 weeks.** If the organism is susceptible, such as **most Streptococcus species, penicillin G** is the agent of choice. For **S aureus, nafcillin** is the drug of choice, often used in combination with **gentamicin** initially for synergy, to help resolve bacteremia. Therapy for intravenous drug users should be directed against *S aureus.* **Vancomycin** is used when **methicillin-resistant** *S aureus* or **coagulase-negative staphylococci** are present. **Ceftriaxone is the usual therapy for the HACEK** group of organisms. Devising a rationale therapy for culture-negative endocarditis may be challenging and depends on the clinical situation.

Table 30–2 DUKE CRITERIA FOR DIAGNOSIS OF ENDOCARDITIS

Major criteria
- Isolation of typical organisms (viridans streptococci, *Staphylococcus aureus,* entero-cocci, *Streptococcus bovis,* or one of the HACEK organisms) from two separate blood cultures, or persistently positive blood cultures with other organisms
- Evidence of endocardial involvement: either echocardiographic evidence of endocarditis, eg, oscillating intracardiac mass, or new valvular regurgitation

Minor criteria
- Predisposing valvular lesion or intravenous drug use
- Fever >100.4°F (38.0°C)
- Vascular phenomena: arterial or septic pulmonary emboli, mycotic aneurysm, Janeway lesions
- Immunologic phenomena: glomerulonephritis, Osler nodes, Roth spots, positive rheumatoid factor
- Positive blood cultures not meeting major criteria

Table 30–3 INDICATIONS FOR SURGICAL MANAGEMENT OF ENDOCARDITIS
Intractable congestive heart failure caused by valve dysfunction >1 serious systemic embolic episode, or large (>10 mm) vegetation with high risk for embolism
Uncontrolled infection, eg, positive cultures after 7 d of therapy
No effective antimicrobial therapy (eg, fungal endocarditis)
Most cases of prosthetic valve endocarditis, especially *S aureus* prosthetic valve infection
Local suppurative complications, eg, myocardial abscess

Table 30–3 summarizes the commonly recognized indications for surgical intervention, that is, valve excision and replacement.

Patients at high risk for developing infective endocarditis benefit from antibiotic prophylaxis prior to dental procedures. The most recent American Heart Association guidelines (2008) specify the following individuals:

- Prosthetic heart valves
- Previous infective endocarditis
- Congenital heart disease (unrepaired cyanotic coronary heart disease [CHD] including palliative shunts and conduits)
- Completely repaired CHD repaired with prosthetic material or device during the first 6 postoperative months
- Repaired CHD with residual defects at the site or adjacent to the site of a prosthetic patch or prosthetic device
- Valve regurgitation caused by a structurally abnormal valve in cardiac transplant recipients

Amoxicillin is the drug of choice for prophylaxis unless the patient is allergic to penicillin or unable to take medications by mouth. Alternatives for use in these situations include ampicillin, cephalosporins, or clindamycin.

Comprehension Questions

30.1   A 68-year-old man is hospitalized with *Streptococcus bovis* endocarditis of the mitral valve and recovers completely with appropriate therapy. Which of the following is the most important next step?

A. Good dental hygiene and proper denture fitting to prevent reinfection of damaged heart valves from oral flora.

B. Repeat echocardiography in 6 weeks to ensure the vegetations have resolved.

C. Colonoscopy to look for mucosal lesions.

D. Mitral valve replacement to prevent systemic emboli such as cerebral infarction.

30.2   A 24-year-old intravenous drug user is admitted with 4 weeks of fever.
       He has three blood cultures positive with *Candida* spp and suddenly
       develops a cold blue toe. Which of the following is the appropriate
       next step?
       A. Repeat echocardiography to see if the large aortic vegetation pre-
          viously seen has now embolized.
       B. Cardiovascular surgery consultation for aortic valve replacement.
       C. Aortic angiography to evaluate for a mycotic aneurysm, which
          may be embolizing.
       D. Switch from fluconazole to amphotericin B.

30.3   A patient with which of the following conditions requires antimicro-
       bial prophylaxis before dental surgery?
       A. Atrial septal defect
       B. Mitral valve prolapse without mitral regurgitation
       C. Previous coronary artery bypass graft
       D. Previous infective endocarditis

ANSWERS

30.1   **C.** Colonoscopy is necessary because a significant number of patients
       with S *bovis* endocarditis have a colonic cancer or premalignant polyp,
       which leads to seeding of the valve by gastrointestinal (GI) flora.
       Heart valves damaged by endocarditis are more susceptible to infec-
       tion, so good dental hygiene is important, but in this case, the organ-
       ism came from the intestinal tract, not the mouth, and the possibility
       of malignancy is most important to address. Serial echocardiography
       would not add to the patient's care after successful therapy, because
       vegetations become organized and persist for months or years without
       late embolization. Prophylactic valve replacement would not be indi-
       cated, because the prosthetic valve is even more susceptible to rein-
       fection than the damaged native valve and would actually increase the
       risk of cerebral infarction or other systemic emboli as a consequence of
       thrombus formation, even if adequately anticoagulated.

30.2   **B.** Fungal endocarditis, which occurs in intravenous drug users or
       immunosuppressed persons with indwelling catheters, frequently gives
       rise to large friable vegetations with a high risk of embolization (often
       to the lower extremities) and is very difficult to cure with antifungal
       medications. Valve replacement usually is necessary. Repeat echocar-
       diography would not add to the patient's care, because the clinical
       diagnosis of peripheral embolization is almost certain, and it would not
       change the management. Medical therapy with any antifungal agent is
       unlikely to cure this infection. Mycotic aneurysms may occur in any
       artery as a consequence of endocarditis and can cause late embolic
       complications, but in this case, the source probably is the heart.

30.3   **D.** Prior endocarditis damages valvular surfaces, and these patients
         are at increased risk for reinfection during a transient bacteremia, as
         may occur during dental procedures or some other GI or genitouri-
         nary tract procedures. All of the other conditions mentioned have a
         negligible risk of endocarditis, the same as in the general population,
         and antibiotic prophylaxis is not recommended by the American
         Heart Association.

Clinical Pearls

> ➤ The diagnosis of infective endocarditis is established by using clinical cri-
> teria, the most important of which are sustained bacteremia and evidence
> of endocardial involvement, usually by echocardiography.
> ➤ Right-sided endocarditis may be difficult to diagnose because it lacks the
> systemic emboli seen in left-sided endocarditis, and the new murmur of
> tricuspid regurgitation is often not heard.
> ➤ Left-sided native valve endocarditis usually is caused by Streptococcal viri-
> dans, *Staphylococcus aureus*, and *Enterococcus*. The large majority of right-
> sided endocarditis is caused by *Staphylococcus aureus*.
> ➤ Valve replacement usually is necessary for persistent infection, recurrent
> embolization, or when medical therapy is ineffective, for example, in cases
> of large vegetations as seen in fungal endocarditis.
> ➤ Culture-negative endocarditis usually is caused by prior administration of
> antibiotics before obtaining blood cultures or by infection with fungi or
> fastidious organisms such as the HACEK group.

REFERENCES

Baddour LM, Wilson WR, Bayer AS, et al. Infective endocarditis: diagnosis, antimicro-
    bial therapy, and management of complications. *Circulation*. 2005;111:3167-3184.
Houpikian P, Raoult D. Blood culture negative endocarditis in a reference center: eti-
    ologic diagnosis of 348 cases. *Medicine*. 2005;84:162-173.
Karchmer AW. Infective endocarditis. In: Fauci AS, Braunwald E, Kasper DL, eds.
    Harrison's Principles of Internal Medicine. 17th ed. New York, NY: McGraw-Hill;
    2008:789-798.
Mylonakis E, Calderwood SB. Infective endocarditis in adults. *N Engl J Med*. 2001;
    345:1318-1330.

Case 31

A 62-year-old man is brought to the clinic for a 3-month history of unintentional weight loss (12 lb). His appetite has diminished, but he reports no vomiting or diarrhea. He does report some depressive symptoms since the death of his wife a year ago, at which time he moved from Hong Kong to the United States to live with his daughter. He denies a smoking history. He complains of a 3-month history of productive cough with greenish sputum. He has not felt feverish. He takes no medications regularly. On examination, his temperature is 100.4°F and respiratory rate 16 breaths per minute. His neck has a normal thyroid gland and no cervical or supraclavicular lymphadenopathy. His chest has few scattered rales in the left mid-lung fields and a faint expiratory wheeze on the right. His heart rhythm is regular with no gallops or murmurs. His abdominal examination is benign, his rectal examination shows no masses, and his stool is negative for occult blood. His chest X-ray is shown in Figure 31–1.

➤ What is the most likely diagnosis?

➤ What is your next step?

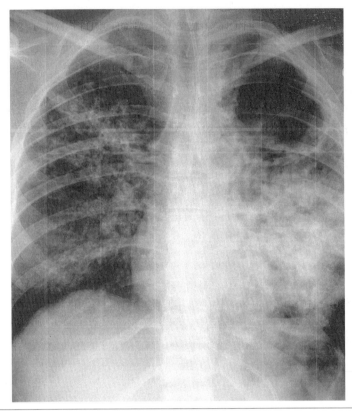

Figure 31–1. Chest X-ray. *Reproduced, with permission, from Fishman AP.* Fishman's Pulmonary Diseases and Disorders. *3rd ed. New York, NY: McGraw-Hill; 1998:2487.*

ANSWERS TO CASE 31:
Tuberculosis (Pulmonary), Cavitary Lung Lesions

Summary: A 62-year-old man from Hong Kong has a 12-lb unintentional weight loss with diminished appetite but no vomiting or diarrhea. On examination, he has a low-grade fever, and there are a few scattered rales in the left mid-lung fields and a faint expiratory wheeze on the right. His chest X-ray shows a cavitary lesion (left lower lobe).

➤ **Most likely diagnosis:** Pulmonary tuberculosis (TB).

➤ **Next step:** Refer him to the hospital for admission so that serial sputum samples can be collected for identification of the organism, and for culture and sensitivities to guide antimicrobial therapy.

ANALYSIS

Objectives

1. Know the natural history and the clinical and radiographic manifestations of primary and reactivation pulmonary TB and of latent TB infection.
2. Understand the methods of diagnosis of TB.
3. Learn treatment strategies for TB.
4. Know the common extrapulmonary sites of TB, including pleurisy, lymphadenitis, miliary, meningeal, genitourinary, skeletal, and adrenal TB.

Considerations

This elderly Asian gentleman has symptoms suggestive of TB, such as weight loss and productive cough. A chest radiograph is essential in helping to establish the diagnosis. His chest X-ray is highly suggestive of TB, but many other diseases may cause cavitary lung lesions, including other infections and malignancies. If the sputum samples do not reveal acid-fast organisms, then further testing, such as bronchoscopy, may be needed to rule out malignancy.

APPROACH TO
Suspected Tuberculosis

DEFINITIONS

LATENT TUBERCULOSIS: Asymptomatic infection of *Mycobacterium tuberculosis*.

PRIMARY TUBERCULOSIS: Development of clinical illness immediately after infection with M *tuberculosis*.

REACTIVATION TUBERCULOSIS: Illness that occurs when latent TB becomes active and infectious after a period of dormancy, such as years after the initial infection.

CLINICAL APPROACH

Pulmonary Tuberculosis

Tuberculosis is a bacterial infection caused by the acid fast bacillus (AFB) M *tuberculosis*, which usually is transmitted through airborne spread of droplets from infected patients with pulmonary TB. The vast majority of cases occur in developing countries, but a resurgence of cases in the United States occurred during the mid-1980s as a consequence of various factors, including human immunodeficiency virus (HIV) infection. Untreated disease can have a 1-year mortality rate of 33% and a 5-year mortality rate as high as 50%.

Often seen in children, **primary pulmonary TB usually affects the middle and lower lung zones.** Lesions form in the periphery with hilar and paratracheal lymphadenopathy. Granulomatous lesions are caused by the inflammatory response of lymphocytes and macrophages. The center of the lesion may become necrotic (caseous necrosis) and liquefied, forming a cavity. Healed lesions are called **Ghon lesions.** Most patients exposed to M *tuberculosis* do not manifest clinical symptoms, but they may have a latent infection. Years later, frequently during times of stress or immunosuppression, TB may reactivate and become symptomatic. **Reactivation TB** usually involves the **apical and posterior segments of the upper lobes** or the superior segments of the lower lobes of the lungs. The course may be rapid (weeks to months), chronic and slowly progressive ("consumption"), or spontaneously remit.

Signs and symptoms are nonspecific and subacute, including **fever, night sweats, malaise, weight loss, and anorexia.** The **cough usually is productive** of purulent sputum and sometimes **streaked with blood.** A lesion may erode into a vessel, causing massive hemoptysis. **Rasmussen aneurysm** is the rupture of a dilated vessel in a cavity. Physical findings can include fever, wasting, rales and rhonchi (if there is a partial bronchial obstruction), pallor, or finger clubbing from hypoxia. Possible laboratory abnormalities are leukocytosis, anemia, and hyponatremia secondary to the syndrome of inappropriate secretion of antidiuretic hormone **(SIADH).**

Extrapulmonary Tuberculosis

The sites, in order of decreasing frequency of occurrence, are the **lymph nodes, pleura, genitourinary tract, bones and joints, meninges, and peritoneum.** Tuberculosis lymphadenitis is common in HIV-infected patients, children, and nonwhite women and generally is **painless adenopathy.** Pleural disease can have an exudative effusion but may require pleural biopsy for diagnosis. Tuberculosis meningitis usually has cerebrospinal fluid with high protein, a lymphocyte predominance (or neutrophils in early infection), and low glucose level. **Adjunctive glucocorticoids** may improve the treatment response in TB meningitis. Genitourinary TB can be asymptomatic or have local symptoms such as dysuria, hematuria, and urinary frequency. It is characterized by the finding of leukocytes in the urine but negative bacterial cultures— **"sterile pyuria."** Skeletal TB affects weight-bearing joints, whereas **Pott disease involves the spine. Miliary TB** occurs by **hematogenous dissemination** with 1- to 2-mm granulomas that resemble millet seeds (hence the name). Adrenal TB can present as adrenal insufficiency.

Diagnosis

The diagnosis of TB is made by combining the history and clinical picture with AFB stains or culture of a specimen (smear or tissue biopsy). When **pulmonary**

TB is suspected, **three samples of early morning sputum** should be obtained while the patient is in isolation. Biopsy material should not be put in formaldehyde. Cultures may take from 4 to 8 weeks on ordinary solid media or 2 to 3 weeks on liquid media. Tuberculosis cases should be reported to the local public health department. Purified protein derivative (PPD) skin testing is useful for screening for latent infection but has a limited role in diagnosing active infection because of frequent false-negative results in this setting. A positive **PPD** is defined by induration after 48 to 72 hours that is **5 mm or greater in patients with HIV, close contacts** of patients with TB, or patients with **chest X-ray findings consistent with TB**. People with other risk factors, such as health-care workers and patients who are immunocompromised for reasons other than HIV, are considered to have a latent infection if the PPD is **10 mm** or more. Everyone else should have less than **15 mm of induration**.

Treatment

The probable resistance pattern of the TB organism, based on the country of origin, may help to guide treatment. For individuals from areas with low drug-resistance, therapy generally starts with a **2-month course of isoniazid (INH), rifampin, and pyrazinamide. Multiple drugs are used to avoid resistance.** Directly observed treatment (watching patients take the medication) should be instituted in all patients in this phase. Subsequently, the patient should receive a 4-month course of INH and rifampin. Pyridoxine is frequently added to the regimen. Drug resistance or intolerable side effects may require alternate therapy, such as with amikacin, ethambutol, or streptomycin. Toxicity for which patients must be monitored includes **hepatitis**, hyperuricemia, and thrombocytopenia. Treatment failure is defined by positive cultures after 3 months or positive AFB stains after 5 months and should be treated by adding two more drugs. **Latent TB infection** should be treated with INH for 9 months, with the goal of preventing reactivation TB later in life.

Comprehension Questions

31.1   A 42-year-old woman from Pakistan is being treated with infliximab for rheumatoid arthritis. After 6 months of therapy, she develops persistent fever, weight loss, and night sweats, and tuberculosis is suspected. Which of the following is the most likely location of the tuberculosis?

   A. Middle and lower lung zones
   B. Pleural space
   C. Apical segment of the upper lung lobes
   D. Cervical or supraclavicular lymph nodes

31.2   A 24-year-old man has been treated with isoniazid, rifampin, and
        pyrazinamide for active pulmonary tuberculosis. After 3 months, he
        states that he is having numbness and tingling of both feet but no back
        pain. He denies taking other medications. Which of the following is
        the most appropriate next step?
        A. CT scan of the lumbar spine.
        B. Initiate pyridoxine.
        C. Continue the tuberculosis agents and monitor for further neuro-
           logical problems.
        D. Initiate a workup for tuberculosis adenopathy compression on the
           femoral nerve.

31.3   A 25-year-old woman is seen in the clinic because her father, who
        recently immigrated from South America, was diagnosed with and has
        been treated for tuberculosis. She denies a cough and her chest radi-
        ograph is normal. A PPD test shows 10 mm of induration. Her only
        medication is an oral contraceptive. Which of the following is the best
        next step?
        A. Oral isoniazid and barrier contraception.
        B. Combination therapy including isoniazid, rifampin, and pyrazinamide.
        C. Observation.
        D. Induce three sputum samples.

31.4   Which of the following tests is the most important to follow for a
        patient receiving isoniazid and rifampin for tuberculosis treatment?
        A. Renal function tests
        B. Liver function tests
        C. Slit-lamp examinations
        D. Amylase and lipase tests

ANSWERS

31.1   **C.** Reactivation tuberculosis (in this case, likely triggered by infliximab)
        usually involves the apical aspects of the lungs. Primary TB infection
        most often affects the middle and lower lung zones. Lymphadenitis
        and pleural infection are the most common extrapulmonary sites of TB,
        but they are less common than pulmonary TB.

31.2   **B.** Pyridoxine (vitamin B_6) is important for preventing the periph-
        eral neuropathy that can complicate isoniazid therapy. If the numb-
        ness were caused by Pott disease, he should have back pain and other
        neurologic findings, such as lower-extremity weakness.

31.3 **A.** Because this woman is a household contact of a patient with active TB, she is among the highest risk group: her skin test would be considered positive with 5 mm induration. She has latent TB infection and should be offered treatment to prevent reactivation TB later in life. Oral contraceptives may reduce drug levels, so barrier contraception might be a better option for her.

31.4 **B.** Drug-induced hepatitis is a common complication of isoniazid and rifampin and requires periodic surveillance. Alcohol use, prior liver disease, and increased age are risk factors.

Clinical Pearls

➤ Reactivation pulmonary tuberculosis most commonly presents radiographically with infiltrates or nodules in the apical and posterior segments of the upper lobes.

➤ Tuberculin skin testing is not a diagnostic test but is a useful screening test for potential contacts of infected persons; the response cutoff for a positive test depends on the patient's level of risk.

➤ Patients with a positive tuberculin skin test and no clinical or radiographic evidence of active disease are said to have *latent tuberculosis infection;* they can be treated with isoniazid to reduce their lifetime risk of developing reactivation tuberculosis.

➤ Individuals with active tuberculosis should be initiated on multiple agents, such as isoniazid, rifampin, and pyrazinamide.

➤ Pyridoxine (vitamin B_6) usually is added to antituberculosis medications to prevent peripheral neuropathy.

REFERENCES

Campbell IA, Bah-Sow O. Pulmonary tuberculosis: diagnosis and treatment. *BMJ.* 2006;332:1194-1197.

Jasmer RM, Nahid P, Hopewell PC. Latent tuberculosis infection. *N Engl J Med.* 2002;347:1860-1866.

Raviglione MC, O'Brian R. Tuberculosis. In: Kasper DL, Braunwald E, Fauci AS, et al, eds. *Harrison's Principles of Internal Medicine.* 17th ed. New York, NY: McGraw-Hill; 2008:1006-1020.

Small PM, Fujiwara PI. Management of tuberculosis in the United States. *N Engl J Med.* 2001;345:189-200.

Case 32

A 42-year-old man complains of 2 days of worsening chest pain and dyspnea. Six weeks ago, he was diagnosed with non-Hodgkin lymphoma with lymphadenopathy of the mediastinum, and he has been treated with mediastinal radiation therapy. His most recent treatment was 1 week ago. He has no other medical or surgical history and takes no medications. His chest pain is constant and unrelated to activity. He becomes short of breath with minimal exertion. He is afebrile, heart rate 115 bpm with a thready pulse, respiratory rate 22 breaths per minute, and blood pressure 108/86 mm Hg. Systolic blood pressure drops to 86 mm Hg on inspiration. He appears uncomfortable and is diaphoretic. His jugular veins are distended to the angle of the jaw, and his chest is clear to auscultation. He is tachycardic, his heart sounds are faint, and no extra sounds are appreciated. The chest X-ray is shown in Figure 32–1.

➤ What is the most likely diagnosis?

➤ What is your next step in therapy?

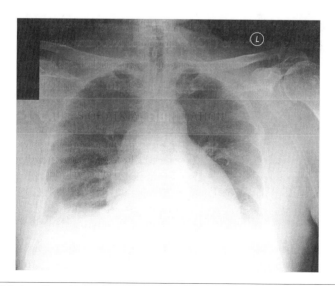

Figure 32–1. Chest X-ray. *Courtesy of Dr. Jorge Albin.*

ANSWERS TO CASE 32:
Pericardial Effusion/Tamponade Caused by Malignancy

Summary: A 42-year-old man with a thoracic malignancy and history of radiotherapy to the mediastinum now presents with chest pain, dyspnea, cardiac enlargement on chest X-ray (which could represent cardiomegaly or pericardial effusion), jugular venous distention, distant cardiac sounds, and pulsus paradoxus.

➤ **Most likely diagnosis:** Pericardial effusion causing cardiac tamponade.

➤ **Next therapeutic step:** Urgent pericardiocentesis or surgical pericardial window.

ANALYSIS

Objectives

1. Recognize pericardial tamponade; know how to check for pulsus paradoxus.
2. Know the features of cardiac tamponade, constrictive pericarditis, and restrictive cardiomyopathy and how to distinguish among them.
3. Understand the treatment of each of these conditions.
4. Know the potential cardiac complications of thoracic malignancies and radiation therapy.

Considerations

The patient described in the scenario, with his thoracic malignancy and history of radiation therapy, is at risk for diseases of the pericardium and myocardium. The jugular venous distention, distant heart sounds, and pulsus paradoxus all are suggestive of cardiac tamponade. All of these conditions can impede diastolic filling of the heart and lead to cardiovascular collapse. The major diagnostic considerations in this case, each with a very different treatment, are pericardial effusion causing cardiac tamponade, constrictive pericarditis, and restrictive cardiomyopathy. Urgent differentiation among these conditions is required, because the treatment is very different and the consequences of these diseases can be immediately fatal. Clinically, the patient's fall in systolic blood pressure with inspiration, pulsus paradoxus, is suggestive of cardiac tamponade, which would be treated by evacuating the pericardial fluid.

APPROACH TO
Suspected Cardiac Tamponade

DEFINITIONS

PERICARDIAL EFFUSION: Fluid that fills the pericardial space, which may be due to infection or malignancy. A rapid accumulating effusion may lead to cardiac compromise.

CARDIAC TAMPONADE: Increased pressure within the pericardial space caused by an accumulating effusion, which compresses the heart and impedes diastolic filling.

CLINICAL APPROACH

Cardiac tamponade refers to increased pressure within the pericardial space caused by an accumulating effusion, which compresses the heart and impedes diastolic filling. Because the heart can only pump out during systole what it receives during diastole, severe restrictions of diastolic filling lead to a marked decrease in cardiac output, which can cause cardiovascular collapse and death. If pericardial fluid accumulates slowly, the sac may dilate and hold up to 2000 mL (producing amazing cardiomegaly on chest X-ray) before causing diastolic impairment. If the fluid accumulates rapidly, as in a hemopericardium caused by trauma or surgery, as little as 200 mL can produce tamponade. The classic description of **Beck triad (hypotension, elevated jugular venous pressure, and small quiet heart)** is a description of **acute tamponade** with rapid accumulation of fluid, as in cardiac trauma or ventricular rupture. If the fluid accumulates slowly, the clinical picture may look more like congestive heart failure, with cardiomegaly on chest X-ray (although there should be no pulmonary edema), dyspnea, elevated jugular pressure, hepatomegaly, and peripheral edema. A high index of suspicion is required, and cardiac tamponade should be considered in any patient with hypotension and elevated jugular venous pressure.

The **most important physical sign** to look for **in cardiac tamponade** is **pulsus paradoxus**. This refers to a **drop in systolic blood pressure during inspiration** of more than 10 mm Hg. Although called "paradoxical," this drop in systolic blood pressure is actually not contrary to the normal physiologic variation with respiration; it is an exaggeration of the normal small drop in systolic pressure during inspiration. Although not a specific sign of tamponade (ie, it is often seen in patients with disturbed intrathoracic pressures during respiration, eg, those with obstructive lung disease), the paradoxical pulse is fairly sensitive for hemodynamically significant tamponade in almost all cases. To test for this, one must use a manual blood pressure cuff that is inflated above systolic pressure and deflated very slowly until the first Korotkoff sound is heard during expiration and then, finally, during both phases of respiration. The difference between these two pressure readings is the pulsus paradoxus. When the pulsus paradoxus is severe, it may be detected by palpation as a diminution or disappearance of peripheral pulses during inspiration.

Constrictive pericarditis is a complication of previous pericarditis, either acute or chronic fibrinous pericarditis. The inflammation with resultant granulation tissue forms a **thickened fibrotic adherent sac** that gradually contracts, encasing the heart and **impairing diastolic filling.** In the past, tuberculosis was the most common cause of this problem but now is rare in the United States. Currently, this is **most commonly caused by radiation therapy, cardiac surgery,** or any cause of acute pericarditis, such as **viral infection, uremia, or malignancy.** The pathophysiology of constrictive pericarditis is similar to that of cardiac tamponade in the restricted ability of the ventricles to fill during diastole because of the thickened noncompliant pericardium.

Because the process is **chronic,** patients with **constrictive pericarditis** generally do not present with acute hemodynamic collapse but rather with **chronic and slowly progressive weakness and fatigue and exertional dyspnea.** Patients commonly have what appears to be right-sided heart failure, that is, chronic lower-extremity edema, hepatomegaly, and ascites. Like patients with tamponade, they have elevated jugular venous pressures, but **pulsus paradoxus usually is absent.** Examination of neck veins shows an increase in jugular venous pressure during inspiration, termed **Kussmaul sign.** This is easy to see because it is the opposite of the normal fall in pressure as a person inspires. Normally, the negative intrathoracic pressure generated by inspiration sucks blood into the heart, but because of the severe diastolic restriction, the blood cannot enter the right atrium or ventricle, so it fills the jugular vein. Another physical finding characteristic of constrictive pericarditis is a **pericardial knock,** which is a high-pitched early diastolic sound occurring just after aortic valve closure. Chest radiography frequently shows cardiomegaly and a calcified pericardium.

Restrictive cardiomyopathy, like the previous diagnoses, is primarily a problem of impaired diastolic filling, usually with preserved systolic function. This is a relatively uncommon problem in the Western world. The **most common causes are amyloidosis,** an infiltrative disease of the elderly, in which an abnormal fibrillar amyloid protein is deposited in heart muscle, or fibrosis of the myocardium following radiation therapy or open heart surgery. In **Africa,** restrictive cardiomyopathy is much more common because of a process called **endomyocardial fibrosis,** characterized by fibrosis of the endocardium along with fever and marked eosinophilia, accounting for up to 25% of deaths due to heart disease.

Clinically, it may be very difficult to distinguish restrictive cardiomyopathy from constrictive pericarditis, and various echocardiographic criteria have been proposed to try to distinguish between them. In addition, magnetic resonance imaging (MRI) can be very useful to visualize or exclude the presence of the thickened pericardium typical of constrictive pericarditis. Nevertheless, it may be necessary to obtain an **endomyocardial biopsy** to make the diagnosis. Differentiation between the two is essential because constrictive pericarditis is a potentially curable disease, whereas very little effective therapy is available for either the underlying conditions or the cardiac failure of restrictive cardiomyopathy. Table 32–1 compares features of cardiac tamponade, acute pericarditis, restrictive cardiomyopathy, and constrictive pericarditis.

Treatment

Treatment of cardiac tamponade consists of relief of the pericardial pressure, either by echocardiographically guided pericardiocentesis or a surgical pericardial window. Resection of the pericardium is the definitive treatment of constrictive pericarditis. There is no effective treatment for restrictive cardiomyopathy.

Table 32–1 FEATURES OF CARDIAC TAMPONADE, ACUTE PERICARDITIS, RESTRICTIVE CARDIOMYOPATHY, AND CONSTRICTIVE PERICARDITIS

DISEASE	PATHOPHYSIOLOGY	CLINICAL FEATURES	ECG FINDINGS
Cardiac tamponade	Increased pressure in pericardial space due to effusion, impeding diastolic filling	Pulsus paradoxus, hypotension, elevated jugular venous distention, small quiet heart	Low voltage diffusely, electrical alternans
Constrictive pericarditis	Inflammation and granulation tissue forms a thickened fibrotic adherent sac, commonly caused by radiation, viral infection, uremia	Absent pulsus paradoxus, Kussmaul sign, pericardial knock Chronic and slow progressive weakness and exertional dyspnea	Low voltage
Acute pericarditis	Acute inflammation of the parietal pericardium and superficial myocardium	Chest pain, fever, pericardial rub	ST-segment elevation, low voltage diffusely
Restrictive cardiomyopathy	Myocardial fibrosis, hypertrophy, or infiltration leading to impaired diastolic filling	No pulsus paradoxus or Kussmaul sign. Progressive exertional dyspnea and dependent edema	

Comprehension Questions

32.1   A 35-year-old woman is noted to have a positive Kussmaul sign.
        Which of the following conditions does she most likely have?
        A. Constrictive pericarditis
        B. Cardiac tamponade
        C. Dilated cardiomyopathy
        D. Diabetic ketoacidosis

32.2   Which of the following is the most sensitive finding in patients with
        cardiac tamponade?
        A. Disappearance of radial pulse during inspiration
        B. Drop in systolic blood pressure more than 10 mm Hg during
           inspiration
        C. Rise in heart rate more than 20 bpm during inspiration
        D. Distant heart sounds

32.3   While awaiting pericardiocentesis, immediate supportive care of a
        patient with cardiac tamponade should include which of the following?
        A. Diuresis with furosemide
        B. Intravenous fluids
        C. Nitrates to lower venous congestion
        D. Morphine to relieve dyspnea

32.4   Which of the following is most likely to cause restrictive cardiomyopathy?
        A. Endomyocardial fibrosis
        B. Viral myocarditis
        C. Beriberi (thiamine deficiency)
        D. Doxorubicin therapy

ANSWERS

32.1   **A.** Kussmaul sign, an increase in neck veins with inspiration, is seen
        with constrictive pericarditis.

32.2   **B.** Pulsus paradoxus is a sensitive although nonspecific sign for cardiac
        tamponade.

32.3   **B.** Patients with cardiac tamponade are preload dependent, and diuretics, nitrates, or morphine may cause them to become hypotensive.

32.4   **A.** Endomyocardial fibrosis is an etiology of restrictive cardiomyopathy, common in developing countries, that is associated with
        eosinophilia. The other disease processes mentioned are causes of
        dilated cardiomyopathy.

Clinical Pearls

➤ Elevated jugular venous pressure and pulsus paradoxus are features of cardiac tamponade.

➤ Kussmaul sign and right-sided heart failure are features of constrictive cardiomyopathy, but pulsus paradoxus is not.

➤ Cardiac tamponade requires urgent treatment by pericardiocentesis or a pericardial window.

➤ Constrictive pericarditis may show calcifications of the pericardium on chest X-ray or thickened pericardium on echocardiography. Definitive therapy is resection of the pericardium.

➤ Restrictive cardiomyopathy is most often caused by amyloidosis or radiation therapy. There is no effective therapy.

REFERENCES

Bertog SC, Thambidorai SK, Parakh K, et al. Constrictive pericarditis: etiology and cause-specific survival after pericardiectomy. *J Am Coll Cardiol*. 2004;43:1445-1452.

McGregor M. Pulsus paradoxus. *N Engl J Med*. 1979;301:480-482.

Spodick DH. Acute cardiac tamponade. *N Engl J Med*. 2003;349:684-690.

Wynne J, Braunwald E. Cardiomyopathy and myocarditis. In: Kasper DL, Braunwald E, Fauci AS, et al, eds. *Harrison's Principles of Internal Medicine*. 17th ed. New York, NY: McGraw-Hill; 2008:1481-1485.

Case 33

A 23-year-old man is the next patient you see in the clinic. Under chief complaint, the nurse has written, "Wants a general checkup." You enter the room and greet a generally healthy appearing young, white man, who seems nervous. He finally admits that he has been worried about a lesion on his penis. He denies pain or dysuria. He has never had any sexually transmitted diseases (STDs) and has an otherwise unremarkable medical history. He is afebrile, and his examination is notable for a shallow clean ulcer without exudates or erythema on the glans penis, which is mildly tender to palpation. There are some small, nontender, inguinal lymph nodes bilaterally.

➤ What is the most likely diagnosis?

➤ What is the likely treatment?

ANSWERS TO CASE 33:

Syphilis

Summary: A 23-year-old healthy man reluctantly requests evaluation of a lesion on his penis. He has never had any STDs and has an otherwise unremarkable medical history. He is afebrile, and his examination is notable for a nontender ulcer on the glans penis with small, nontender inguinal lymph nodes bilaterally.

➤ **Most likely diagnosis:** Chancre of primary syphilis.

➤ **Likely treatment:** Single intramuscular injection of benzathine penicillin G.

ANALYSIS

Objectives

1. Understand the pathogenesis and natural history of *Treponema pallidum* infection.
2. Know the differential diagnosis of genital ulceration and STDs.
3. Learn the treatment of syphilis.

Considerations

This 23-year-old man reluctantly reveals his concern about a nontender ulcer of the penis. Although he has no history of STD, the most common cause of a painless ulcer of the genital area in a young, immunocompetent person is syphilis. The STDs often travel together, so he should be evaluated for other STDs such as chlamydia and human immunodeficiency virus (HIV). Other causes of genital ulcers should also be considered, including chancroid and herpes virus (both usually painful), and a superficially infected skin lesion. Compliance with therapy and follow-up are crucial because syphilitic infections can progress to a chronic form that can lead to aneurysmal dilation of the aorta as well as permanent neurologic changes. He could continue spreading the disease to others, and if he infects women of childbearing age, these women, if infected during pregnancy, could pass the infection to their newborns.

APPROACH TO

Suspected Syphilis

DEFINITIONS

PRIMARY SYPHILIS: Initial lesion of *T pallidum* infection, usually in the form of the nontender ulcer, the chancre.

SECONDARY SYPHILIS: Disseminated infection manifesting in a pruritic, maculopapular diffuse rash that classically involves the **palms and soles,** or the flat moist lesion of **condyloma lata.**

CLINICAL APPROACH

Syphilis is classically called the "great imitator" for its protean manifestations. After a decline in cases over the prior decades, the incidence of syphilis has been increasing since the 1980s. The public health consequences can be grave, so recognizing and correctly treating this disease is of great importance. An estimated 70,000 new cases of syphilis occur every year in the United States. Most occur in young adults in their twenties, and most cases are concentrated in the southern states. The number of cases reached its lowest point in the 1980s; however, the number of cases has increased since then, especially in heterosexuals, young women, and neonates. Some researchers believe this increase may be a result of cocaine use, sex for drugs trade, and perhaps the increased incidence of HIV infections.

Syphilis is caused by the spirochete *T pallidum.* The organism penetrates abraded skin or mucous membranes and then disseminates through the lymphatics and bloodstream to involve almost every organ. Within 1 week to 3 months of inoculation, a chancre usually forms at the site of entrance. Multiple ulcers may form, as in HIV-infected patients, but some patients may not notice the ulceration at all. The **chancre** of syphilis typically is **nonerythematous, with rolled borders and a clean base.** It usually is **painless,** although it may be tender if touched. Other diseases that can cause ulcerations include **chancroid;** however the ulcer in this disease usually is **painful, exudative, with ragged borders and a necrotic base,** and bleeds easily. The lymph nodes can also suppurate in chancroid, unlike in syphilis. The ulcers in **herpes simplex infections typically are painful, grouped vesicles on an erythematous base** that eventually ulcerate.

If untreated, syphilis progresses to a **second stage,** in which the disease disseminates widely, and the patient may present with a **pruritic, maculopapular diffuse rash that classically involves the palms and soles.** Patients also may have these lesions orally, called "mucous patches," and they may suffer constitutional symptoms such as fever, myalgias, and headache. Other typical skin findings include **condyloma lata,** a gray papillomatous lesion found in intertriginous areas, and patchy hair loss.

If still left untreated, the patient will pass into a quiescent, or latent, stage. Although relapses of symptoms of secondary syphilis can occur during this time, they become less frequent over years. Approximately 30% of patients will go on to develop **late-stage syphilis.** The symptoms of this stage result from the destruction of tissue caused by the chronic infection. The immune reaction to the organism causes a proliferative, obliterative endarteritis. In some organs, such as the skin, liver, and bone, these lesions are organized into **granulomas** with an amorphous or coagulated center called **gummas.**

These lesions, in themselves, are benign; however, they can cause organ dysfunction through destruction of normal tissue. In the aorta, the obliterative endarteritis involves the vasa vasorum, which leads to necrosis of the media of the arterial wall. The resulting weakness of the wall leads to the formation of **saccular aneurysmal dilations of the aorta**.

Neurosyphilis is another form of tertiary disease that may occur after secondary disease or from the latent stage. The organism disseminates to the central nervous system (CNS), causing a broad range of neurologic symptoms. In the CNS, it may cause vasculitis, leading to ischemia, stroke, and focal neurologic deficits. Patients may exhibit personality changes or dementia, demyelination of the posterior column with wide-based gait and loss of proprioception (**tabes dorsalis**), or cranial nerve impairment, including the development of the Argyll Robertson pupil (accommodates but does not react to light). Lumbar puncture to exclude neurosyphilis is generally indicated when any patient with syphilis develops neurologic or ocular symptoms or if HIV-infected patients with syphilis are relatively immunosuppressed (CD4 <350) or have a high rapid plasma reagin (RPR) titer (>1:32).

The diagnosis of syphilis is always made indirectly, as the organism has not yet been cultured. Nonspecific serologic tests, such as the RPR and Venereal Disease Research Laboratory (VDRL) tests, which actually are tests for antibodies against lipid antigens that occur as part of the host reaction to *T pallidum*, are fairly sensitive for the detection of disease. However, especially at low titers, they may be nonspecific and may result in false-positive results. Therefore, **confirmatory testing** in the form of specific antibody testing for *T pallidum*, such as the **fluorescent treponemal antibody absorption (FTA-ABS) or microhemagglutination assay for *Treponema pallidum* (MHA-TP)** test, is the next step. **Dark-field microscopy**, in which scrapings from an ulcer are placed under a phase contrast lens to actually identify the organisms, is the classic method of diagnosis but is rarely performed today. Biopsy of lesions, such as those seen in secondary syphilis with special stains, also can identify the organisms. To diagnose CNS disease, a positive cerebrospinal fluid (CSF) VDRL or RPR in the setting of increased CSF leukocytosis and protein counts, sometimes with low glucose levels, is suggestive of CNS involvement. However, false-negative results for VDRL in CSF are common, and the diagnosis is often made on clinical grounds.

Penicillin is the treatment of choice for syphilis. The most effective treatment and regimen, however, are truly unknown, because no therapeutic trials have been performed. However, current recommendations are to treat syphilis based on the stage of presentation (Table 33–1). Individuals with early disease, that is, with primary or secondary syphilis, or those with early latent syphilis (infection for <1 year) may be treated with a single intramuscular injection of benzathine penicillin G, a long-lasting intramuscular (IM) injection. For patients with late disease, that is, latent syphilis of an unknown duration (presumed to be >1 year), or with cardiovascular manifestations or with gummas, treatment is given as three weekly IM injections of benzathine penicillin G.

Table 33–1 TREATMENT OF SYPHILIS BASED ON STAGE

STAGE	CLINICAL MANIFESTATIONS	TREATMENT
Primary disease	Chancre	Single dose of intramuscular penicillin
Secondary disease, early latent (<1 y—no symptoms)	Maculopapular rash involving palms and soles, condyloma lata	Single dose of intramuscular penicillin
Late latent disease (>1 y—no symptoms)	None	Intramuscular penicillin at 1-wk intervals for total of three doses
Tertiary syphilis, neurosyphilis	Various: dementia, focal neurologic deficits, cranial nerve palsies, gummas, aortitis	Intravenous penicillin for 10-14 d

Neurosyphilis is notoriously difficult to treat. Those with CNS disease or patients concurrently infected with HIV and syphilis should receive high doses of intravenous penicillin G for 10 to 14 days or longer. Pregnant women can receive either regimen, and all patients should be followed closely to ensure that their titer falls over the year after treatment. Pregnant women who are allergic to penicillin should be desensitized and then receive penicillin, because this is the only treatment known to prevent congenital infection.

Treponema pallidum infection usually leads to a **positive specific serologic test (FTA-ABS or MHA-TP) for life**, whereas an adequately treated infection will lead to a fall in RPR serology. A **normal response** is considered a **four-fold drop in titers within 3 months** and a **negative or near-negative titer after 1 year**. A suboptimal response may mean inadequate treatment or undiagnosed tertiary disease. In any patient diagnosed with an STD, the possibility that they may have other STDs should be considered. Gonorrheal and chlamydial infections can be asymptomatic, especially in women. HIV is often asymptomatic early in the course of infection, and screening should be recommended to those persons who have histories of high-risk behaviors or who have evidence of other STDs. Hepatitis B and C are also, although less often, transmitted by sexual contact.

Comprehension Questions

33.1   A 25-year-old man presents to your office complaining of left knee and right great toe pain, which started 1 week ago and has not responded to over-the-counter pain relievers. He also has felt feverish and achy, has dysuria, and has developed an eye infection. Approximately 1 month ago, he was seen at an outside clinic and treated for syphilis. On examination, he is afebrile, and both eyes are injected and very sensitive to light. His left knee and the metatarsophalangeal (MTP) joint of his right great toe are swollen and tender. Which of the following is your diagnosis?

A. Gouty arthritis
B. Reactive arthritis (Reiter syndrome)
C. Infectious arthritis
D. Rheumatoid arthritis
E. Syphilis

33.2   As part of normal screening during pregnancy, a 28-year-old G2P1 has a positive RPR with a titer of 1:64 and a positive MHA-TP. She is allergic to penicillin, which causes shortness of breath and "swelling of her tongue." Which of the following treatments do you offer?

A. Erythromycin estolate
B. Doxycycline.
C. Tetracycline.
D. Penicillin after desensitization.
E. Vancomycin.
F. Wait until delivery of the baby before treatment.

33.3   A 23-year-old man is found to have late latent syphilis (RPR 1:64) as part of a workup following his diagnosis with HIV. He is asymptomatic with a CD4 count of 150 and does not remember having lesions or rashes in the past. Prior to starting therapy with penicillin for the syphilis, the patient should undergo which of the following procedures?

A. Lumbar puncture to exclude neurosyphilis
B. Skin biopsy to confirm the diagnosis of syphilis
C. Magnetic resonance imaging (MRI) of his brain and an electroencephalogram (EEG)
D. Skin testing to exclude penicillin allergy
E. Adjustment of his HIV medications to optimize his CD4 count prior to treatment for syphilis

33.4 A 28-year-old woman is noted to have a nontender ulcer of the vulva. A herpes culture is taken of the ulcer scraping, which is negative, and the RPR titer is negative. Which of the following is the next best step?

A. Empiric treatment with doxycycline for *Chlamydia trachomatis*
B. Empiric treatment with acyclovir for herpes simplex virus (HSV)
C. Empiric treatment with azithromycin for *Haemophilus ducreyi*
D. Dark-field microscopy
E. Biopsy for possible vulvar cancer

ANSWERS

33.1 **B.** The triad of uveitis or conjunctivitis, urethritis, and arthritis are characteristics of reactive arthritis or Reiter syndrome. This poorly understood disease is thought to be caused by immune cross-reaction between antigens in infectious organisms and the host connective tissue. Organisms commonly involved include *C trachomatis*, which this patient may have contracted when he contracted syphilis but which may not have been treated. The arthritis typically involves large joints and is both progressive and additive. The uveitis can be difficult to treat; however, the dysuria of the urethritis can be transient. Patients with Reiter syndrome are often HLA-B27–positive.

33.2 **D.** This patient should be desensitized and treated with penicillin, especially because she is pregnant and may pass the disease to her child. Following treatment, her titers should be closely followed and should show at least a fourfold decrease. Treatment of the child after delivery with intravascular (IV) penicillin should be considered.

33.3 **A.** Lumbar puncture to exclude neurosyphilis is generally indicated when any patient with syphilis develops neurologic or ocular symptoms, or if HIV-infected patients with syphilis have a CD4 less than 350 or an RPR more than 1:32.

33.4 **D.** Approximately one-third of patients who have the primary lesion of the chancre will have negative serology and require either dark-field microscopy or biopsy with special stains to identify the spirochetes. The organism is too thin to be visualized by conventional light microscopy. Empiric treatment with penicillin is reasonable if dark-field microscopy is not available. Genital herpes and chancroid should produce painful genital ulcers, and *Chlamydia* should cause nonulcerative cervicitis or urethritis.

Clinical Pearls

> ➤ Syphilitic chancres are generally clean, painless, ulcerative lesions and can be located anywhere on the body where inoculation occurred.
> ➤ The rash of secondary syphilis typically involves the palms and soles.
> ➤ Elevated RPR and VDRL tests are nonspecific and may be falsely positive in several normal conditions (pregnancy) and disease states (systemic lupus erythematosus). Specific treponemal antibody tests, such as the micro-hemagglutination assay for *Treponema pallidum* (MHA-TP) and the fluorescent treponemal antibody absorption (FTA-ABS) test, should be performed for confirmation, but once positive, they usually stay positive for life.
> ➤ A declining RPR titer can be followed to test the efficacy of therapy.
> ➤ Central nervous system involvement can be excluded only through testing of the cerebrospinal fluid.
> ➤ Treatment of syphilis is based on stage: early syphilis can be treated with a single intramuscular injection of penicillin; late latent syphilis can be treated with three weekly injections; and neurosyphilis or tertiary syphilis can be treated with intravenous penicillin for 10 to 14 days.

REFERENCES

Centers for Disease Control and Prevention. 2006 Sexually transmitted diseases treatment guidelines. *Morbidity and Mortality Weekly Report (MMWR)* 55:22.

Lukehaart SA. Syphilis. In: Fauci AS, Braunwald E, Kasper DL, eds. *Harrison's Principles of Internal Medicine*. 17th ed. New York, NY: McGraw-Hill; 2008:1038-1046.

Marra CM, Maxwell CL, Smith SL, et al. Cerebrospinal fluid abnormalities in patients with syphilis: association with clinical and laboratory features. *J Infect Dis*. 2004; 189:369-376.

Case 34

A 58-year-old man comes to see you because of shortness of breath. He has experienced mild dyspnea on exertion for a few years, but more recently he has noted worsening shortness of breath with minimal exercise and the onset of dyspnea at rest. He has difficulty reclining, and, as a result, he spends the night sitting up in a chair trying to sleep. He reports a cough with production of yellowish-brown sputum every morning throughout the year. He denies chest pain, fever, chills, or lower extremity edema. He has smoked about two packs of cigarettes per day since age 15 years. He does not drink alcohol. A few months ago, the patient went to an urgent care clinic for evaluation of his symptoms, and he received a prescription for some inhalers, the names of which he does not remember. He was also told to find a primary care physician for further evaluation. On physical examination, his blood pressure is 135/85 mm Hg, heart rate 96 bpm, respiratory rate 28 breaths per minute, and temperature 97.6°F. He is sitting in a chair, leaning forward, with his arms braced on his knees. He appears uncomfortable with labored respirations and cyanotic lips. His neck was without lymphadenopathy, carotid bruit, or jugular venous distention. He is using accessory muscles of respiration, and chest examination reveals wheezes and rhonchi bilaterally, but no crackles are noted. The anteroposterior diameter of the chest wall appears increased, and he has inward movement of the lower rib cage with inspiration. Cardiovascular examination reveals distant heart sounds but with a regular rate and rhythm. His extremities show no cyanosis, edema, or clubbing.

➤ What is the most likely diagnosis?

➤ What is the next best diagnostic test?

➤ What is the best initial treatment?

ANSWERS TO CASE 34:
Chronic Obstructive Pulmonary Disease

Summary: A 58-year-old smoker has noted worsening shortness of breath with minimal exercise and the onset of dyspnea at rest and difficulty reclining. He reports a productive cough with yellowish-brown sputum every morning throughout the year. He is sitting in a characteristic "tripod" position to facilitate use of accessory muscles of respiration. He appears to have airway obstruction with respiratory distress, with lower chest retractions, and bilateral wheezes and rhonchi. His perioral cyanosis suggests hypoxemia. The anteroposterior diameter of the chest wall appears increased, suggesting hyperinflation. Cardiovascular examination reveals distant heart sounds but no signs of significant cardiac disease.

➤ **Most likely diagnosis:** Chronic obstructive pulmonary disease (COPD) with a serious acute exacerbation.

➤ **Next diagnostic step:** Arterial blood gas to assess oxygenation and acid-base status.

➤ **Best initial treatment:** Oxygen by nasal canula, followed closely by bronchodilators, and steroids for inflammatory component.

ANALYSIS

Objectives

1. Know the definition and etiologies of chronic bronchitis, COPD, and emphysema.
2. Be familiar with spirometry and flow-volume loops for diagnosis of obstructive and restrictive lung diseases.
3. Be familiar with the treatment of chronic stable COPD, as well as management of acute exacerbations, including the indications for ventilatory assistance.

Considerations

This 58-year-old long-time smoker likely has chronic obstructive lung disease. He is now in respiratory distress with labored respirations, cyanosis, and wheezing. The urgent issue is his current respiratory status. Rapid clinical assessment is critical in case this patient is headed toward respiratory failure, perhaps necessitating intubation and mechanical ventilation. An arterial blood gas will quickly provide information regarding the adequacy of oxygenation status (PaO_2) and ventilation ($PaCO_2$).

APPROACH TO
Chronic Obstructive Pulmonary Disease

DEFINITIONS

CHRONIC BRONCHITIS: Clinical diagnosis characterized by excessive secretion of bronchial mucus and productive cough for 3 months or more in at least 2 consecutive years in the absence of any other disease that might account for this symptom.

CHRONIC OBSTRUCTIVE PULMONARY DISEASE (COPD): Disease state characterized by the presence of airflow obstruction caused by chronic bronchitis or emphysema. The airflow obstruction usually is progressive, may be accompanied by airway hyperreactivity, and may be partially reversible. Typically the forced expiratory volume in first second of expiration (FEV_1) will be less than 80% of expected, and some use a staging system of FEV_1/FVC (forced vital capacity) less than 0.7 (mild), 0.3 to 0.5 (moderate), and less than 0.3 (severe).

EMPHYSEMA: Pathologic diagnosis that denotes abnormal, permanent enlargement of air spaces distal to the terminal bronchiole, with destruction of their walls and without obvious fibrosis.

SPIROMETRY: Method of evaluating respiratory flow volumes and flow rates to assess pulmonary function.

FORCED VITAL CAPACITY (FVC): Total volume of air expired after full inspiration. FVC is reduced in restrictive lung disease. Patients with obstructive lung disease usually have normal FVC.

FEV_1: Volume of air expired in the first second during maximal expiratory effort. FEV_1 is reduced in both obstructive lung disease (increased airway resistance) and restrictive lung disease (low vital capacity).

FEV_1/FVC: Percentage of the vital capacity that is expired during the first second of maximal effort.

RESTRICTIVE LUNG DISEASE: Chronic pulmonary disorders characterized by low lung volumes either because of alterations of the lung parenchyma (intrinsic), or chest wall, pleura, respiratory muscles (extrinsic). Typically the FVC is reduced, and FEV_1 is reduced, but the FEV_1/FVC is normal. The diagnosis is best made by a reduced total lung capacity (TLC).

CLINICAL APPROACH

The most common etiology for COPD is inhalation injury, specifically cigarette smoking. Another important cause is α_1-**antitrypsin deficiency**, which is hereditary. The disease may become evident by age 40 years and often occurs without cough or smoking history. Therapy by replacement of α_1-antitrypsin enzyme is available. Characteristically, patients with COPD present with progressively worsening dyspnea (first on exertion, then with activity, then at rest). Patient

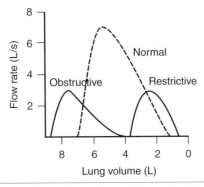

Figure 34–1. Expiratory flow volume loops of normal, obstructive, and restrictive lung disease.

may vary in appearance from a "blue bloater" (chronic bronchitis, overweight, edematous, cyanotic) to a "pink puffer" (emphysema, thin, ruddy cheeks).

Arterial blood gases (ABG) often are normal in the early phase of the disease; however, in more advanced disease, there is evidence of hypoxemia and hypercapnea, Often with a chronic compensated respiratory acidosis as a consequence of CO_2 retention. Such chronic stable patients may have a PaO_2 near 50 mm Hg and a $PaCO_2$ near 50 mm Hg, but a near-normal pH (the "50-50" club). During an acute exacerbation, more severe hypoxemia or hypercapnea, or respiratory acidosis noted on ABG may be an indication of impending respiratory failure and need for ventilatory support.

Spirometry is the most basic, inexpensive, widely valuable pulmonary function test to diagnose pulmonary diseases (Figure 34–1). Spirometric tracings of **forced expiration** (Figure 34–2) and **flow-volume loops** (Figure 34–3) help to identify the type of lung disease (obstructive vs restrictive), as well as potential reversibility of airflow obstruction. **Restrictive lung diseases tend to have lower lung volumes (decreased TLC and VC [vital capacity]), whereas obstructive diseases have larger lung volumes (TLC normal or increased) with decreased expiratory flow rates (reduced FEV_1 to <80% expected, and FEV_1/FVC <0.7)** . Specific parameters help to classify the type and degree of lung dysfunction (Table 34–1). Reduced FEV_1/FVC with minimal response to bronchodilators is the hallmark of COPD.

Management of severe COPD exacerbations focuses simultaneously on relieving airway obstruction and correcting life-threatening abnormalities of gas exchange. Bronchodilators (beta-agonist and anticholinergic agents) are administered via handheld nebulizers; high-dose systemic glucocorticoids accelerate the rate of improvement in lung function among these patients; antibiotics should be given if there is suspicion of a respiratory infection. Controlled oxygen administration with nasal oxygen at low flows or oxygen with Venturi masks will correct hypoxemia without causing severe hypercapnia. Caution must be exercised in patients with chronic respiratory insufficiency whose

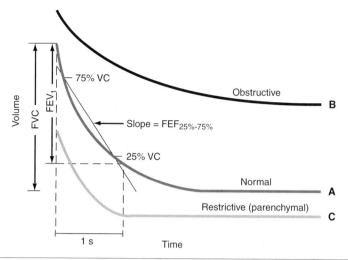

Figure 34–2. Spirographic tracing of fored expiration, comparing normal tracing (A) with that of patients with obstructive (B) and restrictive (C) lung disease. Calculation of FVC, FEV$_1$, and FEF 25%-75% are shown for the normal tracing. The curves are positioned to show the relative starting lung volumes in each of these different conditions. Lung volumes increase to the left on the horizontal axis. VC, vital capacity. *Reproduced, with permission, from Braunwald E, Fauci AS, Kasper KL, et al,* Harrison's Principles of Internal Medicine, *17th ed. New York: McGraw-Hill, 2008: 1586.*

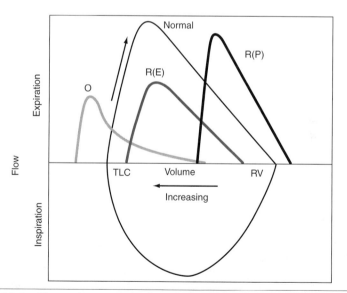

Figure 34–3. Flow-volume curves showing forced inspiratory and expiratory volumes in lung disease: O = obstructive lung disease, eg COPD; R(P) = parenchymal restrictive disease, eg, pulmonary fibroasis; R(E) = extraparenchymal restrictive disease, eg, chest wall deformity, with limitation of both inspiration and expiration. Lung volumes increase to the left on the horizontal axis. TLC, total lung capacity. VC, vital capacity. *Reproduced, with permission, from Braunwald E, Fauci AS, Kasper KL, et al,* Harrison's Principles of Internal Medicine, *17th ed. New York: McGraw-Hill, 2008: 1588.*

Table 34–1 · TREATMENT OF SYPHILIS BASED ON STAGE

	OBSTRUCTIVE LUNG DISEASE	RESTRICTIVE LUNG DISEASE	
Pulmonary Function Tests	Decreased FEV_1 <80% of predicted; FEV_1/FVC <0.7; TLC usually normal or increased; diffusion capacity decreased	Decreased lung volumes: decreased VC and TLC (this is diagnostic hallmark); FEV_1 decreased; normal FEV_1/FVC	
Example of Diseases	**BABE** Bronchiectasis (ie, cystic fibrosis) Asthma Bronchitis (chronic) Emphysema	Extrapulmonary: poor breathing mechanics; **PMS** Poliomyelitis Myasthenia Gravis scoliosis	Pulmonary: poor lung expansion; **PAPI** Pneumonia ARDS Pulmonary edema Interstitial fibrosis

Abbreviations: ARDS, acute respiratory distress syndrome; FEV1, forced expiratory volume in first second; FVC, forced vital capacity; PAPI Pneumonia ARDS Pulmonary edema Interstitial fibrosis; TLC, total lung capacity; VC, vital capacity.

respiratory drive is dependent on "relative hypoxemia"; these individuals may become apneic if excessive oxygen is administered.

Positive-pressure mask ventilation, such as continuous positive airway pressure (CPAP) or biphasic positive airway pressure (BiPAP), offers an alternative to intubation and mechanical ventilation in the treatment of cooperative patients with an acute exacerbation of COPD and severe hypercapnia. Signs of **acute respiratory failure** include **tachypnea** (respiratory rate >40 breaths per minute), **inability to speak** because of dyspnea, **accessory muscle use with fatigue** despite maximal therapy, confusion, restlessness, agitation, lethargy, a rising $PaCO_2$ **level,** and extreme **hypoxemia.** Acute respiratory failure is generally treated with endotracheal intubation with ventilatory support to correct the gas-exchange disorders. Complications of mechanical ventilation include difficulty in extubation, ventilator-associated pneumonia, pneumothorax, and acute respiratory distress syndrome.

Long-term complications of COPD from hypoxemia can cause pulmonary hypertension, secondary erythrocytosis, exercise limitation, and impaired mental functioning. **For patients with COPD who are stable, only** smoking cessation, supplemental oxygen therapy **for patients with chronic hypoxemia, and** lung volume reduction **surgery in selected patients have been shown to alter the natural history of the disease, and provide any reduction in mortality.**

Patients with a resting hypoxemia (PaO_2 <55 mm Hg) generally benefit from home oxygen therapy, which must be utilized at least 18 hours per day. Other therapies such as inhaled bronchodilators (beta agonists and/or anticholinergics) or inhaled glucocorticoids are for symptomatic relief, and to try to reduce the frequency of exacerbations.

Comprehension Questions

34.1 Which of the following are the most likely physical examination findings in a patient with emphysema?
  A. Diffuse expiratory wheezing
  B. Clubbing of the fingers
  C. Bibasilar inspiratory crackles with increased jugular venous pressure (JVP)
  D. Inspiratory stridor
  E. Third heart sound

34.2 Which of the following findings are you most likely to encounter in an 80-year-old woman with severe kyphoscoliosis?
  A. Enlarged overall lung volume (TLC)
  B. Alveolar hypoventilation
  C. Decreased FEV_1/FVC
  D. Increased vital capacity (VC)
  E. ABG with pH 7.48 and $PaCO_2$ of 32 mm Hg.

34.3 A 56-year-old woman admits to a 60-pack-year smoking history. She complains of fatigue and dyspnea with minimal exertion, and a cough that is productive each morning. Which of the following is the most likely finding in this patient?
  A. Normal diffusing capacity of lung for carbon monoxide (DLCO)
  B. Decreased residual volume
  C. Normal to slightly increased forced expiratory volume in first second (FEV_1)
  D. Decreased forced expiratory volume in first second/forced vital capacity (FEV_1/FVC)
  E. Decreased forced vital capacity (FVC)

34.4 Which of the following therapies is most likely to provide the greatest benefit to a patient with chronic stable emphysema and a resting oxygen saturation of 86%?
  A. Inhaled tiotropium daily
  B. Inhaled albuterol as needed
  C. Oral prednisone daily
  D. Supplemental oxygen used at night
  E. Supplemental oxygen used continuously

ANSWERS

34.1   **A.** COPD is characterized by chronic airway obstruction, with most airflow resistance occurring in small airways of the lower respiratory tract, producing expiratory wheezing. Inspiratory stridor would occur with upper airway, usually extrathoracic, obstruction. Clubbing is not generally a feature of COPD and should prompt investigation for another disease process such as a bronchogenic carcinoma. Crackles, elevated JVP, and an S_3 are signs of congestive heart failure.

34.2   **C.** Chest wall deformities can lead to chronic hypoventilation with elevated $PaCO_2$ levels, as well as with recurrent pulmonary infection. The pattern on pulmonary function testing is usually that of a restrictive pattern, with decreased lung volumes and compliance.

34.3   **D.** This patient likely has COPD, based on the smoking history and symptoms. A decrease in the forced expiratory volume in first second/forced vital capacity ratio is the hallmark of airflow obstruction. The FEV_1 is decreased in obstructive, as well as in restrictive, lung disease. The diffusing capacity is typically deceased in COPD as well as intrinsic restrictive lung disease. The DLCO indicates the adequacy of the alveolar-capillary membrane; the residual volume is the volume of air remaining in the lungs after a maximal expiratory effort and is usually increased in COPD due to air trapping.

34.4   **E.** For patients with chronic hypoxemia, supplemental oxygen has a significant impact on mortality, with a greater benefit with continuous usage, rather than intermittent or nocturnal-only usage. Bronchodilators such as tiotropium and albuterol improve symptoms and improve FEV_1, but offer no mortality benefit. Chronic use of oral corticosteroids should be avoided because of unfavorable side effects such as osteoporosis, glucose intolerance, and gastrointestinal (GI) side effects.

Clinical Pearls

➤ Patients with obstructive lung disease have trouble blowing air out (reduced FEV_1/FVC), whereas patients with restrictive lung disease have trouble getting air in (reduced TLC).

➤ The mainstay for treatment of chronic obstructive pulmonary disease exacerbations includes bronchodilators, oxygen, and glucocorticoids, as well as antibiotics if infection is suspected.

➤ Controlled supplemental oxygen along with positive-pressure mask ventilation (biphasic positive airway pressure) may prevent respiratory failure requiring intubation.

➤ Smoking cessation and supplemental oxygen to treat chronic hypoxemia are the only medical therapies shown to decrease mortality among persons with chronic obstructive pulmonary disease.

➤ The hallmark of restrictive lung disease is decreased lung capacities, particularly the TLC but also the FVC.

➤ Whereas in obstructive and restrictive lung disease, the FEV_1 is decreased, the FEV_1/FVC is decreased in obstructive processes and normal in restrictive processes.

REFERENCES

Reilly JJ, Silverman EK, Shapiro SD. Chronic obstructive pulmonary disease. In: Kasper DL, Braunwald E, Fauci AS, et al, eds. *Harrison's Principles of Internal Medicine*. 17th ed. New York, NY: McGraw-Hill; 2008:1635-1643.

Sutherland ER, Chemiak RM. Management of chronic obstructive pulmonary disease. *N Engl J Med*. 2004;350:2689-2697.

Weinberger SE, Rosen IM. Disturbances of respiratory function. In: Fauci AS, Braunwald E, Kasper DL, eds. *Harrison's Principles of Internal Medicine*. 17th ed. New York, NY: McGraw-Hill; 2008:1586-1592.

Case 35

A 37-year-old man presents to your office with the complaint of cough. The cough began approximately 3 months prior to this appointment, and it has become more annoying to the patient. The cough is nonproductive and worse at night, and after exercise. He has had a sedentary lifestyle but recently started an exercise program, including jogging, and says he is having a much harder time with the exertion. He just runs out of breath earlier than he used to previously, and he coughs a great deal. He has not had any fever, blood-tinged sputum, or weight loss. He denies nasal congestion and headaches. He does not smoke and has no significant medical history. His examination is notable for a blood pressure of 134/78 mm Hg and lungs that are clear to auscultation bilaterally, except for an occasional expiratory wheeze on forced expiration. A chest radiograph is read as normal.

➤ What is the most likely diagnosis?

➤ How would you confirm the diagnosis?

ANSWERS TO CASE 35:

Chronic Cough/Asthma

Summary: A 37-year-old nonsmoking man complains of a 3-month history of a nonproductive cough that is worse at night and with exercise. He does not have fevers or other symptoms to suggest infection. He is normotensive, and his lungs are clear to auscultation bilaterally, except for an occasional expiratory wheeze on forced expiration. A chest radiograph is read as normal.

> **Most likely diagnosis:** Reactive airway disease (asthma).

> **Confirmation of diagnosis:** Pulmonary function tests, with methacholine challenge if indicated.

ANALYSIS

Objectives

1. Know the differential diagnosis of chronic cough in adult patients.
2. Understand the stepwise approach to finding the cause of cough in these patients.
3. Learn how to diagnose and treat reactive airway disease (asthma).

Considerations

This is a 37-year-old man who presents with a chronic cough of more than 8-week duration. With the history of exercise intolerance, worsening cough at night, and occasional wheezes on examination, asthma is the most likely diagnosis in this patient. A chest radiograph is important to evaluate for more serious processes such as tumor, infection, or parenchymal abnormality; this is especially true of smokers but also in nonsmokers. A focused history should look for exposure to environmental irritants, medications such as angiotensin-converting enzyme (ACE) inhibitors, or possible underlying disorders such as post-nasal drip or gastroesophageal reflux.

APPROACH TO

Chronic Cough

DEFINITIONS

ACUTE COUGH: Condition for less than 3 weeks, most commonly caused by acute upper respiratory infection but also may be caused by congestive heart failure, pneumonia, and pulmonary embolism.

ASTHMA: Condition of bronchial hyperactivity and smooth muscle hypertrophy leading to a chronic inflammatory condition of the airways associated with widespread bronchospasm that is reversible.

CHRONIC COUGH: Condition for longer than 3 to 8 weeks (case definitions vary), which in a smoker may be suspicious for chronic obstructive pulmonary disease (COPD) or bronchogenic carcinoma; in a nonsmoker with a normal chest radiograph and not taking an ACE inhibitor; may be postnasal drip, gastrophageal reflux disease (GERD), or asthma.

CLINICAL APPROACH

Chronic cough represents a common complaint and a large portion of healthcare dollars. Physiologically, cough serves two main functions: (1) to protect the lungs against aspiration and (2) to clear secretions or other material into more proximal airways to be expectorated from the tracheobronchial tree. Patients with hemoptysis, immunocompromised states, comorbidities such as COPD or cystic fibrosis, current or previous infections such as tuberculosis or human immunodeficiency virus (HIV), and significant symptoms such as weight loss, night sweats, and chills are beyond the scope of this discussion.

Evaluation of chronic cough begins with a detailed history and physical examination, including smoking habits, complete medication list, environmental and occupational exposures, and any history of asthma or obstructive lung disease. Specific questions regarding the precipitating factors, duration, character, and development of the cough should be elicited. Although the physical examination or nature of the cough rarely identifies the cause, meticulous review of the ears, nose, throat, and lungs may suggest a particular diagnosis. For example, a cobblestone appearance of the oropharynx (representing lymphoid hyperplasia) or boggy erythematous nasal mucosa can be consistent with postnasal drip. **End-expiratory wheezing suggests active bronchospasm,** whereas **localized wheezing may be consistent with a foreign body or a bronchogenic tumor.**

In more than 90% of cases, a negative chest radiograph in an immunocompetent nonsmoker guides the physician to one of three diagnoses: **postnasal drip, asthma, or GERD.** In the outpatient setting, the mainstay of diagnosis relates to the response with empiric therapy, and multiple etiologies are addressed in terms of treatment. Often, a definitive diagnosis for chronic cough depends on observing a successful response to therapy. A rational approach includes stopping an ACE inhibitor if present, chest radiograph, and avoiding irritants. If persistent, then three conditions—postnasal drip, asthma, GERD—should be considered. Referral to a pulmonologist is recommended when the diagnostic and empiric therapy options are exhausted. If suspicion for carcinoma is high, a high-resolution computed tomographic (CT) scan of the thorax or bronchoscopy should be actively pursued. A diagnosis of psychogenic cough should be one of exclusion. See Figure 35–1 for example of an algorithm.

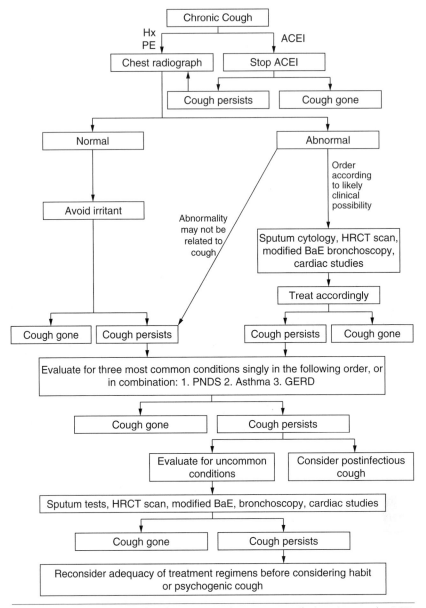

Figure 35–1. Algorithm for diagnosis and treatment of chronic cough. ACEI, angiotensin-converting enzyme inhibitor; BaE, barium esophagography; GERD, gastroesophageal reflux disease; HRCT, high-resolution computed tomography; Hx, history; PE, physical examination; PNDS, postnasal drip syndrome. *Data from Irwin RS, Boulet L-P, Cloutier MM, et al. Managing cough as a defense mechanism and as a symptom: a consensus panel report of the American College of Chest Physicians. Chest. 1998;114(suppl): 133S-181S.*

Postnasal Drip

Postnasal drip syndrome can be attributed to sinusitis and the following types of rhinitis, alone or in combination: nonallergic, allergic, postinfectious, vasomotor, drug-induced, and environmental irritant–induced. Because the symptoms may be nonspecific (eg, frequent throat clearing, nasal discharge, or sensation of liquid in the throat), no definitive diagnostic criteria exist for postnasal drip, and response to therapy confirms the diagnosis. Initial treatment for a nonallergic etiology usually includes combination treatment with a first-generation antihistamine and a decongestant for 3 weeks. For allergic rhinitis, a newer-generation antihistamine, along with a nasal corticosteroid, should be used. If the patient's symptoms do not improve, sinus radiographs may be ordered. Opacification, air-fluid levels, or mucosal thickening could suggest sinusitis, which should be treated with antibiotics.

Asthma

Although wheezing is considered a classic sign of reactive airway disease, cough is often the only symptom. Cough-variant asthma usually presents with a dry cough that occurs throughout the day and night that is worsened by airway inflammation from viral infections of the upper respiratory tract, allergies, cold air, or exercise. Although the history may be suggestive of asthma, the diagnosis should be confirmed with pulmonary function tests. Spirometry can confirm airflow obstruction with reduced FEV_1 and FEV_1/FVC, as well as reversibility with increased FEV_1 after inhalation of beta-agonist. If the diagnosis is in doubt, airway hyperresponsiveness (the fundamental pathophysiologic abnormality in asthma) can be confirmed by reduced FEV_1 after challenge with methacholine or histamine. A positive methacholine challenge is generally defined as reversible obstruction with an increase in FEV_1 of more than or equal to 12% after bronchodilator treatment. Management of asthma should be aimed at bronchodilators for rapid relief of symptoms, and asthma controllers, which inhibit airway inflammation. Initial empiric treatment usually includes inhaled bronchodilators for intermittent bronchospasm as well as inhaled or oral corticosteroids to reduce airway inflammation. Therapy is initiated in a stepwise approach, based on frequency and severity of symptoms (Table 35–1).

Gastroesophageal Reflux Disease

Gastrophageal reflux disease often can be clinically inapparent, and it may be the primary or coexisting cause of the cough, often as a result of aspiration and vagal stimulation. Initial treatment includes lifestyle modification along with medical therapy. Recommendations include a, low-fat diet; elevation of the head of the bed; avoidance of caffeine, alcohol, peppermint, and chocolate; smoking cessation; and weight reduction. If the cough does not resolve with lifestyle changes, daily treatment with an H_2 receptor antagonist such as famotidine, or a proton pump inhibitor such as omeprazole, should be initiated.

Table 35–1 GUIDELINES FOR DIAGNOSIS AND MANAGEMENT OF ASTHMA

CLASSIFICATION	STEP	DAYS WITH SYMPTOMS	NIGHTS WITH SYMPTOMS	DAILY MEDICATION	QUICK RELIEF MEDICATION
Severe persistent	4	Continual	Frequent	High-dose inhaled steroids and long-acting inhaled β_2-agonist; if needed, add oral steroids	Short-acting inhaled β_2-agonist, as needed; oral steroids may be required
Moderate persistent	3	Daily	>1/wk	Low-to-medium–dose inhaled steroids and long-acting inhaled β_2-agonist (preferred) or medium-dose inhaled steroids or low-to-medium–dose inhaled steroids and either leukotriene modifier or theophylline	Short-acting inhaled β_2-agonist, as needed; oral steroids may be required
Mild persistent	2	>2/wk, but <1 time/d	>2/mo	Low-dose inhaled steroids (preferred) or cromolyn, leukotriene modifier, or nedocromil, or sustained-release theophylline to serum concentration of 5-15 μg/mL	Short-acting inhaled β_2-agonist, as needed; oral steroids may be required
Mild intermittent	1	<2/wk	<2/mo	No daily medications	Short-acting inhaled β_2-agonist, as needed; oral steroids may be required

If acid suppression does not resolve the symptoms, a gastric motility stimulant such as metoclopramide can be added.

Patients who remain symptomatic after maximal medical treatment often benefit from 24-hour esophageal pH monitoring to confirm the diagnosis. An esophagogastroduodenoscopy showing esophagitis or an upper gastrointestinal radiographic series demonstrating reflux further supports the diagnosis. Of note, gastrointestinal symptoms may resolve prior to resolution of the cough, and full resolution may require 2 to 3 months of intensive medical therapy.

Comprehension Questions

35.1 A patient with known asthma undergoing therapy with inhaled corticosteroid and intermittent (short-acting) β_2-agonist presents with complaints of nocturnal awakenings secondary to cough and occasional wheezing. This episode occurs three to four times per week. Pulmonary function tests in the past have shown mild obstructive lung disease. Which of the following is the best next step?
A. Oral steroids
B. Leukotriene inhibitors
C. Long-acting β_2-agonists
D. Theophylline
E. Antireflux therapy

35.2 Which of the following is most accurate?
A. Cough caused by captopril may resolve with switching to enalapril.
B. Initial treatment of a chronic cough should include codeine or a similar opiate derivative to suppress the cough.
C. Cough caused by reflux can be effectively ruled out by a negative history of heartburn or dyspepsia.
D. More than one condition often is responsible for causing a chronic cough in a given patient.

35.3 A 22-year-old African American woman presents with fatigue, arthralgias, and a nagging dry cough for the past 6 weeks, but no shortness of breath. On physical examination, her lungs are clear to auscultation, and she has bilateral pretibial tender erythematous raised nodules. Which of the following is your best next step?
A. Chest radiograph
B. High-resolution CT
C. Empiric treatment for postnasal drip
D. Antinuclear antibody
E. Initiation of antituberculosis therapy

35.4   An obese 50-year-old man with a history of asthma returns with com-
        plaints of occasional dyspepsia and nocturnal cough. He wakes up in
        the morning with a sour taste in his mouth. His current medications
        include inhaled corticosteroid and a short-acting β_2-agonist. Which of
        the following should be your next step?
        A. 24-Hour esophageal pH monitoring
        B. Chest radiograph
        C. Initiation of omeprazole
        D. Short course of oral corticosteroids
        E. Initiation of allergy desensitization

ANSWERS

35.1   **C.** Long-acting β_2-agonists are helpful in this situation. The asthma
        would be classified as moderate persistent, and the recommended
        treatment is long-acting β_2-agonists, such as salmeterol, which are
        particularly helpful with nocturnal symptoms.

35.2   **D.** Often more than one condition is responsible for causing a chronic
        cough in a given patient. Cough from ACE inhibitors are class
        dependent, and change to another class of antihypertensives is more
        appropriate. The etiology of chronic cough should be determined prior
        to suppression of the cough because treatment of the underlying con-
        dition is the most effective approach. The GERD may present with the
        sole manifestation of cough, or it may present "silently."

35.3   **A.** The patient has clinical features suggestive of sarcoidosis given
        the new cough, myalgias, and description of erythema nodosum. The
        initial, most cost-effective study is a chest radiograph. Hilar lym-
        phadenopathy with or without interstitial infiltrates would solidify a
        diagnosis of sarcoidosis. A high-resolution CT may be ordered if the
        patient has interstitial lung disease, but it is not the first study of
        choice. Postnasal drip does not explain the patient's other symptoms.
        An antinuclear antibody would not necessarily identify the cause of
        the cough or provide a diagnosis.

35.4   **C.** Initiation of omeprazole, a proton pump inhibitor, dyspepsia and
        the sour taste suggest GERD. Other recommendations include dietary
        modifications and weight reduction. Twenty-four–hour esophageal
        pH monitoring is indicated only if the medications did not help.
        Oral corticosteroids could be a consideration if the clinical scenario
        is more consistent with asthma exacerbation.

Clinical Pearls

➤ A normal chest radiograph excludes most, but not all, of the serious and uncommon causes of chronic cough.

➤ The three most common causes of chronic cough in immunocompetent nonsmokers who are not taking angiotensin-converting enzyme inhibitors are postnasal drip, asthma, and gastroesophageal reflux disease.

➤ Cough caused by ACE inhibitors can occur in patients who have been stable on their medication for some time.

➤ Treatment of asthma is a stepwise process based on frequency of symptoms and response to prescribed medications.

➤ Asthma can be the cause of cough in a patient with normal examination and pulmonary function tests. If suspicion is high, a methacholine challenge, if positive, has a high predictive value.

➤ Definitive diagnosis of the etiology of chronic cough is not always necessary for successful treatment.

REFERENCES

Barnes PJ. Asthma. In: Fauci AS, Braunwald E, Kasper DL, eds. *Harrison's Principles of Internal Medicine*. 17th ed. New York, NY: McGraw-Hill; 2008:1596-1607.

Irwin RS, Bauman MH, Bolser DC, et al. Diagnosis and management of cough executive summary: ACCP evidence-based clinical practice guidelines. *Chest*. 2006; 129(suppl 1): 1S-23S.

Irwin RS, Madison JM. The diagnosis and treatment of cough. *N Engl J Med*. 2000;343:1715-1721.

Morice AH, Kastelik JA. Chronic cough in adults. *Thorax*. 2003;58:901-907.

Williams SG, Schmidt DK, Redd SC, et al. National Asthma Education and Prevention Program. Key clinical activities for quality asthma care. Recommendations of the National Asthma Education and Prevention Program. *MMWR Recomm Rep*. 2003;52(RR-6):1-8.

Case 36

A 63-year-old African American woman is brought to the emergency room for upper arm pain and swelling following a fall at home. The family has noted that for approximately the past 2 months, the patient has become progressively fatigued and absent-minded, and she has developed loss of appetite and weight loss. She has been getting up to urinate several times per night and complains of thirst; however, a test for diabetes in her doctor's office was negative. This morning, she lost her balance because she felt "lightheaded" and fell, landing on her left arm. Physical examination is notable for an elderly, thin woman in mild distress as a result of pain. She is afebrile; her blood pressure is 110/70 mm Hg and heart rate 80 bpm. Her thyroid gland is normal to palpation. Her mucus membranes are somewhat dry and sticky. Heart and lung examinations are normal, and carotid auscultation reveals no bruits. Examination of her extremities is significant only for deformity of the left mid-humerus with swelling. The left radial pulse is 2+ and symmetric. The radiologist calls you to confirm the fracture of the mid-left humerus but also states that there is the suggestion of some lytic lesions of the proximal humerus and recommends a skull film. Serum creatinine level is 2.1 mg/dL, with normal electrolyte and glucose concentrations, but serum calcium level is 13 mg/dL and hemoglobin level is 9.2 g/dL.

➤ What is the most likely diagnosis?

➤ What is the most likely underlying etiology in this patient?

➤ What is your next therapeutic step?

ANSWERS TO CASE 36:
Hypercalcemia/Multiple Myeloma

Summary: A 63-year-old African American woman is evaluated for a humeral fracture sustained during a fall because of lightheadedness. She has a 2-month history of fatigue, absent-mindedness, loss of appetite and weight, and nocturia. Her vital signs are normal, and she appears dehydrated. In addition to the fracture seen on X-ray, she also has lytic lesions of the proximal humerus. She has renal insufficiency, anemia, and hypercalcemia.

➤ **Most likely diagnosis:** Hypercalcemia with pathologic fracture of the left humerus.

➤ **Most likely underlying etiology:** Multiple myeloma.

➤ **Next therapeutic step:** Initial therapy of the hypercalcemia with intravenous (IV) fluids could be started in the emergency room.

ANALYSIS

Objectives

1. Know the clinical presentation and differential diagnosis of hypercalcemia.
2. Know the treatment of symptomatic hypercalcemia.

Considerations

The patient presents with acute confusion, fatigue, and lethargy, all symptoms of hypercalcemia, consistent with the calcium level of 13 mg/dL. The first step in therapy should be intravenous saline to restore volume status and facilitate urinary calcium excretion. Given the rapidity of onset of symptoms, weight loss, age, and presence of lytic bone lesions, the first concern should be for malignancy, such as multiple myeloma, or bony metastases from an undiagnosed cancer. Both serum and urine electrophoresis would help to identify the presence of a monoclonal gammopathy. Normal serum parathyroid hormone (PTH) and parathyroid hormone-related protein (PTHrP) levels would exclude other causes of hypercalcemia (diagnostic algorithm is given in Figure 36–1 and causes of hypercalcemia in Table 36–1). Treatment then can be aimed at the underlying cause (Table 36–2).

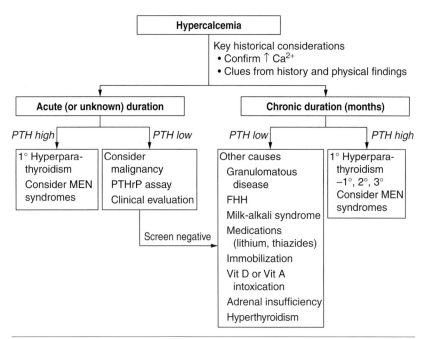

Figure 36–1.   Algorithm for evaluation of patients with hypercalcemia. FHH, familial hypocalciuric hypercalcemia; MEN, multiple endocrine neoplasia; PTH, parathyroid hormone; PTHrP, parathyroid hormone-related protein. *Reproduced, with permission, from Potts JT. Diseases of the parathyroid gland and other hyper- and hypocalcemia disorders. In: Braunwald E, Fauci AS, Kasper DL, et al, eds.* Harrison's Principles of Internal Medicine. *16th ed. New York, NY: McGraw-Hill; 2005:2260.*

Table 36–1 CAUSES OF HYPERCALCEMIA

DISEASE PROCESS	MECHANISM	CLINICAL PRESENTATION	DIAGNOSTIC CRITERIA	TREATMENT
Primary hyperparathyroidism	Elevated parathyroid hormone leading to increased turnover of bone	Solitary adenoma or part of multiple endocrine neoplasia (MEN); nephrolithiasis, peptic ulcers, and mental changes (bones, groans, etc.)	Hypercalcemia, hypophosphatemia, elevated PTH	Medical therapy for mild symptoms; surgery for symptoms of hypercalciuria or osteoporosis
Lithium therapy	Stimulation of PTH	Same as with primary hyperparathyroidism	Same as with primary hyperparathyroidism	Discontinue lithium if symptoms
Malignancy-related hypercalcemia	Local destruction of bone (multiple myeloma or leukemia or lymphoma) or humoral release of PTHrP (solid tumors such as breast, renal, or lung cancer)	Symptoms of hypercalcemia and of the particular cancer	Imaging of bones (either plain film or CT), PTHrP levels, bone marrow biopsy	Treatment of the tumor and control of cancer, biphosphonates, calcitonin

Table 36–1 CAUSES OF HYPERCALCEMIA (CONTINUED)

DISEASE PROCESS	MECHANISM	CLINICAL PRESENTATION	DIAGNOSTIC CRITERIA	TREATMENT
Sarcoidosis (and other granulomatous disorders)	Excess 1,25(OH)$_2$D synthesized in macrophages and lymphocytes	Usually few symptoms	Low PTH levels and elevated 1,25(OH)$_2$D levels	Avoidance of sunlight, decrease vitamin D and calcium intake; glucocorticoids if needed
Excessive vitamin D intake	Increased calcium intestinal absorption and, if severe, bone resorption	Symptoms of hypercalcemia	Low PTH levels, markedly elevated levels of 25(OH)$_2$D, and normal 1,25(OH)$_2$D levels	Glucocorticoids and, if needed, intensive hypercalcemia management
Renal insufficiency	Secondary hyperparathyroidism as a result of partial resistance to PTH effects	Bone pain, pruritus, ectopic calcification, osteomalacia	Elevated renal function tests	Limit dietary phosphate intravenous calcitriol

Abbreviations: CT, computed tomography; PTHrP, parathyroid hormone-related protein; PTH, parathyroid hormone.

Table 36–2 TREATMENT OF HYPERCALCEMIA

TREATMENT	ONSET	ADVERSE EFFECTS
Hydration ± loop diuretic	Acute (effect seen in hours)	Volume overload, electrolyte disturbances
Bisphosphonates	Subacute (1-2 d)	Hypophosphatemia, hypomagnesemia, hypocalcemia, osteonecrosis of jaw
Calcitonin	Acute (hours)	Efficacy short-lived (tachyphylaxis)
Glucocorticoids (effective in cancer-induced hypercalcemia)	Lengthy (days)	Hyperglycemia, osteoporosis, immune suppression
Dialysis (renal insufficiency)	Acute (hours)	Volume shifts, electrolyte disorders, complicated procedure

APPROACH TO

Hypercalcemia

DEFINITIONS

CORRECTED CALCIUM LEVEL: Add 0.8 mg/dL to the serum total calcium for every 1 g/dL of albumin level below 4 g/dL. Example: If the serum calcium level is 9.0 mg/dL and the albumin level is 2.0 g/dL, the corrected calcium level is 10.6 mg/dL.

HYPERCALCEMIA: Elevated serum calcium levels after correction for albumin concentration (normal range approximately 8.8-10.4 mg/dL).

CLINICAL APPROACH

Hypercalcemia

The most common causes of hypercalcemia include malignancies or hyperparathyroidism, accounting for 90% of cases. Other causes include granulomatous disorders such as sarcoid and tuberculosis; less commonly, hypercalcemia may be the presentation of intoxication with vitamin A, vitamin D, or calcium-containing antacids, or may occur as a side effect of therapies with drugs such as lithium or thiazide diuretics. Genetic conditions such as familial hypocalciuric hypercalcemia and hyperparathyroidism as part of a multiple endocrine neoplasia syndrome are less common causes.

The differential diagnosis can be narrowed based on the chronicity of the patient's presentation and the presence or absence of other symptoms and signs. **Primary hyperparathyroidism**, usually caused by a **solitary parathyroid adenoma**, is the most likely cause when hypercalcemia is discovered in an otherwise **asymptomatic** patient on routine laboratory screening. Most patients have no symptoms with mild hypercalcemia less than 12 g/dL, except perhaps some polyuria and dehydration. With levels more than 13 mg/dL, patients begin developing increasingly severe symptoms, including central nervous system (CNS) symptoms (lethargy, stupor, coma, mental status changes, psychosis), gastrointestinal symptoms (anorexia, nausea, constipation, peptic ulcer disease), kidney problems (polyuria, nephrolithiasis, and prerenal azotemia), and musculoskeletal complaints (arthralgias, myalgias, weakness). The **symptoms of hyperparathyroidism** can be remembered as **stones** (kidney), **moans** (abdominal pain), **groans** (myalgias), **bones** (bone pain), and **psychiatric overtones** (mental status changes). Diagnosis can be established by finding hypercalcemia, hypophosphatemia, with inappropriately elevated PTH levels. Patients may be treated surgically with parathyroidectomy if the hypercalcemia is severe (>15 mg/dL), or if less than 50 years old and significantly decreased bone mineral density.

However, a patient presenting with acute onset of **symptomatic hypercalcemia** is more likely to have a **malignancy**. Multiple myeloma, lymphoma, and leukemia all can present with hypercalcemia, as can solid tumors such as breast, lung, and kidney cancers. Some of these cancers cause elevated calcium levels by **stimulating osteoclast activity** through direct bone marrow invasion (multiple myeloma, leukemia, and breast cancer). Others produce **excess 1,25-vitamin D** (lymphomas), whereas others secrete a **parathyroid hormone-related protein** (PTHrP) that binds the PTH receptor (kidney and lung). Cancer-related hypercalcemia can be differentiated from primary hyperparathyroidism by a suppressed PTH level.

Electrolytes, to assess acid-base status, and renal function are important tests to consider. A normal complete blood count (CBC) and peripheral smear would make leukemia a less likely cause. Levels of PTH and specific assays for PTHrP are generally measured. If multiple myeloma is suspected, serum and urine electrophoresis for monoclonal antibody spikes should be examined. Radiographs showing lytic or blastic lesions may be helpful; finally, a bone marrow biopsy may be considered.

Multiple Myeloma

Multiple myeloma is a neoplastic proliferation of plasma cells that usually produce monoclonal immunoglobulin (Ig)A or IgG antibodies. Patients typically present with **lytic bone lesions, hypercalcemia, renal insufficiency, anemia,** and an elevated globulin fraction on serum chemistries, which, if separated by electrophoresis, shows a **monoclonal proliferation** (M-spike). The **diagnosis** of multiple myeloma requires laboratory and clinical criteria: a **monoclonal antibody spike** in the serum or light chains in the urine, and more than **10% clonal plasma cells in the bone marrow, and lytic bone lesions**.

Patients with lower level monoclonal IgA or IgG antibody production without the signs or symptoms of multiple myeloma have what is termed a *monoclonal gammopathy of undetermined significance* (**MGUS**). MGUS is much more common than myeloma, affecting up to 1% of the population more than 50 years of age. Long-term studies demonstrate that approximately 16% of these patients will go on to develop multiple myeloma. Patients with MGUS typically require no therapy. Some patients with myeloma with no bone lesions or other end-organ damage have an indolent course (**"smoldering myeloma"**) and can be **observed without treatment** for many years. **Therapy for symptomatic multiple myeloma** includes a high-dose pulsed **dexamethasone,** often in combination with **chemotherapy** with vincristine/doxorubicin or thalidomide. Some patients may be candidates for autologous stem cell transplant.

Comprehension Questions

36.1   On routine blood work performed for a life insurance application, a 53-year-old woman was found to have a calcium level of 12 mg/dL (normal = 8.8-10.4 mg/dL) and a phosphate level of 2 mg/dL (normal = 3.0-4.5 mg/dL). She is not anemic and has no symptoms. Her medical history is significant for osteoporosis, discovered on a dual-energy X-ray absorptiometry (DEXA) scan performed at the time of her menopause 1 year ago. Which of the following is the most likely cause of her hypercalcemia?

A. Multiple myeloma
B. Parathyroid adenoma
C. Familial hypocalciuric hypercalcemia
D. Multiple myeloma
E. Undiagnosed breast cancer

36.2   A 62-year-old asymptomatic woman is noted to have multiple myeloma and an elevated calcium level, but no bone lesions or end-organ damage. Which of the following therapies is useful for immediate treatment of the hypercalcemia?

A. Bisphosphonates.
B. Erythropoietin.
C. Dexamethasone plus thalidomide.
D. Interferon-a.
E. Observe without treatment since she is asymptomatic.

36.3   A 22-year-old African American woman presents with worsening cough and shortness of breath over 6 weeks, which did not improve with a course of antibiotics or antitussives. Her serum calcium level is found to be 12.5 mg/dL, and a chest X-ray reveals bilateral hilar lymphadenopathy. Which of the following is the most likely diagnosis?
        A. Sarcoidosis
        B. Mycoplasma pneumonia
        C. Acute lymphoblastic leukemia
        D. Squamous cell carcinoma of the lung
        E. Pulmonary embolism

36.4   A 66-year-old man with known metastatic squamous cell carcinoma of the esophagus is brought to the emergency room for increasing lethargy and confusion. He is clinically dehydrated, his serum calcium level is 14 mg/dL, and his creatinine level is 2.5 mg/dL but 1 month ago was 0.9 mg/dL. Which therapy for his hypercalcemia should be instituted first?
        A. Intravenous bisphosphonate
        B. Intravenous furosemide
        C. Glucocorticoids
        D. Intravenous normal saline
        E. Chemotherapy for squamous cell carcinoma

ANSWERS

36.1   **B.** An asymptomatic, most likely chronically elevated calcium level is most likely caused by primary hyperparathyroidism caused due to a parathyroid adenoma. The chronicity of this patient's hypercalcemia can be guessed at because she has osteoporosis and is only 1 year postmenopausal.

36.2   **A.** Bisphosphonates are helpful in controlling hypercalcemia through inhibition of osteoclastic bone reabsorption. Erythropoietin is useful in treating the anemia associated with multiple myeloma, and dexamethasone, in combination with thalidomide, is useful in treatment of the disease itself.

36.3   **A.** Both sarcoidosis and lymphoma can present with cough, dyspnea, and hilar adenopathy on chest X-ray. In approximately 10% of cases, sarcoidosis can cause elevated calcium levels through the production of 1,25-vitamin D that occurs in the macrophages of the granulomas. This can also be seen in granulomas caused by tuberculosis and in lymphoma. Leukemia usually does not present in this manner, although it can cause hypercalcemia. Squamous cell carcinoma of the lung would be unusual in a patient of this age, and the radiographic presentation is atypical.

36.4   **D.** Although all of the other therapies listed may be helpful in the treatment of hypercalcemia, given the clinical findings of dehydration and elevated creatinine level with a history of previously normal renal function, volume expansion with normal saline would correct the dehydration and presumed prerenal azotemia, allowing the kidneys to more efficiently excrete calcium. Other therapies can be added if the response to normal saline alone is insufficient.

Clinical Pearls

> Hypercalcemia that is acutely symptomatic is most likely caused by cancer. Asymptomatic hypercalcemia is most likely caused by primary hyperparathyroidism.

> In primary hyperparathyroidism, serum parathyroid hormone and calcium levels are elevated, and phosphate levels are decreased. In malignancy-related hypercalcemia, the calcium level is high and parathyroid hormone levels are suppressed.

> Symptoms of hyperparathyroidism can be remembered as stones, moans, groans, bones, and psychiatric overtones.

> Monoclonal gammopathy of undetermined significance (MGUS) and symptomatic multiple myeloma are on opposite ends of a spectrum of neoplastic disease of plasmacytes.

> The classic triad of multiple myeloma consists of a bone pain due to lytic lesions, anemia, and renal insufficiency.

REFERENCES

Bataille R, Harousseau J. Multiple myeloma. *N Engl J Med*. 1997;336:1657-1664.

Deftos LJ. Hypercalcemia in malignant and inflammatory diseases. *Endocrinol Metab Clin North Am*. 2002;31:141-158.

Munshi NC, Longo DL, Anderson KC. Plasma cell disorders. In: Kasper DL, Braunwald E, Fauci AS, et al, eds. *Harrison's Principles of Internal Medicine*. 17th ed. New York, NY: McGraw-Hill; 2008:700-707.

Potts JT. Diseases of the parathyroid gland and other hyper- and hypocalcemic disorders. In: Fauci AS, Braunwald E, Kasper DL, eds. *Harrison's Principles of Internal Medicine*. 17th ed. New York, NY: McGraw-Hill; 2008:2377-2396.

Case 37

A 48-year-old woman calls 911 and is brought to the emergency room complaining of a sudden onset of dyspnea. She reports she was standing in the kitchen making dinner, when she suddenly felt as if she could not get enough air, her heart started racing, and she became lightheaded and felt as if she would faint. She denied chest pain or cough. Her medical history is significant only for gallstones, for which she underwent a cholecystectomy 2 weeks previously. The procedure was complicated by a wound infection, requiring her to stay in the hospital for 8 days. She takes no medications regularly, only for acetaminophen as needed for pain at her abdominal incision site.

On examination, she is tachypneic with a respiratory rate of 28 breaths per minute, oxygen saturations 84% on room air, heart rate 124 bpm, and blood pressure 118/89 mm Hg. She appears uncomfortable, diaphoretic, and frightened. Her oral mucosa is slightly cyanotic, her jugular venous pressure is elevated, and her chest is clear to auscultation. Her heart rhythm is tachycardic but regular with a loud second sound in the pulmonic area, but no gallop or murmur. Her abdominal examination is benign, with a clean incision site without signs of infection. Her right leg is moderately swollen from mid-thigh to her feet, and her thigh and calf are mildly tender to palpation. Laboratory studies including cardiac enzymes are normal, her electrocardiogram (ECG) reveals only sinus tachycardia, and her chest X-ray is interpreted as normal.

➤ What is the most likely diagnosis?

➤ What is the most appropriate diagnostic step?

ANSWERS TO CASE 37:
Pulmonary Embolism

Summary: A 48-year-old woman is brought to the hospital for very acute onset of dyspnea and is found to be tachypneic, tachycardic, and hypoxemic. On physical examination, she has elevated jugular venous pressure and a loud pulmonic closure sound, perhaps signifying acutely elevated pulmonary pressures. All of these findings, especially the hypoxemia despite a clear chest radiograph, strongly suggest a pulmonary embolism (PE), most likely caused by a lower-extremity deep venous thrombosis (DVT), a late complication of her recent hospitalization and relative immobilization.

> **Most likely diagnosis:** Pulmonary embolism.

> **Most appropriate diagnostic step:** Chest computed tomography (CT) with intravenous contrast, or other imaging study as indicated.

ANALYSIS

Objectives

1. Understand the factors that predispose patients to develop thromboembolic disease.
2. Recognize the clinical presentation of PE.
3. Know the strategies to diagnose PE.
4. Understand the goals and methods of treatment of thromboembolism.

Considerations

Pulmonary embolism (PE) embolism is a difficult diagnosis to establish because of the nonspecificity of presenting signs and symptoms, and the probabilistic nature of the most common noninvasive diagnostic tests. In patients with suspected PE, initial treatment is supportive to maintain adequate oxygenation and hemodynamic stability, and efforts are undertaken to try to diagnose the PE or other cause of the patient's symptoms. Often, a series of diagnostic tests is necessary to determine the likely diagnosis. Specific treatment of PE may include thrombolysis or surgical embolectomy for unstable patients and initiation of anticoagulation as a long-term measure to prevent recurrence.

APPROACH TO
Suspected Pulmonary Embolism

DEFINITION

DEEP VENOUS THROMBOSIS (DVT): Blood clot in the deep venous system that usually affects the lower extremities or pelvic veins.

CLINICAL APPROACH

Etiology and Risk Factors

Successful treatment and management of PE requires a combination of clinical suspicion and appropriate use of diagnostic tools. Pulmonary emboli usually arise from deep venous thrombi and occasionally from less common sources, including air, fat, amniotic fluid, or tumor thrombus. More than 100 years ago, Rudolf **Virchow postulated three factors** that predispose to venous thrombus: **local trauma to vessel wall, a state of hypercoagulability, and venous stasis.** Genetic predisposition to hypercoagulability accounts for approximately 20% of PEs. **The most common inherited conditions** are the **factor V Leiden mutation** and the **prothrombin gene mutations.** Malignancy is also a predisposing condition for deep venous thrombosis. These neoplastic cells are thought to generate thrombin or to synthesize various procoagulants. Even surgery has been found to significantly increase the risk of PE as late as 1 month postoperatively.

Pathophysiology

When venous thrombi dislodge from their site of formation, they may embolize to the pulmonary arteries causing PE. The **deep proximal lower-extremity veins** are the **most common site of clot formation resulting in PE**, although thromboses in pelvic, calf, and upper-extremity veins may also embolize. Obstruction to the pulmonary artery causes platelets to release vasoactive agents such as serotonin, thereby elevating pulmonary vascular resistance. The resulting increase in alveolar dead space and subsequent redistribution of blood flow create areas of V/Q mismatch and impair gas exchange. Reflex bronchoconstriction causes increasing airway resistance. This cascade can result in pulmonary edema, hemorrhage, or loss of surfactant, further decreasing lung compliance. As pulmonary vascular resistance increases, right-heart wall tension rises, resulting in dilation and dysfunction that ultimately may impair left heart function. **Progressive right heart failure is the usual cause of death from PE.**

Clinical and Nonimaging Evaluation

Pulmonary embolism (PE) can often mimic other cardiopulmonary diseases, making the diagnosis challenging. Acute onset of dyspnea is the most common symptom of PE, whereas tachypnea is the most frequently observed sign. Severe dyspnea accompanied by syncope, hypotension, or cyanosis may indicate massive PE, whereas pleuritic pain, cough, or hemoptysis may suggest a smaller more peripheral embolus causing infarction of lung tissue. Classic findings on physical examination include tachycardia and signs of right ventricular dysfunction, including bulging neck veins, left parasternal lift, accentuated pulmonic component of the second heart sound, and systolic murmur that increases with inspiration. Findings suggestive of DVT include pain, swelling, and erythema to the lower extremity, particularly the back of the leg below the knee. Some patients complain of calf tenderness.

Nonimaging diagnostic tools include laboratory tests and ECG. The serum D-dimer enzyme-linked immunosorbent assay (ELISA) is elevated (>500 ng/mL) in more than 95% of patients with PE, reflecting the breakdown of fibrin and thrombolysis. Although the D-dimer ELISA has a high negative predictive value and thus is useful in excluding PE, it lacks specificity. Elevations may be seen in patients with myocardial infarction, pneumonia, heart failure, cancer, or sepsis. Abnormalities on the ECG may be useful in the evaluation of PE; the most frequent finding is T-wave inversions in the anterior leads (especially V_1 through V_4). Other common findings are sinus tachycardia, new-onset atrial fibrillation, and an S wave in lead I, a Q wave in lead III, and an inverted T wave in lead III ($S_1Q_3T_3$).

Imaging Modalities

Radiologic studies are critical in the diagnosis of PE and DVT. A chest X-ray is the first study indicated in a symptomatic patient with new-onset dyspnea. A normal or near-normal chest X-ray is the most common finding in PE, sometimes with nonspecific abnormalities, such as atelectasis. In general, **acute onset of hypoxemia in a patient with a normal chest X-ray should be interpreted as PE until otherwise proven.** Classic abnormalities associated with PE include Westermark sign (nonspecific prominence of the central pulmonary artery with decreased pulmonary vascularity), Hampton hump (peripheral wedge-shaped density above the diaphragm), and Palla sign (enlargement of the right descending pulmonary artery). The chest radiograph probably is more important in identifying other significant pulmonary parenchymal disease (pneumonia, pulmonary edema) and cardiac disease (cardiomyopathy) as the cause of the respiratory symptoms.

Chest CT with intravenous contrast is now the principal imaging modality to diagnose suspected pulmonary embolism. Current generation multidetector-row spiral CT can acquire high-resolution images in a single breath hold, and can visualize small branch artery emboli. In addition, the chest CT has the additional benefit of imaging other abnormalities such as pneumonia, aortic abnormalities, or pulmonary masses that may not have been apparent on routine chest radiograph, and which may provide an alternative diagnosis for the patient's symptomatology. The main caveat in the use of CT is the image quality, and the experience of the center in interpreting this type of scan. In general, however, CT has been shown to be at least as accurate as the previously accepted standard imaging modality, ventilation/perfusion (V/Q) lung scanning.

In patients in whom a CT with radiocontrast cannot be obtained or is contraindicated (advanced renal insufficiency, severe contrast allergy), a **V/Q scan** remains a useful tool. A normal scan, or a low-probability scan with a low clinical suspicion for PE effectively excludes the diagnosis.

For any imaging modality, the most accurate diagnosis will be achieved in combination with the clinical suspicion. The **Wells score** is a useful clinical calculator to clinically estimate pretest probability of PE. A point score less than 4 with a negative D-dimer assay indicates a low probability for PE. A score of 2 to 6 points indicates moderate probability, and more than 7 points is high probability. (See Figure 37-1)

If the CT and/or V/Q scan are nondiagnostic, yet the clinical suspicion remains high, other imaging modalities may be obtained. A **lower-extremity venous ultrasound** demonstrating an acute DVT in a patient with signs and symptoms of PE would be sufficient to diagnose and treat PE (especially since the treatment with anticoagulation is the same). It should be noted, though, that a normal ultrasound does not exclude the diagnosis of PE, since most patients with PE do not have evidence of residual DVT, and in many cases because the clot has already embolized.

Other imaging studies such as **contrast-enhanced magnetic resonance imaging (MRI)** or **echocardiography** (especially transesophageal echocardiography) may be used when the clinical suspicion remains high, but other diagnostic studies are inconclusive. Figure 37–2 gives a diagnostic algorithm for suspected PE.

Treatment

Treatment options can be categorized in terms of primary and secondary therapy based on different management goals. **Primary therapy** consists of clot dissolution or **thrombolysis or removal of clot by surgical embolectomy** and usually is reserved for patients with a high risk for adverse outcomes if the clot remains, that is, those with **right-heart failure or hypotension.**

For patients who are normotensive with normal RV function, treatment is with **anticoagulation,** with the goal of **secondary prevention** of thrombus extension or recurrence. Anticoagulation does not dissolve existing thrombus, but allows for endothelialization and organization, which begins within days of treatment. Immediate anticoagulation should be initiated with intravenous **unfractionated heparin** (UFH), subcutaneous **low-molecular-weight**

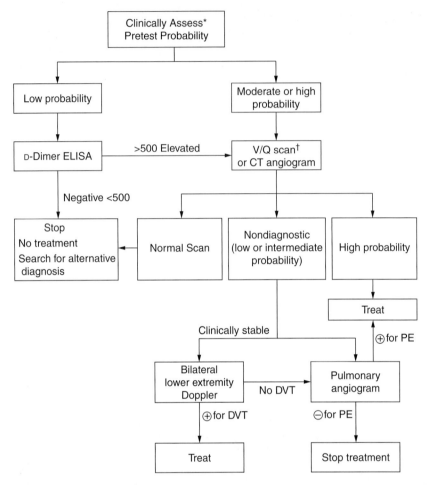

Figure 37–1. Diagnostic algorithm for suspected pulmonary embolism. DVT, deep venous thrombosis; ELISA, enzyme-linked immunosorbent assay; PE, pulmonary embolism; V/Q, ventilation/perfusion.

heparin (LMWH) enoxaparin or tinzaparin, or the direct factor Xa inhibitor **fondaparinux.** While UFH requires a continuous infusion and frequent laboratory monitoring every 4 to 6 hours, LMWH and fondaparinux provide rapid onset of action, predictable dose response, and no laboratory monitoring is generally required.

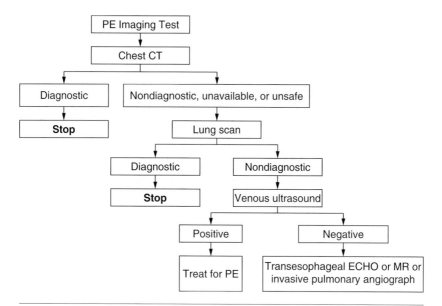

Figure 37–2. Diagnostic algorithm for patients with suspected pulmonary embolism. *Modified, with permission, from Braunwald E, Fauci AS, Kasper KL, et al, Harrison's Principles of Internal Medicine, 17th ed. New York: McGraw-Hill, 2008: 1655.*

Patients can then be started on the oral vitamin K antagonist **warfarin**. It may cause an initial paradoxical prothrombotic state, so requires overlap with UFH, LMWH, or fondaparinux when beginning therapy. Because its biologic effect is unpredictable, warfarin requires routine monitoring of the prothrombin time, standardized across laboratories as the international normalized ratio (**INR**). The target therapeutic INR is usually 2.5. When initiating warfarin therapy, the usual course is to use UFH, LMWH, or fondaparinux for at least 5 days while overlapping with warfarin until the INR has been therapeutic for 2 consecutive days. **The duration of treatment relates to the risk of recurrence.** One factor in assessing this risk is whether the DVT or PE was provoked (ie, occurred due to a readily identifiable and transient event such as trauma or surgery) or unprovoked. For provoked DVT of the calf or upper extremity, 3 months of anticoagulation is recommended. Six months is recommended for patients with provoked proximal leg DVT, or PE. For patients with idiopathic or unprovoked DVT or PE, or with ongoing risk factors, such as malignancy or antiphospholipid syndrome, the duration of therapy is controversial, but indefinite anticoagulation may be required.

Inferior vena cava filter placement to prevent recurrent PE is recommended when there is active bleeding or other contraindication to anticoagulation, or recurrent DVT or PE despite therapeutic anticoagulation.

Comprehension Questions

37.1   A 35-year-old woman complains of calf tenderness and acute dyspnea.
       The arterial blood gas reveals P_{O_2} (partial pressure of oxygen) of 76 mm Hg.
       Which of the following is the most common physical examination
       finding of pulmonary embolism?
       A. Wheezing
       B. Increased pulmonary component of the second heart sound
       C. Tachypnea
       D. Calf swelling
       E. Pulmonary rales

37.2   A 39-year-old man is noted to have a deep venous thrombosis without
       any known risk factors. He notes that his brother also developed a pul-
       monary embolism at age 45 years, and his mother developed a "clot in
       the leg" when she was in her thirties. Which of the following is the
       most likely inherited disorder in this patient?
       A. Protein S deficiency
       B. Antithrombin III deficiency
       C. Factor V Leiden mutation
       D. Antiphospholipid antibody syndrome
       E. Familial malignancy syndrome

37.3   A 54-year-old woman is noted to have cervical cancer and presents
       with significant vaginal bleeding with a hemoglobin level of 7 g/dL.
       Her left leg is swollen, which on Doppler investigation reveals a deep
       venous thrombosis. Which of the following is the best treatment for
       the thrombus?
       A. Intravenous unfractionated heparin
       B. Fractionated subcutaneous heparin
       C. Subcutaneous unfractionated heparin
       D. Oral warfarin (Coumadin)
       E. Vena cava filter

ANSWERS

37.1   **C.** Tachypnea is the most common physical sign associated with pul-
       monary embolus.

37.2   **C.** Factor V Leiden mutation is the most common hereditary
       thrombophilia.

37.3   **E.** Cervical cancer with significant vaginal bleeding is a relative con-
       traindication for anticoagulation. Thus, a vena cava filter is the most
       appropriate choice in this patient.

Clinical Pearls

➤ Acute onset of dyspnea or hypoxemia with a normal chest X-ray should be considered a pulmonary embolism until proven otherwise.
➤ Diagnosis of pulmonary embolism is usually established using imaging tests such as chest CT considered in the light of clinical pretest probability.
➤ The primary therapy of DVT or PE is anticoagulation, with the goal of preventing recurrence.

REFERENCES

Goldhaber SZ. Deep venous thrombosis and pulmonary thromboembolism. In: Kasper DL, Braunwald E, Fauci AS, et al, eds. *Harrison's Principles of Internal Medicine.* 17th ed. New York, NY: McGraw-Hill; 2008:1651-1657.

Stein PD, Fowler SE, Goodman LR, et al. Multidetector computed tomography for acute pulmonary embolism. *N Engl J Med.* 2006;354:2317-2327.

Van Belle A, Buller HR, Huisman MV, et al. Effectiveness of managing suspected pulmonary embolism using an algorithm combining clinical probability, D-dimer testing, and computed tomography. *JAMA.* 2006;295:172-179.

Wells PS, Anderson DR, Rodger M, et al. Derivation of a simple clinical model to categorize patients probability of pulmonary embolism: increasing the models utility with the SimpliRED D-dimer. *Thromb Haemost.* 2000;83(3):416-420.

Case 38

A 68-year-old woman is brought to the emergency room after coughing up several tablespoons of bright red blood. For the previous 3 to 4 months, she has had a chronic nonproductive cough but no fevers. More recently, she has noticed some scant blood-streaked sputum. On review of her symptoms, she reports increased fatigue, decreased appetite, and a 25-lb weight loss in the past 3 months. She denies chest pain, fever, chills, or night sweats. The patient has smoked one pack of cigarettes per day for the past 35 years. She drinks two martinis every day and has not had any significant mental illness. She worked in a library for 35 years and has no history of occupational exposures. She does not take any medication except for one aspirin per day.

The patient is a thin woman who is mildly anxious, alert, and oriented. Her blood pressure is 150/90 mm Hg, heart rate 88 bpm, respiratory rate 16 breaths per minute, and temperature 99.2°F. Neck examination reveals no lymphadenopathy, thyromegaly, or carotid bruit. The chest has scattered rhonchi bilaterally, but there are no wheezes or crackles. Cardiovascular examination reveals a regular rate and rhythm, without rubs, gallops, or murmurs. The abdomen is benign with no hepatosplenomegaly. Examination of her extremities reveals no cyanosis; there is finger clubbing. Neurologic examination is normal.

➤ What is your next step?

➤ What is the most likely diagnosis?

ANSWERS TO CASE 38:

Hemoptysis, Lung Cancer

Summary: A 68-year-old female smoker has expectorated bright red blood. She has had a chronic nonproductive cough and, more recently, some blood-streaked sputum. She reports increased fatigability, reduced appetite, and unintentional weight loss. She has no fever, chills, or night sweats to suggest infection. On examination, her chest reveals scattered rhonchi bilaterally without wheezes or crackles. She has clubbing of the fingers.

> ➤ **Next step:** Chest X-ray film, posteroanterior and lateral.
> ➤ **Most likely diagnosis:** Lung cancer.

ANALYSIS

Objectives

1. Know the differential diagnosis of hemoptysis.
2. Be familiar with the risk factors for and the clinical presentation of lung cancer (including superior vena cava [SVC] syndrome and Horner syndrome).
3. Know the workup of the solitary pulmonary nodule.
4. Be familiar with the general principles of treatment of lung cancer.

Considerations

The most likely diagnosis in this case is lung cancer. On physical examination, there was finger clubbing, an enlargement of the terminal digital phalanges with loss of the nail bed angle. In pulmonary disease, clubbing of fingers is most commonly seen in patients with lung cancer or with chronic septic conditions, such as bronchiectasis or lung abscess. She will require imaging studies such as a chest X-ray and likely a computed tomography (CT) of the chest, and if abnormalities are seen, a biopsy procedure to establish a tissue diagnosis. In the meantime, she will benefit from rest and cough suppression to minimize her hemoptysis, which may be acutely life-threatening, if massive bleeding.

APPROACH TO

Hemoptysis

DEFINITIONS

MASSIVE HEMOPTYSIS: More than 100 to 600 mL blood loss that is coughed up within 24-hour period.

HORNER SYNDROME: Symptoms are ptosis, loss of pupillary dilation (miosis), and loss of sweating on the ipsilateral side (anhydrosis) caused by compression of the superior cervical ganglion and resultant loss of sympathetic innervation.

SUPERIOR VENA CAVA (SVC) SYNDROME: Obstruction of venous drainage, usually by external compression of the SVC, leading to edema of the face, neck, and upper part of the torso often with formation of collateral veins on the upper chest.

CLINICAL APPROACH

Hemoptysis is defined as an expectoration of blood from the respiratory tract. It is an alarming symptom, both because it may be a manifestation of a serious underlying diagnosis, such as malignancy, and because massive hemoptysis can fill up alveolar air spaces and cause asphyxiation. Hemoptysis, particularly if in large quantity or recurrent, is a potentially fatal event requiring an immediate search for the cause and precise location of the bleeding. Hemoptysis must be differentiated from hematemesis and from blood originating in the nasopharynx. **Currently, the most common causes of hemoptysis in the United States are bronchitis and lung cancer.** In prior eras, the most common causes have been tuberculosis, lung abscess, and bronchiectasis. History is an important diagnostic step: blood-streaked purulent sputum suggests bronchitis; **chronic copious sputum production suggests bronchiectasis. Hemoptysis with an acute onset of pleuritic chest pain and dyspnea** suggests a **pulmonary embolism.** Every patient with hemoptysis should undergo a chest X-ray to look for a mass lesion, evidence of bronchiectasis, or parenchymal disease. If the chest radiograph reveals a pulmonary mass, the patient should undergo fiberoptic bronchoscopy to localize the site of bleeding and to visualize and attempt to biopsy any endobronchial lesion. Patients with massive hemoptysis require measures to maintain their airway and to prevent spilling blood into unaffected areas of the lungs. These patients should be kept at rest with suppression of cough. If the bleeding is localized to one lung, the affected side should be placed in a dependent position so that bleeding does not flow into the contralateral side. They may also require endotracheal intubation and rigid bronchoscopy for better airway control and suction capacity.

Risk Factors for Lung Cancer

Primary lung cancer, or bronchogenic carcinoma, is the leading cause of cancer deaths in both men and women. Approximately 85% of lung cancers of all cell types are linked to smoking. Of the 15% of lung cancers that are not related to smoking, the majority are found in women for reasons that are unknown. Thoracic radiation exposure as well as exposure to environmental toxins such as asbestos or radon are also associated with increased risk of developing lung caner.

Clinical Presentation of Lung Cancer

Only 5% to 15% of patients with lung cancer are asymptomatic when diagnosed. In these cases, a lung nodule usually is found incidentally on chest X-ray or CT.

Tumors that are endobronchial present with cough or with hemoptysis. Chest pain is also a possible symptom of lung cancer and suggests the neoplastic invasion of the chest wall. Symptoms of weight loss, malaise, and fatigue usually develop later in the disease course. Malignant serosanguineous pleural effusion is common. **Horner syndrome** is caused by the invasion of the cervicothoracic sympathetic nerves and occurs with apical tumors **(Pancoast tumor).** Phrenic nerve invasion may cause diaphragmatic paralysis. SVC obstruction is produced by direct extension of the tumor or by compression from the neighboring lymph nodes. **SVC syndrome** has a dramatic clinical presentation and requires urgent care.

Once a patient presents with symptoms or radiographic findings suggestive of lung cancer, the next steps are as follows:

1. Tissue diagnosis to establish malignant diagnosis and histologic type
2. Staging to determine resectability or curative potential
3. Cancer treatment: surgery, radiotherapy, or chemotherapy

Lung Cancer Classification

Histologically, primary lung cancer can be divided into two major categories with important therapeutic implications: **small cell lung cancer** (SCLC), and **non–small cell lung cancer** (NSCLC), as well as miscellaneous types. An NSCLC is further divided into three types: squamous cell carcinoma, adenocarcinoma, and large cell carcinoma. Together SCLC and NSCLC constitute 95% of primary lung cancers, with NSCLC being three to four times more common than SCLC (relative frequency NSCLC 75%, SCLC 25%).

Squamous cell cancer usually does not metastasize early. It usually is a central/hilar lesion with local extension that may present with symptoms caused by bronchial obstruction, such as atelectasis and pneumonia. It may present on chest X-ray as a cavitary lesion; **squamous cell cancer is by far the most likely to cavitate.** It may also produce PTH (parathyroid hormone)-like hormone and present with hypercalcemia. **Adenocarcinoma** and large cell cancer are peripheral lesions. Adenocarcinoma metastasizes early, especially to the CNS, bones, and adrenal glands. **Adenocarcinoma has the least association with smoking** and a stronger association with pulmonary scars/fibrosis. **Large cell cancer** usually is a peripheral lesion and tends to metastasize to the CNS and mediastinum, **causing SVC syndrome or hoarseness as a consequence of laryngeal nerve paralysis.** If the patient has a history of asbestos exposure, then squamous cancer, adenocarcinoma, and mesothelioma should all be considered. Small cell cancer, previously called oat-cell, is made up of cells of neuroendocrine origin. It is extremely aggressive but is more likely to respond to chemotherapy than NSCLC. The primary lesion is usually central. Eighty percent of patients have metastasis at the time of diagnosis, so its treatment usually is different from that of other lung cancers. Contrary to other lung cancers, cavitation never occurs in small cell cancer. SCLC can cause the syndrome of inappropriate secretion of antidiuretic hormone (SIADH), ectopic adrenocorticotropic hormone (ACTH) production, and Eaton-Lambert syndrome. Table 38–1 lists typical characteristics of various cell types, including thoracic location, tendency to cavitate, and association with extrapulmonary or paraneoplastic manifestations.

SCLC is initially very responsive to chemotherapy and radiation therapy, but unfortunately, most SCLC relapses. Additionally, SCLC has almost always spread at time of diagnosis, so surgical treatment with curative intent is not possible. In contrast, NSCLC is much less responsive to chemotherapy or to radiation, but tumors that are localized at time of diagnosis may be treated effectively surgically, or with radiation therapy. NSCLC includes several histologic subtypes—squamous cell carcinoma, adenocarcinoma, and large cell carcinoma—but they all have similar prognoses at similar stages, and are treated similarly.

Table 38–1 LUNG CANCER CHARACTERISTICS

	SMALL CELL	SQUAMOUS CELL	ADENOCARCINOMA	LARGE CELL
Location	Central	Central	Peripheral	Peripheral
Associated with smoking	Yes	Yes	Often not associated	Yes
Cavitation	Rare	Most likely		
Metastases	Early	Late	Early	Late
Extrapulmonary manifestations	SIADH, ectopic ACTH, Eaton-Lambert, Cushing, peripheral neuropathy	Hypercalcemia	Thrombophlebitis	SVC syndrome or hoarseness

Abbreviations: ACTH, adrenocorticotropic hormone; SIADH, syndrome of inappropriate secretion of antidiuretic hormone; SVC, superior vena cava.

General Principles of Treatment

Treatment of lung cancer is performed with either curative or palliative intent.

The treatment of lung cancer consists of surgical resection, chemotherapy, and/or radiation therapy in different combinations, depending on the tissue type and extent of the disease.

The SCLC is nearly always metastatic at time of diagnosis and, therefore, not eligible for surgical resection. It is staged as either **limited-stage** disease, that is, disease confined to one hemithorax that can be treated within a radiotherapy port, or **extensive-stage** disease, that is, contralateral lung involvement or distant metastases. Patients with untreated SCLC have a grim prognosis, with survival measured in weeks. With treatment, survival can be prolonged, and approximately 20% to 30% of patients with limited-stage disease can be cured with radiotherapy and chemotherapy. The prognosis for relapsed patients, though, is very poor.

Once the diagnosis of NSCLC is made, the next step is to stage the disease by the TNM (tumor, node, and metastasis) system (size, local spread of tumor, node involvement, and metastatic spread; Table 38–2). Patients with NSCLC who are stage I or II, or some with IIIA, may be candidates for curative resection

---

Table 38–2 SUMMARY OF STAGING

Staging of lung cancer is based on the TNM system. T is for tumor size or extension to adjacent tissues; N is for nodal involvement; and M is for distant metastases.

Stage I: Tumor is without nodal involvement or distant metastasis.
IA: Tumor <3 cm without extension to adjacent tissues.
IB: Tumor either (1) is >3 cm or (2) invades visceral pleura, causes atelectasis of less than entire lung, or extends at least 2 cm from carina.

Stage II: Tumor is without distant metastasis.
IIA: Tumor <3 cm with ipsilateral hilar and/or ipsilateral bronchial nodal involvement.
IIB: (1) Stage IB with involvement of ipsilateral hilar or bronchial nodes or
(2) tumor invading chest wall, diaphragm, mediastinal pleura, pericardium, or (3) tumor with atelectasis of entire lung or extending within 2 cm of carina.

Stage III: Tumor is without distant metastasis.
IIIA: (1) Tumor invading chest wall, diaphragm, mediastinal pleura, pericardium, or tumor with atelectasis of entire lung, or tumor extending within 2 cm of carina with ipsilateral hilar or bronchial nodal involvement, or (2) tumor with involvement of ipsilateral mediastinal and/or subcarinal nodes.
IIIB: (1) Involvement of contralateral nodes or of scalene or supraclavicular nodes (either side), or (2) tumor invading mediastinum, heart or great vessels, trachea/esophagus, vertebral body or carina, or (3) tumor with malignant pleural or pericardial effusion, or (4) satellite tumor nodules within same lobe as primary tumor.

Stage IV: Distant metastasis (including tumor nodules in different lobe from primary tumor).

and radiotherapy. The next decision point is whether the patient can withstand an operation. Because most lung cancer occurs in older patients who have been smokers, they frequently have underlying cardiopulmonary disease and require preoperative evaluation, including pulmonary function testing, to predict whether they have sufficient pulmonary reserve to tolerate a lobectomy or pneumonectomy.

Solitary Pulmonary Nodule

The solitary pulmonary nodule is defined as a nodule surrounded by normal parenchyma. Approximately 35% of solitary pulmonary nodules are malignant. Proper management of a solitary nodule in an individual patient depends on a variety of elements: age, risk factors, presence of calcifications, and size of the nodule. The presence and type of calcification on a solitary pulmonary nodule can be helpful. "Popcorn" and "bull's-eye" calcifications suggest a benign process, whereas absence of calcification increases the likelihood of malignancy. In low-risk patients (ie, age 35 years and younger and nonsmokers), a solitary calcified nodule can be followed with serial chest CT, and is considered benign after 2 years if there is no growth. The risk of malignancy in such patients is less than 1%. High-risk patients require a more aggressive approach: bronchoscopy with biopsy of the lesion is highly recommended to sort out benign from malignant lesions. The size of the nodule is another important factor, because the likelihood of malignancy increases with size. Lesions more than 2.5 cm in diameter are highly suspicious for malignancy.

Comprehension Questions

38.1 A 67-year-old long-time smoker with chronic obstructive pulmonary disease presents with 3 days of headaches and plethoric swelling of his face and right arm. Which of the following is the most likely diagnosis?
   A. Angioedema
   B. Hypothyroidism
   C. Superior vena cava syndrome
   D. Trichinosis

38.2 A 64-year-old woman comes to your office complaining of hoarse voice for 4 months. She has not had fever, sore throat, or a cough. On examination, she has expiratory wheezes in her left mid-lung fields. Which of the following is the best next step?
   A. Prescribe antibiotics for bronchitis.
   B. Order a chest X-ray.
   C. Advise gargling with salt-water solution.
   D. Prescribe an albuterol inhaler.

38.3   A 33-year-old woman who is a nonsmoker has lost 30 lb and has a
        cough. She is noted to have a lung mass on chest radiograph. Which
        of the following lung cancers is the most likely cell type?
        A. Squamous cell
        B. Adenocarcinoma
        C. Small cell
        D. Large cell

38.4   A 52-year-old man presents with dyspnea, and chest X-ray shows a hilar
        mass with ipsilateral pleural effusion. Which of the following is the
        best next step?
        A. CT scan of the chest, head, and abdomen for cancer staging.
        B. Pulmonary function testing to evaluate pulmonary reserve to eval-
           uate for pulmonectomy.
        C. Obtain a specific tissue diagnosis by biopsy of the hilar mass.
        D. Initiate palliative radiation because the patient is not a candidate
           for curative resection.

ANSWERS

38.1   **C.** The patient has features of SVC syndrome, caused by compression
        of the SVC, almost always by a thoracic malignancy. Urgent diagnosis
        and treatment are mandatory because of impaired cerebral venous
        drainage and resultant increased intracranial pressure or possibly fatal
        intracranial venous thrombosis. Angioedema, hypothyroidism, and
        trichinosis all may cause facial swelling, but not the plethora or swelling
        of the arm.

38.2   **B.** This patient has chronic hoarseness and unilateral wheezing. This
        suggests an intrathoracic mass causing bronchial obstruction and
        impairment of the recurrent laryngeal nerve, causing vocal cord
        paralysis. Thus, an imaging study of the chest is essential.

38.3   **B.** Ninety percent of patients with lung cancer of *all* histologic types
        have a smoking history. The most common form of lung cancer found
        in nonsmokers, young patients, and women is adenocarcinoma.

38.4   **C.** Tissue diagnosis is essential for proper treatment of any malignancy
        and should always be the first step. Once a specific tissue diagnosis is
        obtained, the cancer is staged for prognosis and to guide therapy, that
        is, is there a possibility of curative resection? Questions for this patient
        include the tissue type, location of spread, and whether the pleural
        effusion is caused by malignancy.

Clinical Pearls

➤ Most patients with hemoptysis require evaluation with bronchoscopy. Massive hemoptysis may result in death by asphyxiation.

➤ Lung cancer is the leading cause of cancer deaths in men and women.

➤ A solitary pulmonary nodule in a nonsmoker younger than 35 years can be followed radiographically. For other patients, a biopsy, whether bronchoscopic, percutaneous, or surgical, is necessary.

➤ Steps in management of a patient with suspected lung cancer include tissue diagnosis, staging, preoperative evaluation, and treatment with surgery, radiotherapy, or chemotherapy.

➤ Small cell lung cancer usually is metastatic at the time of diagnosis and not resectable. Non–small cell lung cancer is curable by resection if it is stage I or II disease and some stage IIIA.

REFERENCES

Libby DM, Smith JP, Altorki NK, et al. Managing the small pulmonary nodule discovered by CT. Chest. 2004;125:1522-1529.

Minna JD, Schill JH. Neoplasms of the lung. In: Kasper DL, Braunwald E, Fauci AS, et al, eds. Harrison's Principles of Internal Medicine. 17th ed. New York, NY: McGraw-Hill; 2008:551-562.

Thompson AB, Teschler H, Rennard SI. Pathogenesis, evaluation, and therapy for massive hemoptysis. Clin Chest Med. 1992;13:69-82.

Weinberge SE, Lipson DA. Cough and hemoptysis. In: Fauci AS, Braunwald E, Kasper DL, eds. Harrison's Principles of Internal Medicine. 17th ed. New York, NY: McGraw-Hill; 2008:225-228.

Case 39

A 44-year-old man presents with sudden onset of shaking chills, fever, and productive cough. He was in his usual state of good health until 1 week ago, when he developed mild nasal congestion and achiness. He otherwise felt well until last night, when he became fatigued and feverish, and he developed a cough associated with right-side pleuritic chest pain. His medical history is remarkable only for his 15-pack per year smoking habit. In your office, his vital signs are normal except for a temperature of 102°F. His oxygen saturation on room air is 100%. He is comfortable, except when he coughs. His physical examination is unremarkable except for bronchial breath sounds and end-inspiratory crackles in the right lower lung field.

➤ What is your diagnosis?

➤ What is your next step?

ANSWERS TO CASE 39:

Community-Acquired Pneumonia

Summary: A 44-year-old healthy man presents with sudden onset of shaking chills, fever, and productive cough. He also complains of right-sided pleuritic chest pain. He is febrile to 102°F, but not tachypneic, and is normotensive with good oxygenation. His physical examination is unremarkable except for bronchial breath sounds and end-inspiratory crackles in the right lower lung field, and there is a right lower lobe consolidation on X-ray.

➤ **Most likely diagnosis:** Community-acquired pneumonia.

➤ **Next step:** Oral antibiotic therapy, pain relievers, antipyretics, and cough suppressants for relief of symptoms. Close outpatient follow-up (in 1-2 weeks).

ANALYSIS

Objectives

1. Know the causative organisms in community-acquired pneumonia and the appropriate therapeutic regimens.
2. Understand the clinical criteria indicating inpatient versus outpatient therapy.
3. Discuss the role of radiologic and laboratory evaluation in the diagnosis of pneumonia.
4. Understand the difference between aspiration pneumonitis and aspiration pneumonia.

Considerations

This previously healthy 44-year-old man has clinical and radiographic evidence of a focal consolidation of the lungs, which is consistent with a bacterial process, such as infection with *Streptococcus pneumoniae*. The specific causative organism is usually not definitively established, so you will need to initiate empiric antimicrobial therapy, and risk stratify the patient to determine whether he can safely be treated as an outpatient or requires hospitalization.

APPROACH TO
Suspected Pneumonia

DEFINITIONS

PNEUMONIA: An infection of the lung parenchyma, which may be caused by bacteria, viruses, fungi, or rarely protozoa.

COMMUNITY-ACQUIRED PNEUMONIA: An infection of the alveoli, distal airways, and interstitium of the lungs that occurs outside the hospital setting, affecting individuals of all ages.

CLINICAL APPROACH

Pneumonia is an infection of the lung parenchyma. Patients may present with any of a combination of cough, fever, pleuritic chest pain, sputum production, shortness of breath, hypoxia, and respiratory distress. Certain clinical presentations are associated with particular infectious agents. For example, the "typical" pneumonia is often described as having a sudden onset of fever, cough with productive sputum, often associated with pleuritic chest pain, and possibly **rust-colored sputum.** This is the classic description of pneumococcal pneumonia. The **"atypical" pneumonia** is characterized as having a **more insidious onset, with a dry cough,** prominent extrapulmonary symptoms such as **headache, myalgias, sore throat,** and a chest radiograph that appears much worse than the auscultatory findings. This type of presentation usually is attributed to *Mycoplasma pneumoniae.* Although these characterizations are of some diagnostic value, it is very difficult to reliably distinguish between typical and atypical organisms based on clinical history and physical examination as the cause of a specific patient's pneumonia. Therefore, pneumonias are typically classified according to the immune status of the host, the radiographic findings, and the setting in which the infection was acquired, in an attempt to identify the most likely causative organisms and to guide initial empiric therapy.

Typical **community-acquired pneumonia,** as opposed to nosocomial or hospital-acquired pneumonia, is most commonly caused by *S pneumoniae, Moraxella catarrhalis,* or *Haemophilus influenzae.* Viruses, such as influenza and adenovirus, can also cause pneumonia. Atypical pneumonia, which is characterized by a more insidious onset, a dry cough, muscle aches, headaches, and sore throat, typically is caused by M *pneumoniae.* However, other organisms, such as *Legionella* (typically associated with preceding gastrointestinal symptoms) and *Chlamydia pneumoniae,* should be considered. In a patient with specific risk factors, *Chlamydia psittaci* (bird exposure), coccidiomycosis (travel to the American southwest), or histoplasmosis (endemic to the Mississippi Valley) may be the cause. In a patient with acquired immunodeficiency syndrome (AIDS) or immunosuppression, *Pneumocystis carinii* should be added to the differential diagnosis. Tuberculosis is a possibility in patients with a history suggestive of exposure or predisposition (eg, those with AIDS) to this disease.

Those with hospital- or nursing home–acquired infection, termed **nosocomial pneumonia,** should have antibiotic coverage for gram-negative organisms. An inability to perform basic hygiene leads to colonization of the oral cavity with enteric gram-negative bacteria such as *Escherichia coli.* In these cases, the patient's normal defenses against pulmonary infection are often compromised. A patient's level of consciousness may be depressed; he may be intubated or unable to cough efficiently, leading to an increased risk for pulmonary infection.

Once the clinical diagnosis of pneumonia has been made, the next step is to try to **risk stratify** the patients, to decide which patients can be treated safely as outpatients with oral antibiotics, and which require hospitalization. In 1997, Fine and colleagues described a prediction rule that accurately identified those patients with community-acquired pneumonia who had a low risk for death or other adverse outcomes (Table 39-1). Patients younger than 50 years without these medical problems or physical examination findings have an approximately 0.1% risk of death and a 5.1% risk of hospitalization over the next 30 days. Patients in the lowest risk class usually can be safely treated as outpatients with oral antibiotics. Patients who are hypoxemic, are hemodynamically unstable, or have multiple risk factors have poor prognoses and usually require hospitalization.

Although outpatients usually are diagnosed and empiric treatment is begun based on clinical findings, further diagnostic evaluation is important in hospitalized patients. Chest radiography is important to try to define the cause and extent of the pneumonia and to look for complications, such as parapneumonic effusion or lung abscess. Unless the patient cannot mount an immune response, as in severe neutropenia, or the process is very early, **every patient with**

Table 39-1 RISK STRATIFICATION OF PNEUMONIA

History consistent with high risk
- Age >50 y
- History of cancer
- Congestive heart failure
- Cerebrovascular disease
- Renal or liver disease

Physical findings of high risk
- Altered mental status
- Tachycardia (≥125 bpm)
- Tachypnea (>30 breaths per minute)
- Hypotension (<90 mm Hg systolic)
- Temperature <95°F (35°C) or >104°F (40°C)

pneumonia will have a visible pulmonary infiltrate. The pattern of infiltration can yield diagnostic clues.* Diffuse interstitial infiltrates are common in *P carinii* pneumonia and viral processes. Conversely, pleural effusions are almost never seen in *P carinii* pneumonia. Bilateral apical infiltrate suggests tuberculosis. Appearance of **cavitation** suggests a necrotizing infection such as *Staphylococcus aureus*, tuberculosis, or gram-negative organisms such as *Klebsiella pneumoniae*. Serial chest radiography of inpatients usually is unnecessary, because many weeks are required for the infiltrate to resolve; serial chest radiography typically is performed if the patient does not show clinical improvement, has a pleural effusion, or has a necrotizing infection.

Microbiologic studies, such as sputum Gram stain and culture, and blood cultures are important to try to identify the specific etiologic agent causing the illness. However, use of sputum Gram stain and culture is limited by the frequent contamination by upper respiratory flora as the specimen is expectorated. However, if the sputum appears purulent and it is minimally contaminated (>25 polymorphonuclear cells and <10 epithelial cells per low-power field), the diagnostic yield is good. Additionally, blood cultures can be helpful, because 30% to 40% of patients with pneumococcal pneumonias are bacteremic. Serologic studies can be performed to diagnose patients who are infected with organisms not easily cultured, for example, *Legionella*, *Mycoplasma*, or *C pneumoniae*.

Finally, fiberoptic bronchoscopy with bronchoalveolar lavage often is performed in seriously ill or immunocompromised patients, or in those patients who are not responding to therapy, to try to obtain a specimen from the lower respiratory tract for routine Gram stain and culture, as well as more sophisticated testing, such as direct fluorescent antibody testing for various organisms, for example, *Legionella*.

Initially, empiric treatment is based upon the most common organisms given the clinical scenario. For outpatient therapy of **community-acquired pneumonia**, macrolide antibiotics, such as **azithromycin**, or antipneumococcal **quinolones**, such as gatifloxacin or levofloxacin, are good choices for treatment of *S pneumoniae*, *Mycoplasma*, and other common organisms. **Hospitalized patients** with community-acquired pneumonia usually are treated with an **intravenous third-generation cephalosporin plus a macrolide** or with an antipneumococcal quinolone. For immunocompetent patients with hospital-acquired or ventilator-associated pneumonias, the causes include any of the organisms that can cause community-acquired pneumonia, *Pseudomonas aeruginosa*, or *S aureus*, as well as more gram-negative enteric bacteria and oral anaerobes. Accordingly, the initial antibiotic coverage is broader and includes an antipseudomonal *beta*-lactam, such as piperacillin or cefepime, plus an aminoglycoside, and may include clindamycin.

---

*Infection with *Streptococcus pneumoniae* classically presents with a dense lobar infiltrate, often with an associated parapneumonic effusion.

For immunocompromised patients, such as AIDS patients, the spectrum of potential pathogens is much broader and includes *P carinii* pneumonia, unusual bacteria such as *Rhodococcus equi*, tuberculosis, as well as fungal organisms such as *Histoplasma* or *Cryptococcus*. It should be remembered, however, that even in AIDS patients, the most common cause of pneumonia is *S pneumoniae*. If an AIDS patient presents with an acute onset of fever and a productive cough with purulent sputum, pneumococcal pneumonia is the most likely diagnosis.

Two other commonly confused pulmonary syndromes deserve mention at this point. **Aspiration pneumonitis** is a chemical injury to the lungs caused by aspiration of acidic gastric contents into the lungs. Because of the high acidity, gastric contents are normally sterile, so this is not an infectious process but rather a chemical burn that causes a severe inflammatory response, which is proportional to the volume of the aspirate and the degree of acidity. This inflammatory response can be profound and produce respiratory distress and a pulmonary infiltrate that is apparent within 4 to 6 hours and typically resolves within 48 hours. Aspiration of gastric contents is most likely to occur in patients with a depressed level of consciousness, such as those under anesthesia or suffering from a drug overdose, or after a seizure.

Aspiration pneumonia, by contrast, is an infectious process caused by inhalation of oropharyngeal secretions that are colonized by bacterial pathogens. It should be noted that many healthy adults frequently aspirate small volumes of oropharyngeal secretions while sleeping (this is the primary way that bacteria gain entry to the lungs), but usually the material is cleared by coughing, ciliary transport, or normal immune defenses so that no clinical infection results. However, any process that increases the volume or bacterial organism burden of the secretion or impairs the normal defense mechanisms can produce clinically apparent pneumonia. This is most commonly seen in elderly patients with dysphagia, such as stroke victims, who may aspirate significant volumes of oral secretions, and those with poor dental care. The affected lobe of the lung depends upon the patient's position: in recumbent patients, the posterior segments of the upper lobes and apical segments of the lower lobes are most common. In contrast to aspiration pneumonitis, where aspiration of vomitus may be witnessed, the aspiration of oral secretions typically is silent and should be suspected when any institutionalized patient with dysphagia presents with respiratory symptoms and pulmonary infiltrate in a dependent segment of the lung.

Antibiotic therapy for aspiration pneumonia is similar to that of other pneumonias, that is, it should cover typical respiratory pathogens such as *S pneumoniae* and *H influenzae*, as well as gram-negative organisms and oral anaerobes. Treatment for aspiration pneumonitis, because it usually is not infectious, is mainly supportive. Antibiotics are often added if secondary bacterial infection is suspected because of failure to improve within 48 hours, or if the gastric contents are suspected to be colonized because of acid suppression or bowel obstruction.

Comprehension Questions

39.1 A 65-year-old cigarette smoker with a history of hypertension and mild congestive heart failure presents to the emergency room with worsening cough, fever, and dyspnea at rest. The illness began 1 week ago with fever, muscle aches, abdominal pain, and diarrhea, with nonproductive cough developing later that week and rapidly becoming worse. Therapy for which of the following atypical organisms must be considered in this case?

A. *Chlamydia pneumoniae*
B. *Mycoplasma pneumoniae*
C. *Legionella pneumophila*
D. *Coccidiomycosis*
E. *Aspergillus fumigatus*

39.2 An 85-year-old nursing home resident with a history of congestive heart failure has dementia such that she requires assistance in all activities of daily life. She has a 3-day history of fever and productive cough. Chest X-ray reveals a right middle lobe consolidation. Which of the following is the most appropriate initial antibiotic choice?

A. Oral amoxicillin
B. Intravenous linezolid
C. Intravenous cefepime
D. Oral azithromycin

39.3 A 56-year-old man is brought into the emergency room intoxicated with alcohol. He has repeated bouts of emesis and is found choking. Lung examination reveals some crackles in the right lung base. Which of the following is the most appropriate management?

A. Initiate azithromycin.
B. Initiate corticosteroid therapy.
C. Initiate haloperidol therapy.
D. Observation with follow-up chest radiograph.

ANSWERS

39.1 **C.** *Legionella* typically presents with myalgias, abdominal pain, diarrhea, and severe pneumonia.

39.2 **C.** This nursing home resident would be considered to have a nosocomial rather than community-acquired infection, with a higher incidence of gram-negative infection. Her age and comorbid medical conditions place her at high risk, requiring hospitalization for intravenous antibiotics such as a third-generation cephalosporin.

39.3 **D.** Antibiotic therapy is generally not indicated for aspiration pneumonitis, but patients need to be observed for clinical deterioration.

Clinical Pearls

> ➤ It is difficult to reliably distinguish clinically between typical and atypical causes of pneumonia. Therefore, diagnosis and empiric treatment of pneumonia are based upon the setting in which it was acquired (community acquired or nosocomial) and the immune status of the host.
> ➤ Clinical criteria, such as patient age, coexisting illnesses, tachycardia, and tachypnea, can be used to risk stratify patients with pneumonia to decide who can be treated as an outpatient and who requires hospitalization.
> ➤ Although initial antibiotic therapy is empiric, the etiologic agent frequently can be identified based on chest radiography, blood cultures, or sputum Gram stain and culture.
> ➤ Aspiration pneumonitis is a noninfectious chemical burn caused by inhalation of acidic gastric contents in patients with a decreased level of consciousness, such as seizure or overdose.
> ➤ Aspiration pneumonia is pulmonary infection caused by aspiration of colonized oropharyngeal secretions and is seen in patients with impaired swallowing, such as stroke victims.

REFERENCES

Fine MJ, Auble TE, Yealy DM, et al. A prediction rule to identify low-risk patients with community-acquired pneumonia. *N Engl J Med*. 1997;336:243-250.

Halm EA, Teirstein AS. Management of community-acquired pneumonia. *N Engl J Med*. 2002;347:2039-2045.

Marik P. Aspiration pneumonitis and aspiration pneumonia. *N Engl J Med*. 2001; 344:665-671.

Case 40

A 58-year-old woman comes to the office after a near-fainting spell she experienced 1 day ago. She was outside playing tennis when she vomited and felt lightheaded. She spent the rest of the day lying down with mild, diffuse, abdominal pain and nausea. She had no fever or diarrhea. She reports several months of worsening fatigue, mild, intermittent, generalized abdominal pain, and loss of appetite with a 10- to 15-lb unintentional weight loss. Her medical history is significant for hypothyroidism for which she takes levothyroxine. She takes no medications. On examination, her temperature is 99.8°F, heart rate 102 bpm, blood pressure 89/62 mm Hg, and normal respiratory rate. She does become lightheaded, and her heart rate rises to 125 bpm upon standing with a drop in systolic blood pressure to 70 mm Hg. She is alert and well tanned, with hyperpigmented creases in her hands. Her chest is clear, and her heart rhythm is tachycardic but regular. On abdominal examination, she has normal bowel sounds and mild diffuse tenderness without guarding. Her pulses are rapid and thready. She has no peripheral edema. Initial laboratory studies are significant for Na 121 mEq/L, K 5.8 mEq/L, HCO_3 16 mEq/L, glucose 52 mg/dL, and creatinine 1.0 mg/dL.

➤ What is the most likely diagnosis?

➤ What is your next step?

ANSWERS TO CASE 40:
Adrenal Insufficiency

Summary: A 58-year-old woman presents with orthostatic hypotension, intermittent chronic abdominal pain, and constitutional symptoms such as fatigue and unintentional weight loss. She also has hyponatremia, hyperkalemia, acidosis, and hypoglycemia. All of this patient's clinical features are consistent with acute adrenal insufficiency. The most common cause of adrenal insufficiency is idiopathic autoimmune destruction.

➤ **Most likely diagnosis:** Primary adrenal insufficiency.

➤ **Next step:** After drawing a cortisol level, immediate administration of intravenous saline with glucose and stress doses of corticosteroids.

ANALYSIS

Objectives

1. Know the presentation of primary and secondary adrenal insufficiency and of adrenal crisis.
2. Know the most common causes of primary and secondary adrenal insufficiency.
3. Know the treatment of adrenal insufficiency.

Considerations

This patient has a low-grade fever, which may be a feature of adrenal insufficiency, or it may signify infection, which can precipitate an adrenal crisis or produce a similar clinical picture. It is important to diagnose and treat any underlying infection. Because of the adrenal insufficiency and the aldosterone deficiency, she has volume depletion and hypotension. Thus, intravenous replacement with normal saline is critical.

APPROACH TO
Suspected Adrenal Insufficiency

DEFINITIONS

ADDISON DISEASE: Long-term insufficient function of the adrenal cortex leading to underproduction of corticosteroids.

ACTH STIMULATION TEST: An examination to evaluate the cortisol level after an intravascular (IV) injection of adrenocorticotropic hormone (ACTH). A normal individual should have an increase in cortisol whereas a patient with adrenal insufficiency will have no response or a limited one.

CLINICAL APPROACH

Etiology

Primary adrenal insufficiency (**Addison disease**) refers to adrenal failure to destruction or infiltration of the adrenal glands. The **most common cause in the United States is autoimmune destruction** of the **adrenal glands**. The most common cause worldwide is tuberculous adrenalitis. Other causes include chronic granulomatous infections (histoplasmosis, coccidiomycosis), bilateral adrenal hemorrhage (usually in the setting of sepsis with disseminated intravascular coagulation [DIC]), adrenal metastases (commonly from lung, breast, or stomach cancers), or X-linked adrenoleukodystrophy, a genetic disorder with adrenal and neurologic manifestations. Patients with acquired immunodeficiency syndrome (AIDS) often develop adrenal involvement as a result of infection with cytomegalovirus (CMV) or *Mycobacterium avium– intracellulare*. In primary adrenal insufficiency, the glands themselves are destroyed so that the patient becomes deficient in cortisol and aldosterone. Primary adrenal insufficiency is a relatively uncommon disease seen in clinical practice. A **high level of suspicion**, particularly in individuals who have suggestive signs or symptoms, or who are susceptible by virtue of associated autoimmune disorders or malignancies must be maintained. The nonspecific symptoms might be otherwise missed for many years until a stressful event leads to crisis and death.

Secondary adrenal insufficiency is adrenal failure caused by a lack of adrenocorticotropic hormone (ACTH) stimulation from the pituitary gland. It can be caused by an autoimmune, infiltrative, metastatic disease of the pituitary. The **most common reason, however, is chronic exogenous administration of corticosteroids**, which can suppress the entire hypothalamic-pituitary-adrenal axis. Because of the widespread use of corticosteroids, secondary adrenal insufficiency is relatively common. In secondary adrenal insufficiency, the renin-angiotensin system usually is able to maintain near-normal levels of aldosterone so that the patient is deficient only in cortisol.

Clinical Features

The clinical presentation depends on the relative deficiency of glucocorticoids and mineralocorticoids, ACTH excess, and other associated disorders. **Acute adrenal insufficiency**, or Addisonian crisis, may present with **weakness, nausea, vomiting, abdominal pain, fever, hypotension, and tachycardia**. Laboratory findings may **include hyponatremia, hyperkalemia, metabolic acidosis**, azotemia as a consequence of aldosterone deficiency, and hypoglycemia and eosinophilia as a consequence of cortisol deficiency. Patients with adrenal insufficiency may go into crisis when stressed by infection, trauma, or surgery.

The **clinical features may appear identical to those of septic shock**; the only clues that the cause is adrenal disease may be the hypoglycemia (blood sugar is often elevated in sepsis) and profound **hypotension, which may be refractory to administration of pressors** but is reversed almost immediately when steroids are given.

Chronic adrenal insufficiency has nonspecific clinical features, such as **malaise, weight loss, chronic fatigue, and gastrointestinal symptoms such as anorexia, nausea, and vomiting.** A patient may have hypoglycemia and postural hypotension as a result of volume depletion. **Hyperpigmentation** is seen over time in primary adrenal insufficiency caused by elevated melanocyte-stimulating hormone production from the pituitary as a byproduct of high ACTH levels. It is typically seen as generalized hyperpigmentation of skin and mucous membranes. It is increased in sun-exposed areas or over pressure areas, such as elbows and knees, and may be noted in skin folds. In secondary adrenal insufficiency, patients are deficient in cortisol because of a lack of ACTH from the pituitary, but aldosterone production is maintained by the renin-angiotensin system. Therefore, volume depletion and hyperkalemia are not present, and the patient will not manifest the typical hyperpigmentation.

Diagnosis

Cortisol levels show a diurnal variation. Cortisol levels are high in the morning and low as the day progresses, and levels should be elevated in stressful situations such as acute medical illness, surgery, or trauma. A **morning plasma cortisol level** less than or equal to 5 µg/dL in an acutely ill patient is definitive evidence of adrenal insufficiency. Conversely, a random cortisol level more than 20 µg/dL usually is interpreted as evidence of intact adrenal function. **The ACTH stimulation test** is used to confirm primary adrenal insufficiency. Synthetic ACTH (cosyntropin) 250 µg is administered intravenously, and serum cortisol levels are measured at baseline and then at 30- and 60-minute intervals. An increase in the cortisol level of 7 µg/dL or a maximal stimulated level more than 18 µg/dL is considered normal and indicates intact adrenal function. If cosyntropin stimulation testing indicates probable adrenal insufficiency, ACTH levels can then be measured to distinguish between primary (high ACTH) and secondary (low ACTH) adrenal failure.

The insulin–glucose tolerance test is the gold standard for testing the entire hypothalamic-pituitary axis. It is based on the principle that if a stressful situation is induced (in this case, hypoglycemia), the ACTH level should rise with a consequent increase in cortisol levels. Computed tomography (CT) scan and magnetic resonance imaging (MRI) are helpful in evaluating adrenal and pituitary disease after biochemical confirmation.

Treatment

Treatment of Addisonian crisis includes **intravenous 5% glucose with normal saline** to correct volume depletion and hypoglycemia and administration of

corticosteroid therapy. Hydrocortisone usually is given intravenously at doses of 100 mg every 6 to 8 hours, or it can be given as a bolus followed by a continuous infusion. At high doses, the hydrocortisone provides both glucocorticoid and mineralocorticoid activity. A cortisol level should be drawn before treatment to confirm the diagnosis. Causes of the acute crisis should be identified and treated; in particular, there should be a **search for infection**.

Long-term treatment of patients with primary adrenal insufficiency includes replacement doses of glucocorticoids (eg, hydrocortisone 25-30 mg/d) and mineralocorticoids (eg, fludrocortisone 0.1-0.2 mg/d). Patients with secondary adrenal insufficiency still produce aldosterone, as mentioned earlier, so only glucocorticoids must be replaced. In both cases, to prevent the long-term complications of glucocorticoid excess (diabetes, hypertension, obesity, osteoporosis, cataracts), patients should not be overtreated. Stress doses of steroids should be given for intercurrent illnesses. Patients should wear a medical alert bracelet.

Comprehension Questions

40.1   Which of the following is the most common cause of secondary adrenal insufficiency?
A. Autoimmune process
B. Surgical excision
C. Hemorrhagic shock
D. Exogenous corticosteroids
E. ACTH failure due to panhypopituitarism

40.2   A 30-year-old woman takes prednisone 15 mg/d for systemic lupus erythematosus. She is admitted to the hospital for a cholecystectomy. Which of the following is the most important intervention for her?
A Hydrocortisone intravenously before surgery and every 6 hours for 24 hours.
B. Double the prednisone the night before and hold her steroids the day of the surgery.
C. Use of cyclophosphamide in lieu of corticosteroids for 2 weeks following surgery to promote wound healing.
D. Cancel the surgery and use lithotripsy to break up the stones.

40.3   A 30-year-old woman who is 12 weeks postpartum is noted to have adrenal insufficiency and a very distinct tan, although she hardly ventures outside. Which of the following is the most likely etiology?
A. Long-term steroid use
B. Sheehan syndrome (pituitary insufficiency)
C. Brain tumor
D. Autoimmune adrenal destruction

ANSWERS

40.1   **D.** Long-term steroid use, with secondary suppression of pituitary secretion of ACTH, is the most common cause of secondary adrenal insufficiency. Autoimmune adrenalitis is the most common cause of primary adrenal insufficiency.

40.2   **A.** A stress dose of corticosteroids is important to prevent adrenal insufficiency before surgery.

40.3   **D.** Hyperpigmentation occurs as a result of increased melanocyte-stimulating factor, a byproduct of ACTH, and occurs in primary adrenal insufficiency. Secondary causes of adrenal insufficiency such as Sheehan syndrome result in low ACTH levels and do not cause the "tanned" appearance.

Clinical Pearls

➤ Primary adrenal insufficiency presents with weakness, fatigue, abdominal pain with vomiting, hyperpigmentation, and hyponatremia with hypotension, which may be refractory to pressors.

➤ Treatment of adrenal crisis is immediate administration of salt (saline), sugar (glucose), and steroids (hydrocortisone).

➤ The most common causes of primary adrenal insufficiency in the United States are autoimmune destruction, metastatic disease, and infectious causes (eg, cytomegalovirus in advanced acquired immunodeficiency syndrome). The most common cause worldwide is tuberculosis.

➤ Secondary adrenal insufficiency is the most common form of the illness and usually is a result of suppression of the hypothalamic-pituitary axis by exogenous corticosteroids.

REFERENCES

Aron DC, Findling JW, Tyrrell B, et al. Glucocorticoids and adrenal androgens. In: Greenspan FS, Gardner DG, eds. *Basic and Clinical Endocrinology*. 6th ed. New York, NY: Lange Medical Books/McGraw-Hill; 2001:334-377.

Oelkers W. Adrenal insufficiency. *N Engl J Med*. 1996;335:1206-1212.

Williams GH, Dluhy RG. Disorders of the adrenal cortex. In: Fauci AS, Braunwald E, Kasper DL, eds. *Harrison's Principles of Internal Medicine*. 17th ed. New York, NY: McGraw-Hill; 2008:2247-2269.

Case 41

A 57-year-old man comes to the office complaining of malaise for several weeks. He says that he has not been feeling well for some time, with fatigue, depressed mood, loss of appetite, and a 20-lb unintentional weight loss. In addition, he has been bothered by generalized itching of his skin and has tried moisturizing lotions and creams without improvement. He denies fevers, abdominal pain, nausea, vomiting, or diarrhea. He does think his stools have been lighter in color recently. He has no other medical history and takes no medications except for a multivitamin. He drinks alcohol occasionally and smokes cigars.

On examination, he is afebrile, with heart rate 68 bpm and blood pressure 128/74 mm Hg. He has a flat affect and a somewhat disheveled appearance. He has noticeable icterus of his sclera and skin. His chest is clear, and his heart rhythm is regular without murmurs. His abdomen is soft and nontender with active bowel sounds, a liver span of 10 cm, and no splenomegaly or masses. His skin has a few excoriations on his arms and back, but no rashes or telangiectasias.

Blood is obtained for laboratory analysis; the results are available the next day. His serum albumin is 3.1 g/dL, alkaline phosphatase 588 IU/L, total bilirubin 8.5 mg/dL, direct bilirubin 6 mg/dL, alanine aminotransferase (ALT) 175 IU/L, and aspartate aminotransferase (AST) 140 IU/L. His hemoglobin level is 13.5 g/dL. Prothrombin time (PT) is 15 seconds, and partial thromboplastin time (PTT) is 32 seconds.

➤ What is the most likely diagnosis?

➤ What is the next step?

ANSWERS TO CASE 41:

Painless Jaundice, Pancreatic Cancer

Summary: A 57-year-old man presents with pruritus, weight loss, and light-colored stools. He is found to be jaundiced with markedly elevated alkaline phosphatase level and conjugated hyperbilirubinemia. All of these findings point toward cholestasis. The light-colored, or acholic, stools suggest the cholestasis is most likely caused by biliary obstruction. The absence of abdominal pain makes gallstone disease less likely.

> **Most likely diagnosis:** Biliary obstruction, most likely caused by malignancy.

> **Next step:** Imaging procedure of his biliary system, either ultrasonography or computed tomographic (CT) scan.

ANALYSIS

Objectives

1. Know the causes and evaluation of a patient with unconjugated hyperbilirubinemia.
2. For a patient with conjugated hyperbilirubinemia, be able to distinguish between hepatocellular disease and biliary obstruction.
3. Understand the evaluation of a patient with cholestasis.
4. Know the treatment and complications of biliary obstruction.

Considerations

In patients with jaundice, one must try to distinguish between hepatic and biliary disease. In the patient with suspected biliary obstruction, without the pain typically associated with gallstones, one should be suspicious of malignancy or strictures. In the case presented, the clinical picture is worrisome for a malignant cause of biliary obstruction, such as pancreatic cancer.

APPROACH TO

Painless Jaundice

DEFINITIONS

CHOLESTASIS: Deficient bile flow that can result from intrahepatic disease or extrahepatic obstruction.

CONJUGATED BILIRUBIN (DIRECT-REACTING BILIRUBIN): Bilirubin that has entered the liver and has been enzymatically bound to glucuronic acid forming bilirubin monoglucuronide or diglucuronide.

JAUNDICE OR ICTERUS: Yellowing of the skin or whites of the eyes, indicating hyperbilirubinemia.

UNCONJUGATED BILIRUBIN (INDIRECT-REACTING BILIRUBIN): Bilirubin that has not been enzymatically bound to glucuronic acid by the liver and is in the serum reversibly and noncovalently bound to albumin.

CLINICAL APPROACH

Jaundice, or icterus, is the visible manifestation of **hyperbilirubinemia** and usually can be noticed by physical examination when the serum bilirubin level exceeds 2.0 to 2.5 mg/dL. Traditional instruction regarding the jaundiced patient divides the mechanism of hyperbilirubinemia into prehepatic (excessive production of bilirubin), intrahepatic, or extrahepatic (as in biliary obstruction). For most patients with jaundice, it probably is more clinically useful to think about hepatic or biliary diseases that cause conjugated hyperbilirubinemia, because they represent the most clinically important causes of jaundice.

The term **unconjugated hyperbilirubinemia** is used when the conjugated (or direct-reacting fraction) does not exceed 15% of the total bilirubin. It is almost always caused by hemolysis, or Gilbert syndrome. In these conditions, the serum bilirubin level almost always is less than 5 mg/dL, and there is usually no other clinical signs of liver disease. In addition, there should be no bilirubinuria (only conjugated bilirubin can be filtered and renally excreted). Hemolysis usually is clinically apparent, as in sickle cell disease or autoimmune hemolytic anemia. **Gilbert syndrome** is a benign condition caused by a deficiency of hepatic enzymatic conjugation of bilirubin, which results in intermittent unconjugated hyperbilirubinemia, usually with a total bilirubin less than 4gm/dL, often precipitated by events such as stress, fasting, and febrile illnesses. It is associated with no liver dysfunction and requires no therapy.

Conjugated hyperbilirubinemia almost always reflects either hepatocellular disease or biliary obstruction. These two conditions can be differentiated by the pattern of elevation of the liver enzymes. Elevation of serum AST and ALT levels are characteristic of hepatocellular disease as a result of the inflammation/destruction of the hepatocytes and the release of these enzymes into the blood. The serum alkaline phosphatase level is elevated in cholestatic disease as a consequence of inflammation, destruction, or obstruction of the intrahepatic or extrahepatic bile ducts with relative sparing of the hepatocytes. The serum AST and ALT levels may be mildly elevated in cholestasis but usually not to the levels seen in primary acute hepatocellular disease. Other tests, such as serum albumin or PT, generally reflect the capacity of hepatocytes to synthesize proteins such as clotting factors. When they are abnormal, they most often reflect hepatocellular disease. Table 41–1 summarizes the liver test patterns seen in various categories of hepatobiliary disorders.

Table 41–1 LIVER LAB FINDINGS IN HEPATOBILIARY DISORDERS

TYPE OF DISORDER	BILIRUBIN	AMINOTRANSFERASES	ALKALINE PHOSPHATASE	ALBUMIN	PROTHROMBIN TIME
Hemolysis/Gilbert syndrome	Normal to 5 mg/dL 85% due to indirect fractions. No bilirubinuria	Normal	Normal	Normal	Normal
Acute hepatocellular necrosis (viral and drug hepatitis, hepatotoxins, acute heart failure)	Both fractions may be elevated. Peak usually follows aminotransferases. Bilirubinuria.	Elevated, often >500 IU/L; ALT >AST	Normal to <3 times normal elevation	Normal	Usually normal if >5 times above control and not corrected by vitamin K; suggests poor prognosis
Chronic hepatocellular disorders	Both fractions may be elevated. Bilirubinuria.	Elevated, but usually <300 IU/L	Normal to <3 times normal elevation	Often decreased	Often prolonged; fails to correct with parenteral vitamin K

Table 41–1 LIVER TEST PATTERNS IN HEPATOBILIARY DISORDERS (CONTINUED)

TYPE OF DISORDER	BILIRUBIN	AMINOTRANSFERASES	ALKALINE PHOSPHATASE	ALBUMIN	PROTHROMBIN TIME
Intra- and extra-hepatic cholestasis (obstructive jaundice)	Both fractions may be elevated. Bilirubinuria	Normal to moderate elevation Rarely >500 IU/L	Elevated, often >4 times normal elevation	Normal, unless chronic	Normal; if prolonged, will correct with parenteral vitamin K
Infiltrative diseases (tumor, granulomata); partial bile duct obstruction	Usually normal	Normal to slight elevation	Elevated, often > 4 times normal elevation Fractionate, or confirm liver origin with 5'-nucleotidase or gamma-glutamyl transpeptidase	Normal	Normal

Reproduced, with permission, from Braunwald E, Fauci AS, Kasper KL, et al, eds. Harrison's Principles of Internal Medicine. 17th ed. New York, NY: McGraw-Hill; 2008:1926.

The patient discussed in this case has a pattern consistent with cholestasis, and the first diagnostic test in a patient with cholestasis usually is an ultrasound. It is noninvasive and is very sensitive for detecting stones in the gallbladder as well as intrahepatic or extrahepatic biliary ductal dilation. The **most common cause of biliary obstruction in the United States is gallstones**, which may become lodged in the common bile duct. However, obstructing stones causing jaundice usually are associated with epigastric or right upper quadrant colicky pain. Extrahepatic dilatation without evidence of stones warrants further study with CT or endoscopic retrograde cholangiopancreatography (ERCP) to detect occult stones or strictures, and exclude malignant causes of common bile duct and pancreatic duct obstruction including cholangiocarcinoma, pancreatic cancer, and ampullary cancer (ampulla of Vater).

Other possible causes include strictures, which can result from prior biliary surgery, prior inflammatory conditions such as pancreatitis (rarely), inflammatory diseases of the biliary tree, and infection in the setting of acquired immunodeficiency syndrome (AIDS). The two most important primary conditions are **primary sclerosing cholangitis** and **primary biliary cirrhosis**. Table 41–2 compares features of these two entities.

The complications of biliary obstruction include development of acute cholangitis as a result of ascending infection, or secondary hepatic cirrhosis, if the obstruction is chronic or recurrent. The patient in this case scenario has painless jaundice, liver enzymes consistent with a cholestatic process, and light-colored stools, suggesting obstruction of bile flow into the intestine. Because he has no history of abdominal or biliary surgery that might have caused a stricture, malignancy is the most likely cause of his biliary obstruction. The most common malignancy to present in this way is **pancreatic cancer**. The patient should undergo an imaging procedure of his abdomen, including a right upper quadrant ultrasound to evaluate the biliary tree, as well as a CT scan or magnetic resonance imaging (MRI) to visualize the pancreas. Endoscopic ultrasound with fine-needle aspiration is highly accurate in establishing a tissue diagnosis.

Pancreatic cancer is the fifth leading cause of cancer death in the United States. Peak incidence is in the seventh decade of life, with two-thirds of cases occurring in persons older than 65 years. There is a slight male predominance and a higher incidence in the black population. The median survival is 9 months, with an overall 5-year survival rate of 3%. Clinically apparent metastatic disease is found in 80% of patients at the time of diagnosis. For patients without obvious metastases, the best hope for cure is surgical resection by pancreaticoduodenectomy (Whipple procedure), which in experienced hands has a perioperative mortality rate less than 5%. Even when the cancer is considered to be respectable, there is a high rate of recurrence, so many treatment programs include neoadjuvant chemotherapy. Alternate palliative therapy includes pancreatic and common bile duct stenting to relieve the obstruction.

Table 41–2 COMPARISON OF PRIMARY SCLEROSING CHOLANGITIS AND PRIMARY BILIARY CIRRHOSIS

	YOUNGER MALES	OLDER FEMALES
Disease	Primary sclerosing cholangitis	Primary biliary cirrhosis
Location of Disease	Larger intra- and extrahepatic ducts	Smaller intrahepatic bile ducts
Associated Conditions	Ulcerative colitis	Autoimmune diseases such as rheumatoid arthritis
Serologic Markers	None	Antimitochondrial antibody (AMA)
Complications	Stricture; infection (cholangitis); cholangiocarcinoma	Cirrhosis

Comprehension Questions

For the following questions (41.1 to 41.4) choose the one diagnosis (A-F) that best matches with the most likely clinical situation.

    A. Hemolysis
    B. Alcoholic hepatitis
    C. Gilbert disease
    D. Pancreatic cancer
    E. Gallstones
    F. Primary sclerosing cholangitis

41.1   A 38-year-old man with a 12 pack of beer per day alcohol history presents with jaundice, ascites, and dark urine. His laboratory results are AST 350 U/mL, ALT 150 U/mL, alkaline phosphatase 120 U/mL, total bilirubin 25 mg/dL, direct bilirubin 12 mg/dL, and albumin 2.1 g/dL.

41.2   A 40-year-old moderately obese woman presents with abdominal pain after eating and mild scleral icterus. Her laboratory results are AST 200 U/L, ALT 150 U/L, alkaline phosphatase 355 U/L, total bilirubin 3.5 mg/dL, direct bilirubin 1.8 mg/dL, and albumin 3.5 g/dL.

41.3   A 25-year-old man presents with 3 days of scleral icterus but has been
         otherwise feeling well. His laboratory results are AST 45 U/L, ALT 48 U/L,
         alkaline phosphatase 100 U/L, total bilirubin 3.2 mg/dL, direct biliru-
         bin 0.2 mg/dL, and albumin 3.5 g/dL . Complete blood count and
         lactate dehydrogenase (LDH) are normal.

41.4   A 32-year-old man with a 5-year history of episodic bloody diarrhea
         and abdominal cramping pain presents with scleral icterus and fever.
         His laboratory results are AST 100 U/L, ALT 125 U/L, alkaline
         phosphatase 550 U/L, total bilirubin 5.5 mg/dL, direct bilirubin 3.0 mg/dL,
         and albumin 2.9 g/dL.

ANSWERS

41.1   **B.** The patient's laboratory results show a conjugated hyperbiliru-
         binemia with evidence of hepatocellular disease (hypoalbuminemia,
         ascites). The AST and ALT levels show the 2:1 ratio consistent with
         alcohol-related liver disease.

41.2   **E.** The patient's laboratory results show a conjugated hyperbiliru-
         binemia consistent with an obstructive pattern. She has the risk fac-
         tors for gallstones (middle age, female, obese) and has symptoms of
         postprandial abdominal pain.

41.3   **C.** The patient's laboratory results show an unconjugated hyper-
         bilirubinemia without other abnormality. He is otherwise healthy
         without symptoms of systemic disease or hemolytic anemia. No treat-
         ment is necessary.

41.4   **F.** The patient's laboratory results show a conjugated hyperbilirubinemia
         with an obstructive pattern. The history is consistent with inflamma-
         tory bowel disease, which is associated with primary sclerosing
         cholangitis. The initial evaluation should include ultrasonography to
         rule out gallstones; if negative, ERCP could confirm the diagnosis by
         demonstrating multiple strictures of the extrahepatic bile ducts.
         Treatment options include stenting of the larger bile duct strictures
         and immunosuppression to slow the progression of the disease.

Clinical Pearls

➤ Unconjugated hyperbilirubinemia usually is caused by hemolysis or Gilbert syndrome.

➤ Conjugated hyperbilirubinemia is commonly caused by hepatocellular disease, with elevated aspartate aminotransferase and alanine levels, or biliary obstruction, with elevated alkaline phosphatase level.

➤ An imaging procedure such as ultrasonography is the initial study of choice in a patient with cholestasis to evaluate for intrahepatic or extra-hepatic biliary obstruction.

➤ The most common causes of biliary obstruction are gallstones, which are painful if obstructing, and strictures or neoplasms, which are often painless.

➤ The prognosis for pancreatic cancer is very poor; the best hope for cure is resection by a pancreaticoduodenectomy (Whipple procedure).

REFERENCES

Brugge WR, Dam JV. Medical progress: pancreatic and biliary endoscopy. *N Engl J Med*. 1999;341:1808-1916.

Kosuri K, Muscarella P, Bekaii-Saab TS. Updates and controversies in the treatment of pancreatic cancer. *Clin Adv Hematol Oncol*. 2006;4:47-54.

Pratt DS, Kaplan MM. Evaluation of liver function. In: Kasper DL, Braunwald E, Fauci AS, et al, eds. *Harrison's Principles of Internal Medicine*. 17th ed. New York, NY: McGraw-Hill; 2008:1923-1926.

Wolkoff AW. The Hyperbilirubinemias. In: Fauci AS, Braunwald E, Kasper DL, eds. *Harrison's Principles of Internal Medicine*. 17th ed. New York, NY: McGraw-Hill; 2008:1927-1931.

Case 42

While seeing patients in your preceptor's clinic, you have the opportunity to meet and examine one of her long-time patients, a 46-year-old woman who presents for her yearly physical examination. She has been fine and has no complaints today. Her medical history is notable only for borderline hypertension and moderate obesity. Last year her fasting lipid profile was acceptable for someone without known risk factors for coronary artery disease. Her mother and older brother have diabetes and hypertension. At prior visits, you see that your preceptor has counseled her on a low-calorie, low-fat diet and recommended that she start an exercise program. However, the patient says she has not made any of these recommended changes. With her full-time job and three children, she finds it difficult to exercise, and she admits that her family eats out frequently. Today her blood pressure is 140/92 mm Hg. Her body mass index (BMI) is 27 kg/m². Her examination is notable for acanthosis nigricans at the neck but otherwise is normal. A Papanicolaou (Pap) smear is performed, and a mammogram is offered. The patient has not eaten yet today, so on your preceptor's recommendation, a fasting plasma glucose test is performed, and the result is 140 mg/dL.

➤ What is your diagnosis?

➤ What is your next step?

ANSWERS TO CASE 42:

Type 2 Diabetes Diagnosis and Management

Summary: A 46-year-old woman presents for her yearly physical examination. Her medical history is notable only for borderline hypertension and moderate obesity. She has a family history of diabetes and hypertension. The patient has not followed the recommended lifestyle changes. Today, her blood pressure is 140/92 mm Hg, and her BMI is 27 kg/m². Her examination is notable for acanthosis nigricans at the neck, suggesting insulin resistance. A fasting plasma glucose level is 140 mg/dL, which is consistent with diabetes mellitus.

> ➤ **Most likely diagnosis:** Given her hypertension, obesity, family history, and the finding of acanthosis nigricans, this patient most likely has type 2 diabetes. Diabetes is defined by the American Diabetes Association as a fasting plasma glucose more than or equal to 126 mg/dL.

> ➤ **Next step:** The fasting glucose level should be repeated to confirm the diagnosis. If the next result is less than 126 mg/dL, then an oral glucose tolerance test should be performed.

ANALYSIS

Objectives

1. Know the diagnostic criteria for type 2 diabetes.
2. Understand the initial medical management of diabetes.
3. Understand cardiovascular risk modification in diabetic patients.
4. Understand the prevention of microvascular complications of diabetes.

Considerations

If this patient's diagnosis of diabetes is confirmed, she will require patient education, lifestyle modification, and medical therapy to prevent acute and chronic complications of diabetes. Strict glycemic control can reduce the incidence of microvascular complications such as retinopathy and nephropathy. In addition, patients with diabetes are among the highest at risk for cardiovascular disease, so risk factor modifications, such as smoking cessation and lowering of cholesterol, are essential. **Diabetes confers the same level of risk for coronary events, such as heart attack, as in patients with established coronary artery disease.** Thus, in this patient, the target blood pressure is less than 130/80 mm Hg, and the target low-density lipoprotein (LDL) cholesterol is less than 100 mg/dL.

APPROACH TO
Suspected Diabetes Mellitus

DEFINITIONS

TYPE 1 DIABETES: Caused by what is believed to be an autoimmune destruction of the pancreatic beta cells and complete loss of endogenous insulin production. The presentation of this type of diabetes usually is acute, with hyperglycemia and metabolic acidosis. These patients are dependent upon exogenous insulin delivery.

TYPE 2 DIABETES: Heterogenous syndrome of insulin resistance caused by genetic factors and/or obesity and relative insulin deficiency. Oral medications to enhance endogenous insulin production or improve insulin sensitivity are useful. Exogenous insulin may be used when oral medications are no longer sufficient for adequate glycemic control.

CLINICAL APPROACH

As the prevalence of obesity increases in the American population, so does the prevalence of type 2 diabetes, especially in children and teenagers. Ninety percent of all new cases of diabetes diagnosed in the United States are type 2, and it is estimated that this disease affects approximately 7% of the population older than 45 years. **Diabetes is the leading cause of blindness, renal failure, and nontraumatic amputations of the lower extremities.** It is a major risk factor in patients with coronary artery disease, peripheral vascular disease, and stroke.

Type 2 diabetes is believed to have a prolonged asymptomatic phase. During these years of asymptomatic hyperglycemia, however, organ damage begins to occur. Therefore, several organizations recommend screening of certain high-risk populations. The **risk factors** for diabetes include obesity or overweight, defined as BMI more than 25 kg/m^2; other signs of an insulin-resistance syndrome or "metabolic" syndrome, such as hypertension or low high-density lipoproteins (HDLs) and triglycerides more than 250 mg/dL; first-degree relative with diabetes; history of gestational diabetes; or being a member of a high-risk ethnic group, including African Americans, Hispanics, American Indians, Asian Americans, or Pacific Islanders. Screening should begin at age 45 years and repeated every 3 years. Children with risk factors can be considered for screening at age 10 years and every 2 years thereafter.

Most patients with type 2 diabetes mellitus are insulin resistant and hyper-insulinemic for years before developing overt diabetes, are able to maintain normoglycemia for a long time, first develop postprandial hyperglycemia, and later develop both postprandial and fasting hyperglycemia (ie, hyper-glycemia all the time). Thus, a **glucose tolerance test** to detect postprandial hyperglycemia would be the most sensitive test for diabetes mellitus but is time consuming and difficult to perform in a clinical practice. The **fasting plasma glucose** is the most specific test. **Hemoglobin A$_{1c}$ (HbA$_{1c}$)** is not a recommended screening/diagnostic test because of the lack of standardization between laboratories, but it is useful for monitoring glycemic control once diagnosis is established (Table 42–1). **Tests should be confirmed by a separate measurement on another day.**

By using these tests, patients can be classified into one of three categories: normal, impaired glucose tolerance/impaired fasting glucose (ie, "prediabetic"), or diabetic. Increased risk for microvascular complications of hyperglycemia is seen at a fasting glucose more than 126 mg/dL. Increased risk for macrovascular complications is seen at a fasting glucose more than 110 mg/dL. Once diabetes is diagnosed, therapy is instituted with three major goals.

1. Prevention of acute complications of hyperglycemia (eg, diabetic ketoacidosis or nonketotic hyperosmolar hyperglycemia) or hypoglycemia
2. Prevention of long-term complications of hyperglycemia, for example, microvascular disease such as retinopathy or nephropathy
3. Prevention of long-term complications of macrovascular disease, for example, cardiovascular or cerebrovascular disease

The foundation of diabetes therapy is **dietary and lifestyle modifications**. Randomized trials show that even small amounts of weight loss can lower blood pressure and improve glucose control. Patients should be given instruction in nutrition and encouraged to change sedentary lifestyles. Exercise that the patient finds enjoyable and possible should be encouraged. However, most people with diabetes will eventually require medications, and most patients

Table 42–1 TESTS FOR DIAGNOSING DIABETES			
TEST	NORMAL	IMPAIRED FASTING GLUCOSE/IMPAIRED GLUCOSE TOLERANCE ("PREDIABETES")	DIABETES
Fasting plasma glucose	<100 mg/dL	100-126 mg/dL	>126 mg/dL
Random glucose			>200 mg/dL (plus symptoms of diabetes)
Oral glucose tolerance test (75-g load)	2-h <140 mg/dL	140-200 mg/dL	>200 mg/dL

will eventually require a combination of at least two medications. The United Kingdom Prospective Diabetes Study (UKPDS) followed almost 5000 patients over 20 years and compared intensive blood glucose control to conventional therapy in the prevention of **macrovascular** (coronary artery disease) and **microvascular** (retinopathy, nephropathy, and neuropathy) complications. Intensive therapy, with an HbA_{1c} less than or equal to 7%, resulted in fewer microvascular complications, but there was no significant differences in macrovascular complications between the two groups. Patients in the intensive therapy group had more episodes of hypoglycemia, so intensive therapy may not be appropriate for elderly patients or those patients with other comorbid conditions.

The UKPDS randomized patients to begin treatment with either sulfonylureas or insulin therapy. A subgroup of overweight patients was started on metformin. In the end, those on insulin tended to gain more weight each year; otherwise, there were no differences between the groups. This has been interpreted to mean that any of these medications is an appropriate first choice in newly diagnosed diabetic patients. However, obese persons may benefit from metformin, as it has some effects on appetite and is associated with modest weight loss. Sulfonylureas are very inexpensive and effective. Other medications developed since the UKPDS may be added if needed (Table 42–2). If possible, introduction of insulin may be delayed because it leads to weight gain, which may worsen insulin resistance.

When diabetes is diagnosed, other cardiovascular risk factors should be assessed. Blood pressure and lipid levels should be measured. With regard to lipid therapy, the cardiovascular risk in those with diabetes is equivalent to those with known coronary artery disease, so the desired LDL threshold is less than 100 mg/dL. Those with higher LDL levels should undergo dietary modification or be started on a statin.

The desired blood pressure threshold also is lower, with a goal of less than 130/80 mm Hg. Several randomized trials have demonstrated a **benefit for angiotensin-converting enzyme (ACE) inhibitors** and **angiotensin receptor blockers (ARBs)** in preventing the progression of proteinuria and kidney disease. Patients who already have renal insufficiency or heavy proteinuria (>1-2 g/d) have an even lower target blood pressure of 120/75 mm Hg.

Other routine care in diabetic patients includes frequent physician visits, at least every 3 to 6 months depending on their glucose control, at least yearly ophthalmologic examinations to screen for retinopathy, semiannual dental visits to prevent periodontal disease, and yearly urine screens to detect microalbuminuria. Hemoglobin A_{1c} should be checked at least every 3 to 6 months, depending on the patient's glucose control. This test allows the physician to know the general glucose control over the preceding 2 to 3 months. Patients without neuropathy should have a foot examination yearly to detect early neuropathic changes; however, those with neuropathy should be examined every 3 months and be instructed on daily self-examination and prevention of injury.

Table 42–2 MEDICATIONS AVAILABLE IN THE UNITED STATES FOR TREATMENT OF TYPE 2 DIABETES

MEDICATION	MECHANISM OF ACTION/INDICATIONS	SPECIAL CONSIDERATIONS	COST
Insulin	Supplements patient's own insulin production	Must check blood glucose frequently to monitor therapy and prevent complications	$-$$$
Sulfonylurea	Augments patient's own insulin production, works at the pancreatic beta cells	Can cause hypoglycemia; can accumulate in renal insufficiency and cause prolonged hypoglycemia; best for young patients with fasting plasma glucose <300 mg/dL	$-$$
Metformin	Decreases gluconeogenesis in the liver; decreases insulin resistance	In patients with renal insufficiency or liver dysfunction may cause lactic acidosis	$-$$
Alpha-glucosidase	Inhibits breakdown of complex carbohydrates in the GI tract	Can cause GI distress, and must be taken twice a day with meals; dose-dependent hepatotoxicity	$$
Pioglitazone; rosiglitazone	Promote skeletal muscle glucose uptake and decrease insulin resistance	Hepatotoxicity; edema	$$-$$$
Repaglinide	Nonsulfonylurea but works in a similar manner; rapid onset of action; monotherapy or in combination with metformin	Caution in elderly and in patients with renal or hepatic insufficiency; must dose twice a day with meals	$$

Comprehension Questions

42.1 A patient comes in for a fasting plasma glucose test. On two separate occasions, the result has been 115 mg/dL and 120 mg/dL. Which of the following is the most appropriate next step?

A. Reassurance that these are normal blood sugars.

B. Recommend weight loss, an American Diabetes Association diet, and exercise.

C. Diagnose diabetes mellitus and start a sulfonylurea agent.

D. Recommend cardiac stress testing.

E. Obtain stat arterial blood gas and serum ketone levels.

42.2 A 45-year-old obese Hispanic woman presents for follow-up of her diabetes. She currently takes glipizide (sulfonylurea) 10 mg twice per day, and her fasting morning glucose runs approximately 170 to 200 mg/dL. Her last HbA_{1c} was 7.9. She states that she conscientiously follows her diet and that she walks 30 minutes to 1 hour daily. Which of the following is the best next step in her care?

A. Add an insulin pump.

B. Add metformin.

C. Add NPH (neutral protamine Hagedorn) insulin.

D. Hospitalize her urgently.

42.3 A 75-year-old woman with diabetes for approximately 20 years, diabetic retinopathy, and diabetic nephropathy with creatinine level 2.2 mg/dL is brought into the office by her daughter for follow-up. The patient currently takes a sulfonylurea for her diabetes and an ACE inhibitor for her proteinuria. Her daughter reports that, on three occasions in the past 2 weeks, her mother became sweaty, shaky, and confused, which resolved when she was given some orange juice. Which of the following conditions is most likely to be contributing to these episodes?

A. Excess caloric oral intake

B. Interaction between the ACE inhibitor and the sulfonylurea agents

C. Worsening renal function

D. Hyperglycemic amnesia

ANSWERS

42.1 **B.** By diagnostic criteria, this patient falls into the definition of impaired fasting glucose. Although she does not yet meet the criteria for diabetes, she is at greater risk for developing diabetes in the future and for macrovascular disease. Interventions such as weight loss will decrease her insulin resistance, and following a diet lower in simple sugars and fats may place less stress on her pancreas and increase the time to development of outright diabetes.

42.2   **B.** Because this patient is obese and young, after reviewing her meal plan and exercise schedule, adding metformin is the next best step. Although insulin is just as beneficial in controlling blood sugar levels and vascular complications, it may be associated with weight gain, and most patients prefer to be maintained on oral agents rather than injections, if possible.

42.3   **C.** Sulfonylureas have long half-lives and can cause prolonged hypoglycemia in elderly patients as well in those with **renal insufficiency**. Another method, such as insulin, may be more appropriate in this patient, as well as less-intensive control, aiming for an HbA_{1c} of 8% instead of 7%.

Clinical Pearls

➤ Type 2 diabetes has a prolonged asymptomatic stage during which microvascular disease (eg, retinopathy or nephropathy) can occur. Physicians should have a high index of suspicion and screen those patients with risk factors.

➤ Tight glycemic control (hemoglobin A_{1c} <7.0%) reduces the incidence and progression of microvascular complications of diabetes.

➤ The major cause of morbidity and mortality in patients with type 2 diabetes mellitus is macrovascular disease: coronary artery disease, stroke, and peripheral vascular disease.

➤ Aggressive treatment of other cardiovascular risk factors (hypertension, hyperlipidemia, smoking cessation) is necessary to reduce the incidence of macrovascular complications.

REFERENCES

American Diabetes Association. Standards of medical care for patients with diabetes mellitus. *Diabetes Care*. 2008;31(suppl 1): 12S-54S.

Baldeweg S, Yudkin J. Implications of the UKPDS. *Prim Care*. 1999;26:809-827.

Powers AC. Diabetes mellitus. In: Fauci AS, Braunwald E, Kasper DL, eds. *Harrison's Principles of Internal Medicine*. 17th ed. New York, NY: McGraw-Hill; 2008:2275-2304.

Case 43

An 18-year-old adolescent female is brought to the emergency room by her mother because the daughter seems confused and is behaving strangely. The mother reports the patient has always been healthy and has no significant medical history, but she has lost 20 lb recently without trying and has been complaining of fatigue for 2 or 3 weeks. The patient had attributed the fatigue to sleep disturbance, as recently she has been getting up several times at night to urinate. This morning, the mother found the patient in her room, complaining of abdominal pain, and she had vomited. She appeared confused and did not know that today was a school day.

On examination, the patient is slender, lying on a stretcher with eyes closed, but she is responsive to questions. She is afebrile, and has a heart rate 118 bpm, blood pressure 125/84 mm Hg, with deep and rapid respirations at the rate of 24 breaths per minute. Upon standing, her heart rate rises to 145 bpm, and her blood pressure falls to 110/80 mm Hg. Her funduscopic examination is normal, her oral mucosa is dry, and her neck veins are flat. Her chest is clear to auscultation, and her heart is tachycardic with a regular rhythm and no murmur. Her abdomen is soft with active bowel sounds and mild diffuse tenderness, but no guarding or rebound. Her neurologic examination reveals no focal deficits.

Laboratory studies include serum Na 131 mEq/L, K 5.3 mEq/L, Cl 95 mEq/L, CO_2 9 mEq/L, blood urea nitrogen (BUN) 35 mg/dL, creatinine 1.3 mg/dL, and glucose 475 mg/dL. Arterial blood gas reveals pH 7.12 with P_{CO_2} 24 mm Hg and P_{O_2} 95 mm Hg. Urine drug screen and urine pregnancy test are negative, and urinalysis shows no hematuria or pyuria, but 3+ glucose and 3+ ketones. Chest radiograph is read as normal, and plain film of the abdomen has nonspecific gas pattern but no signs of obstruction.

➤ What is the most likely diagnosis?

➤ What is your next step?

ANSWERS TO CASE 43:

Diabetic Ketoacidosis

Summary: An 18-year-old adolescent female presents with unintentional weight loss, nocturia, and polyuria, with hyperglycemia that likely represents new-onset diabetes mellitus. She is hypovolemic as a result of osmotic diuresis and has an anion gap metabolic acidosis, which is primarily caused by ketoacids. Her mental status and abdominal pain probably are manifestations of the metabolic acidosis and hyperosmolarity.

➤ **Most likely diagnosis:** Diabetic ketoacidosis (DKA).

➤ **Next step:** Aggressive hydration to improve her volume status and insulin therapy to resolve the ketoacidosis.

ANALYSIS

Objectives

1. Know how to diagnose patients with anion gap metabolic acidosis.
2. Be able to differentiate DKA, nonketotic hyperosmolar hyperglycemia, and alcoholic ketoacidosis.
3. Understand the principles of DKA management: restoration of volume, electrolyte replacement, resolution of ketosis, and control of hyperglycemia.
4. Learn the complications of DKA and of improper management.

Considerations

DKA occurs as a result of severe insulin deficiency and may be the initial presentation of diabetes mellitus, as in this patient. In all patients with DKA, one must be alert for precipitating factors, such as infection, pregnancy, or severe physiologic stressors, such as myocardial infarction. Careful management and close monitoring will be required to correct fluid and electrolyte deficits and to prevent complications such as hypokalemia and cerebral edema.

APPROACH TO

Suspected Diabetic Ketoacidosis

DEFINITIONS

DIABETIC KETOACIDOSIS: A syndrome of hyperglycemia, anion gap metabolic acidosis, and ketone bodies in the serum, caused by insufficient insulin levels.

KUSSMAUL RESPIRATIONS: Deep and rapid breathing, represent hyperventilation in an attempt to generate a respiratory alkalosis to compensate for the metabolic acidosis.

CLINICAL APPROACH

Diabetic ketoacidosis is a clinical syndrome that results when the **triad of anion gap metabolic acidosis, hyperglycemia, and ketosis** is present and is caused by a significant insulin deficiency. It is a medical emergency, with an overall mortality rate less than 5% if patients receive prompt and appropriate medical treatment. The majority of episodes are preventable, and many of the deaths also are preventable with proper attention to detail during management.

Pathophysiology

In the normal physiologic state, there is a fine balance between anabolic and catabolic hormones. In the fed state, anabolic actions of insulin predominate. Glycogenesis, lipogenesis, and protein synthesis all are increased. This results in storage of energy reserves in the form of triglycerides and glycogen.

In the fasting state, insulin serves to inhibit lipolysis, ketogenesis, gluconeogenesis, glycogenolysis, and proteolysis. These effects are critical in controlling the rate of breakdown of energy stores under the influence of catabolic hormones. **Glucagon is the most important catabolic hormone.** In the fasting state, it maintains normal glucose levels by stimulating hepatic gluconeogenesis and glycogenolysis.

Diabetes is the condition of relative or absolute insulin deficiency. When there is a severe insulin deficiency and a relative excess of glucagon, lipolysis is enhanced, causing release of free fatty acids. Oxidation of the fatty acids produces ketones, such as acetoacetate and beta-hydroxybutyrate, which are organic acids and often referred to as **ketoacids.** The excess of these ketoacids can produce a life-threatening metabolic acidosis. In addition, hyperglycemia produces an osmotic diuresis, which causes severe volume depletion, and electrolyte deficiencies by washing extracellular sodium, potassium, magnesium, phosphate, and water out of the body. The combination of acidosis, hypovolemia, and electrolyte deficiencies can lead to **cardiovascular collapse, the most common cause of death in DKA**.

Clinical Presentation

Patients with diabetes have an underlying impairment in glucose metabolism and, when challenged by a stress, an increase in insulin requirements. If they are unable to meet these insulin requirements, DKA may result. **The most common precipitating events are infections** such as pneumonia or urinary tract infection, vascular disorders such as myocardial infarction, or other stressors such as trauma. Diabetic ketoacidosis may be the presentation of new-onset diabetes, or it can occur in patients with established diabetes because of

failure to use insulin for whatever reason or because of use of other medications (eg, glucocorticoids) that interfere with insulin action.

An episode of DKA evolves over a short period of time, typically less than
24 hours. The patient with DKA has the signs and symptoms of hyperglycemia,
acidosis, and dehydration. Polyuria, polydipsia, weight loss, visual blurring, and
decreased mental status are related to hyperglycemia and osmotic diuresis.
Nausea, vomiting, abdominal pain, fatigue, malaise, and shortness of breath may
be related to the acidosis.

Typical signs include reduced skin elasticity, dry mucus membranes,
hypotension, and tachycardia related to volume depletion. **Kussmaul respirations**, deep and rapid breathing, represent hyperventilation in an attempt to
generate a respiratory alkalosis to compensate for the metabolic acidosis. One
may also note the fruity breath odor typical of ketosis.

Laboratory Diagnosis

Laboratory values show hyperglycemia (usually >250 mg/dL), acidosis
(pH <7.3), anion gap (usually >15 mmol/L), and ketonemia. The most
important laboratory parameters are the degree of acidosis, the anion gap, and
the serum potassium level.

Patients with a very low pH less than 7.0 are severely acidotic and have a
worse prognosis. The lower pH is a result of the higher concentration of
ketoacids, which are estimated using the anion gap. The first step in evaluating any patient with metabolic acidosis should be calculation of the **anion
gap**. This concept is based on the principle of electrical neutrality, that is, all
the cations must equal all the anions. The anion gap estimates those negatively charged particles that are not routinely measured and can be calculated
using the following calculation:

$$\text{Anion Gap} = [Na] - [Cl + HCO_3]$$

The normal anion gap is 10 to 12 mmol/L. When it is elevated, there is an
excess of unmeasured anions, which typically occurs because of one of the four
causes, which are listed in Table 43–1.

Lactic acidosis can be a result of severe tissue hypoxia, as in septic shock or
carbon monoxide poisoning, or a result of hepatic failure and subsequent
inability to metabolize lactate. Ketoacidosis most commonly occurs as an acute
complication of uncontrolled diabetes, but it also can be seen in starvation and
alcoholism (discussed later). The ingested toxins may be organic acids themselves, such as salicylic acid, or have acidic metabolites, such as formic acid
from methanol. Renal failure leads to an inability to excrete organic acids as
well as inorganic acids such as phosphates (often without an anion gap).

In patients with DKA, total-body potassium stores are depleted because of
urinary losses, and potassium replacement will always be necessary. Initially, the
measured serum potassium levels may be high despite the total-body deficit
because of acidosis resulting in movement of potassium from the intracellular
to the extracellular compartment. As the acidosis is corrected and with the

Table 43-1 CAUSES OF HIGH ANION GAP METABOLIC ACIDOSIS

Lactic acidosis
Ketoacidosis
• Diabetic
• Alcoholic
• Starvation
Toxins
• Ethylene glycol
• Methanol
• Salicylates
Renal failure (acute or chronic)

Reproduced, with permission, from DuBose TD. Acidosis and alkalosis. In: Braunwald E, Fauci AS, Kasper KL, et al, eds. Harrison's Principles of Internal Medicine. 16th ed. New York, NY: McGraw-Hill; 2005:265.

administration of insulin, which drives potassium intracellularly, **serum potassium levels will fall rapidly.**

The serum sodium level can be variable. Hyperglycemia causes water to move extracellularly, which can lead to hyponatremia. Similarly, phosphate levels can be variable in the presence of body store deficits with the extracellular movement of phosphate caused by catabolic state. Blood urea nitrogen (BUN) and creatinine levels are elevated, reflecting dehydration. Serum acetoacetate may cause a false elevation in serum creatinine level because of interference with the assay.

Management

The goal of treatment is restoration of metabolic homeostasis with correction of precipitating events and biochemical deficits, which consists of the following:

1. Replacement of fluid losses with improvement of circulatory volume
2. Correction of hyperglycemia and, in turn, plasma osmolality
3. Replacement of electrolyte losses
4. Clearance of serum ketones
5. Identification and treatment of precipitating cause and complications

Close monitoring of the patient is important. A flow sheet recording vital signs, input and output, insulin dosage, and metabolic progress is important. Serum glucose concentration should be measured every 1 hour, and levels of serum electrolytes and phosphate must be assessed every 3 to 5 hours. Urinalysis, urine and blood cultures, ECG, and chest X-ray should be obtained to identify precipitating factors and complications. Other investigations should be pursued as symptoms and signs warrant.

Fluids

All patients with DKA are volume depleted as a consequence of osmotic diuresis as well as from other ongoing losses, such as vomiting. Hydration improves renal perfusion and cardiac output, facilitating glucose excretion. Rehydration may also diminish insulin resistance by decreasing levels of counterregulatory hormones and hyperglycemia. Sudden reduction in hyperglycemia can lead to vascular collapse with shift of water intracellularly. To avoid this, initial replacement fluid should be isotonic normal saline (NS) to correct circulatory volume deficit. **Over the first hour, 1 to 2 L of NS should be infused.** Following this, total-body water deficit is corrected at the rate of 250 to 500 mL/h, depending on the state of hydration. The composition of fluid should be tailored according to serum sodium and chloride measurements.

Hydration should be gentler in patients with congestive heart failure or end-stage renal disease because such patients can easily get fluid overload.

Insulin

The goal of therapy is a glucose reduction of 80 to 100 mg/dL/h. Use of continuous low-dose intravenous infusion of insulin is recommended because it reduces episodes of hypoglycemia and hypokalemia, and it allows a more controlled reduction of serum glucose and osmolality. Intramuscular and subcutaneous routes can be used if tissue perfusion is adequate.

Insulin treatment may be initiated as an **intravenous bolus** of 0.1 to 0.15 U/kg. This should be followed by a **continuous infusion of 0.1 U/kg/h with hourly serum glucose determinations**. If blood glucose fails to decline at the desired rate, volume status should be reassessed, and insulin infusion should be titrated. The rate of infusion should be decreased to 0.05 U/Kg/h when the blood glucose level decreases to 250 to 300 mg/dL. **Glucose levels fall more quickly than ketosis resolves.** Insulin is necessary for resolution of the ketoacidosis and can be coadministered with a glucose infusion until the anion gap is resolved. A 5% to 10% dextrose solution should be added to the hydrating solution when plasma glucose is less than 300 mg/dL. One can judge the resolution of ketoacidosis when the bicarbonate is more than 18 mEq/L, the anion gap is less than 12, the patient feels better, and the vital signs are stabilized. **Serial determination of serum ketone levels is not clinically useful** in measuring response to therapy. Laboratory tests measure acetoacetate and acetone, but not beta-hydroxybutyrate. With the administration of insulin, beta-hydroxybutyrate is first oxidized to acetoacetate, so measured ketone levels may actually increase with effective therapy. Instead, one should be guided by normalizing the anion gap when making decisions about the rate of insulin infusion. Subcutaneous insulin should be given approximately 30 minutes before stopping insulin infusion to avoid rebound acidosis.

Bicarbonate

Bicarbonate therapy is controversial and should not be given to ketoacidotic patients unless their arterial pH is less than 7.0 or other indications, such as cardiac instability or severe hyperkalemia, are present. Bicarbonate therapy can cause worsening hypokalemia, paradoxical central nervous system acidosis, and delay in ketone clearance.

Electrolytes

In DKA, there is total-body deficit of potassium, phosphate, and magnesium. Patients frequently have hyperkalemia as a result of acidosis, insulin deficiency, and hypertonicity that cause a shift of potassium extracellularly. During treatment, plasma potassium concentration will fall as the metabolic abnormalities are corrected. Potassium should be added to initial intravenous fluids once the concentration is less than 5 mEq/L. Once adequate urine output is established, 20 to 40 mEq of potassium should be added to each liter of fluid. The goal is to maintain potassium in the range of 4 to 5 mEq/L. Cardiac monitoring is recommended in the presence of hypokalemia or hyperkalemia.

Phosphate replacement should be given to patients if serum phosphate concentrations less than 1 mg/dL and to patients with moderate hypophosphatemia with concomitant hypoxia, anemia, or cardiorespiratory compromise. Careful monitoring of the serum calcium level is necessary with phosphate administration.

Magnesium and calcium can be supplemented as needed.

Precipitating Causes

It is important to correct precipitating factors in order to restore metabolic balance. Identifiable sources of infection should be treated aggressively. Possible presence of ischemia and infarction should be evaluated and treated appropriately with help from specialists as needed.

Complications

Cerebral edema, acute respiratory distress syndrome, thromboembolism, fluid overload, and acute gastric dilatation are rare, but serious, complications of DKA.

Prevention

The major precipitating factors in the development of DKA are inadequate insulin treatment and infection. These events can be prevented by patient education and effective communication with a health-care team. Sick-day management regarding dosing of insulin, blood glucose monitoring, avoiding prolonged fasting, and preventing dehydration should be addressed. Socioeconomic barriers contribute to the high rates of admission for DKA. Appropriate allocation of health-care resources toward preventive strategies is needed.

Other metabolic complications of deranged carbohydrate metabolism deserve mention at this point. The first is **hyperosmolar nonketotic diabetic coma**. This condition occurs mainly in patients with type 2 diabetes, who become profoundly dehydrated because of osmotic diuresis. However, these patients have sufficient insulin action to prevent the development of ketoacidosis. They may present with glucose levels more than 1000 mg/dL, serum osmolarity more than 320 to 370 osm, and neurologic symptoms ranging from confusion to seizures to coma. Compared to patients with DKA, they have a much larger fluid deficit, and therapy is primarily volume resuscitation with NS. Insulin is also used to reverse hyperglycemia but usually is given in lesser doses than is required for clearance of ketosis in DKA.

Alcoholic ketoacidosis develops in chronic alcoholics who are malnourished and have depleted glycogen stores, and is often seen in the setting of binge drinking, which may shift the ratio of the reduced form of nicotinamide adenine dinucleotide (NADH) to nicotinamide adenine dinucleotide (NAD), inhibiting gluconeogenesis. They develop an anion gap metabolic acidosis as a result of ketoacidosis and lactic acidosis. They present with the same symptoms of acidosis as do DKA patients, for example, abdominal pain, nausea, and vomiting, but with low, normal, or slightly elevated glucose levels (in contrast to DKA, in which the glucose level usually is markedly elevated). Treatment is administration of volume in the form of NS and glucose solution. Insulin administration typically is unnecessary.

Comprehension Questions

43.1   Which of the following most likely will lead to a non–anion gap acidosis?
    A. Diarrhea
    B. Lactic acidosis
    C. Diabetic ketoacidosis
    D. Ethylene glycol ingestions

43.2   An 18-year-old adolescent male is noted to be in diabetic ketoacidosis with pH 7.20 and serum glucose level 400 mg/dL. Which of the following is the most accurate statement regarding this patient's potassium status?
    A. Likely to have a potassium level less than 3.0 mEq/L
    B. Likely to have a potassium level more than 5 mEq/L
    C. Likely to have a total-body potassium deficit regardless of the serum level
    D. Serum level is likely to increase with correction of the acidosis

43.3   Which of the following is the most important first step in the treatment of diabetic ketoacidosis?
    A. Replacement of potassium
    B. Intravenous fluid replacement
    C. Replacement of phosphorus
    D. Antibiotic therapy

ANSWERS

43.1 **A.** Diarrhea leads to bicarbonate loss and usually does not affect the anion gap.

43.2 **C.** Total-body potassium usually is depleted regardless of the serum level.

43.3 **B.** The basic tenets of treating DKA include intravenous fluid, insulin to control the glucose level, correction of metabolic disturbances, and identification of the underlying etiology.

Clinical Pearls

➤ All patients with diabetic ketoacidosis are volume depleted and require significant replacement of salt solution and, later, free water in the form of glucose solutions.

➤ Despite sometimes elevated potassium concentrations, all patients with diabetic ketoacidosis have a total-body potassium deficit and will require substantial potassium replacement.

➤ Glucose levels fall more quickly than ketones resolve. Continuous insulin therapy is necessary for resolution of the ketoacidosis and can be coadministered with a glucose infusion until the anion gap is resolved.

➤ Cerebral edema can result from overly rapid correction of hyperglycemia or possibly from rapid administration of hypotonic fluids.

➤ Occurrence of diabetic ketoacidosis requires a precipitating cause, either insulin deficiency or a physiologic stressor such as infection.

REFERENCES

Delaney MF. Diabetic ketoacidosis and hyperglycemic hyperosmolar nonketotic syndrome. *Endocrinol Metab Clin North Am.* 2000;129:683-705.

Fishbein HA, Palumbo PJ. Acute metabolic complications in diabetes. In: Maureen I. Harris ed. *Diabetes in America.* Bethesda, MD: National Diabetes Data Group, NIH; 1995:283-291.

Kitabchi AE. Management of hyperglycemic crises in patients with diabetes. *Diabetes Care.* 2001;24:131-153.

Magee MF. Management of decompensated diabetes. *Crit Care Clin.* 2001;117:75-107.

Powers AC. Diabetes mellitus. In: Fauci AS, Braunwald E, Kasper DL, eds. *Harrison's Principles of Internal Medicine.* 17th ed. New York, NY: McGraw-Hill; 2008: 2275-2304.

Quinn L. Diabetes emergencies in the patient with type 2 diabetes. *Nurs Clin North Am.* 2001;136:341-359.

Case 44

A 37-year-old previously healthy woman presents to your clinic for unintentional weight loss. Over the past 3 months, she has lost approximately 15 lb without changing her diet or activity level. Otherwise, she feels great. She has an excellent appetite, no gastrointestinal complaints except for occasional loose stools, a good energy level, and no complaints of fatigue. She denies heat or cold intolerance. On examination, her heart rate is 108 bpm, blood pressure 142/82 mm Hg, and she is afebrile. When she looks at you, she seems to stare, and her eyes are somewhat protuberant. You note a large, smooth, nontender thyroid gland, a 2/6 systolic ejection murmur on cardiac examination, and her skin is warm and dry. There is a fine resting tremor.

➤ What is the most likely diagnosis?

➤ How could you confirm the diagnosis?

➤ What are the options for treatment?

ANSWERS TO CASE 44:

Thyrotoxicosis/Graves Disease

Summary: A 37-year-old woman presents with weight loss without anorexia, tachycardia, borderline hypertension, exophthalmos, and a smooth, nontender goiter.

➤ **Most likely diagnosis:** Thyrotoxicosis/Graves disease.

➤ **Confirming the diagnosis:** A low serum thyroid-stimulating hormone (TSH) level and an increased free thyroxine (T_4) level with this clinical presentation would be confirmatory of hyperthyroidism. However, other tests that would define the etiology would be thyroid-stimulating immunoglobulins or diffusely elevated uptake of radioactive iodine on thyroid scan.

➤ **Treatment options:** Antithyroid drugs, radioactive iodine ablation, or less commonly, surgical ablation of the thyroid.

ANALYSIS

Objectives

1. Understand the clinical presentation of thyrotoxicosis.
2. Be able to discuss the causes of hyperthyroidism, including Graves disease and toxic nodule.
3. Learn the complications of thyrotoxicosis, including thyroid storm.
4. Understand the evaluation of a patient with a thyroid nodule.
5. Know the available treatment options for Graves disease and outcomes of treatment.

Considerations

This 37-year-old woman has unintentional weight loss, loose stools, and warm skin, all symptoms of hyperthyroidism. Her thyroid gland is diffusely enlarged and nontender, and she has exophthalmus (protuberant eyes), which is consistent with Graves disease. This is a systemic disease with many complications that affect the entire body, including osteoporosis and heart failure. Treatment can include elimination of the excess thyroid hormone, but definitive therapy may include radioactive (or, less commonly, surgical) ablative therapy.

APPROACH TO
Hyperthyroidism

DEFINITIONS

HYPERTHYROIDISM: Hypermetabolic condition that results from the effect of excessive amounts of thyroid hormones produced by the thyroid gland itself. Because almost all cases of thyrotoxicosis are caused by thyroid over-production, these terms are often used synonymously.

THYROTOXICOSIS: Usually used as a general term for the state of thyroid hormone excess from any source, for example, exogenous ingestion.

CLINICAL APPROACH

Hyperthyroidism affects numerous body systems.

Neuromuscular system: Nervousness, tremors, and brisk reflexes are common. Inability to concentrate, proximal muscle weakness, emotional lability, and insomnia might be present.

Cardiac system: Wide pulse pressure, flow heart murmurs, and tachycardia usually are present. Atrial fibrillation is present in 10% to 20% of patients. Long-standing thyrotoxicosis can cause cardiomegaly and result in high-output heart failure.

Gastrointestinal system: Despite increased food intake, weight loss is common. Hyperdefecation usually is present as a result of increased gastrointestinal motility, but diarrhea is rare.

Eyes: Retraction of the upper eyelid as a consequence of increased sympathetic tone gives some patients a wide-eyed stare. Lid lag might be found on physical examination (sclera can be seen above the iris as the patient looks downward). Exophthalmos is distinctive of Graves disease.

Skin: The skin is warm, moist, and velvety, with fine hair texture and alopecia. Sweating usually is present as a consequence of vasodilation and heat dissipation.

Reproductive system: Hyperthyroidism impairs fertility in women and may cause oligomenorrhea. The sperm count in men is reduced. Impotence and gynecomastia might be present.

Metabolism: Weight loss is a common finding, especially in older patients who develop anorexia. However, sometimes, especially in young adults, weight gain can occur as a consequence of markedly increased caloric intake. Many patients develop an aversion to heat and a preference for cold temperatures.

Apathetic hyperthyroidism: Older patients with hyperthyroidism may lack typical adrenergic features and present instead with depression or apathy, weight loss, atrial fibrillation, worsening angina pectoris, or congestive heart failure.

Thyroid Storm

Thyroid storm is a dangerous condition of decompensated thyrotoxicosis. The patient has **tachycardia** (>140 bpm), **fever** (104-106°F), **agitation, delirium, restlessness or psychosis, vomiting, and/or diarrhea**. It usually results from long-neglected severe hyperthyroidism to which a complicating event (intercurrent illness: infection, surgery, trauma, or iodine load) is added. Treatment includes supportive care with fluids, antibiotics if needed, and specific treatment directed at the hyperthyroidism: large doses of antithyroid medications to block new hormone synthesis, iodine solution to block the release of thyroid hormone, propranolol to control the symptoms induced by the increased adrenergic tone, and glucocorticoids to decrease T_4 to triiodothyronine (T_3) conversion.

Etiology of Thyrotoxicosis

Graves disease is the most common cause of hyperthyroidism (80%) and usually is seen in women, especially between the ages of 30 and 50 years. It is an autoimmune disease caused by autoantibodies that activate the TSH receptor of the thyroid follicular cell, stimulating thyroid hormone synthesis and secretion as well as thyroid gland growth. In the pregnant patient, these antibodies cross the placenta and can cause neonatal thyrotoxicosis. The disease might follow a relapsing and remitting course.

 Graves disease is marked by **goiter** (enlarged thyroid gland), thyroid bruit, **hyperthyroidism, ophthalmopathy, and dermopathy**. These features are variably present. Ophthalmopathy is characterized by inflammation of extraocular muscles, orbital fat, and connective tissue, resulting in proptosis (exophthalmos), sometimes with impairment of eye muscle function (diplopia), and periorbital edema. Ophthalmopathy can progress even after treatment of thyrotoxicosis. Graves dermopathy is characterized by raised hyperpigmented orange peel texture papules. The most common site is the skin overlying the shins (pretibial myxedema). A low serum TSH will confirm the diagnosis. The degree of elevation of serum free T_4 and free T_3 levels can give an estimate of the severity of the disease. Tests that might be helpful in determining the etiology of thyrotoxicosis are the levels of thyroid-stimulating immunoglobulin (TSI), which is elevated in Graves, and a thyroid uptake and scan, which will reveal a diffusely elevated iodine uptake in our patient.

 Treatment options for Graves disease are medications, radioactive iodine, or surgery. Medications include **beta-blockers** such as propranolol (which are used for symptom relief) and **antithyroid drugs** such as **methimazole** and **propylthiouracil**. The antithyroid drugs work mainly by decreasing the production of thyroid hormone. They can be used for short-term (prior to treatment with radioactive iodine or surgery) or long-term (1-2 years) treatment, after which the chance for remission is 20% to 30%. Possible side effects are rash, allergic reactions, arthritis, hepatitis, and agranulocytosis. **Radioactive iodine** is the treatment of choice in the United States. It is administered as an oral solution of sodium ^{131}I that is rapidly concentrated in thyroid tissue, inducing damage that results in ablation of the thyroid, depending on the dose, within 6 to 18 weeks. At least 30% of patients will become hypothyroid in the first year after treatment and 3% each year after that, requiring thyroid hormone supplementation. Radioactive iodine is contraindicated in pregnancy, and women of reproductive age are advised to postpone pregnancy for 6 to 12 months after treatment. Graves ophthalmopathy might be exacerbated by radioactive iodine treatment, so glucocorticoids can be used to prevent this in selected patients.

Subtotal thyroidectomy usually is reserved for large goiters with obstructive symptoms (dyspnea, dysphagia). Possible complications include laryngeal nerve injury and hypoparathyroidism (due to removal of parathyroids or compromise of the vascular supply to them).

For our patient, treatment with radioactive iodine or antithyroid medications seems the most reasonable way to proceed, and a discussion regarding her options and our recommendations should take place after the diagnosis is confirmed.

Other causes of thyrotoxicosis include the following:

Toxic multinodular goiter: Found mainly in elderly and middle-age patients. Treatment consists of radioactive iodine or surgery. Radioactive iodine uptake is normal to increased, and the scan reveals irregular thyroid lobes and a heterogenous pattern.

Autonomous hyperfunctioning adenoma ("hot nodule" or Plummer disease): Hyperthyroidism usually is not present unless the nodule is more than 3 cm. The iodine scan looks like the flag of Japan: it demonstrates the hot nodule as having increased uptake (dark) and the rest of the gland with suppressed uptake (white). Hot nodules are almost never malignant. Cold nodules (no increased thyroid hormone production and no demonstration of local uptake if thyroid scan is performed) have a 5% to 10% risk of malignancy, so fine-needle aspiration, surgical removal, or ultrasonographic follow-up is needed for these nodules.

Thyroiditis: Caused by destruction of thyroid tissue and release of preformed hormone from the colloid space. Subacute (de Quervain) thyroiditis is an inflammatory viral illness with thyroid pain and tenderness. The hyperthyroid phase lasts for several weeks to months, followed by recovery. Treatment with nonsteroidal anti-inflammatory medications and beta-blockers usually is sufficient, but in severe cases, glucocorticoids might be used. Other forms include postradiation, postpartum, subacute (painless thyroiditis), and amiodarone-induced thyroiditis. In thyroiditis, the radioactive iodine uptake is invariably decreased.

Medications: Excessive ingestion of thyroid hormone (factitious or iatrogenic), amiodarone, and iodine load.

Other conditions, such as TSH-secreting pituitary adenoma, hydatidiform moles, choriocarcinomas secondary to secretion of human chorionic gonadotropin (hCG), ovarian teratomas, and metastatic follicular thyroid carcinomas, are rare causes of thyrotoxicosis.

Comprehension Questions

44.1   A 44-year-old woman is noted to be nervous and has heat intolerance.
       Her thyroid gland is diffusely enlarged, nontender, with an audible
       bruit. Her TSH level is very low. Which of the following is the most
       likely etiology?
       A. Lymphocytic thyroiditis
       B. Hashimoto thyroiditis
       C. Graves disease
       D. Multinodular toxic goiter

44.2   Which of the following distinguishes hyperthyroidism from thyroid
       storm?
       A. Tachycardia to heart rate 120 bpm
       B. Weight loss
       C. Fever and delirium
       D. Large goiter

44.3   A 58-year-old woman is noted to have Graves disease, and has a small
       goiter. Which of the following is the best therapy?
       A. Long-term propranolol
       B. Lifelong oral propylthiouracil (PTU)
       C. Radioactive iodine ablation
       D. Surgical thyroidectomy

ANSWERS

44.1   **C.** Graves disease is the most common cause of hyperthyroidism in
       the United States. It often includes the thyroid gland features described,
       as well as the distinctive eye findings.

44.2   **C.** Thyroid storm is an exaggeration of hyperthyroid features with
       extreme tachycardia (heart rate >140 bpm), fever, and central nerv-
       ous system dysfunction, such as confusion or coma. It is a medical
       emergency with a high mortality.

44.3   **C.** Radioactive iodine is the definitive treatment for Graves disease.
       Surgery is indicated for obstructive symptoms or for women during
       pregnancy.

Clinical Pearls

➤ The most common cause of thyrotoxicosis is Graves disease. No other diagnosis is likely if the patient has bilateral proptosis and a goiter.

➤ In patients with Graves disease, thyrotoxic symptoms may be treated with antithyroid medication or by thyroid gland ablation by radioactive iodine or surgery, but the ophthalmopathy may not improve.

➤ Graves disease may remit and relapse; in patients treated medically, one-third to half will become asymptomatic within 1 to 2 years.

➤ After radioablation, most patients with Graves disease become hypothyroid and will require thyroid hormone supplementation.

➤ Hyperfunctioning thyroid nodules (excessive thyroid hormone production, suppressed thyroid-stimulating hormone, "hot" on radionuclide scan) almost never are malignant.

➤ Most "cold" thyroid nodules are not malignant, but fine-needle aspiration should be used to evaluate the need for surgical excision.

REFERENCES

Davies DF, Larsen TF. Thyrotoxicosis. In: Wilson JD, Foster DW, Kronenberg HM, et al, eds. *Williams Textbook of Endocrinology*. 9th ed. Philadelphia, PA: WB Saunders; 2003:372-421.

Hershman JM. Hypothyroidism and hyperthyroidism. In: Lavin N, ed. *Manual of Endocrinology and Metabolism*. Boston, MA: Little Brown; 2002:396-409.

Jameson LJ, Weetman AP. Disorders of the thyroid gland. In: Fauci AS, Braunwald E, Kasper DL, eds. *Harrison's Principles of Internal Medicine*. 17th ed. New York, NY: McGraw-Hill; 2008:2224-2247.

McDermott MT. Thyroid emergencies. In: *Endocrine Secrets*. Philadelphia, PA: Hanley and Belfus; 2002:302-305.

Singer PA. Thyroiditis. In: Lavin N, ed. *Manual of Endocrinology and Metabolism*. Boston, MA: Little Brown; 2002:386-395.

Case 45

A 32-year-old woman presents to the emergency room complaining of productive cough, fever, and chest pain for 4 days. She was seen 2 days ago in her primary care physician's office with the same complaints, was diagnosed clinically with pneumonia, and was sent home with oral azithromycin. Since then, her cough has diminished in quantity. However, the fever has not abated, and she still experiences left-sided chest pain, which is worse when she coughs or takes a deep breath. In addition, she has started to feel short of breath when she walks around the house. She has no other medical history. She does not smoke, and has no history of occupational exposure. She has not traveled outside of the United States and has no sick contacts.

On physical examination, her temperature is 103.4°F, heart rate 116 bpm, blood pressure 128/69 mm Hg, respiratory rate 24 breaths per minute and shallow, and pulse oximetry 94% saturation on room air. Physical examination is significant for decreased breath sounds in the lower half of the left lung fields posteriorly, with dullness to percussion about halfway up. There are a few inspiratory crackles in the mid-lung fields, and her left side is clear to auscultation. Her heart is tachycardic but regular with no murmurs. She has no cyanosis. Figure 45–1 shows her chest X-ray films.

➤ What is your most likely diagnosis?

➤ What is your next step?

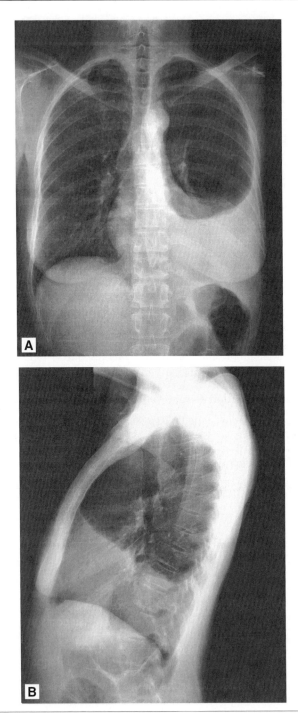

Figure 45–1.   A: Posteroanterior film showing a left-side pleural effusion. **B:** Lateral chest film of the same patient. *Courtesy of Dr. Jorge Albin.*

ANSWERS TO CASE 45:
Pleural Effusion, Parapneumonic

Summary: A 32-year-old previously healthy woman comes in with a clinical diagnosis of community-acquired pneumonia that has not improved with outpatient treatment. She has diminished breath sounds and dullness to percussion on the left side of her chest, suggesting a large left-sided pleural effusion, which is confirmed by chest radiography. The effusion likely is caused by infection in the adjacent lung parenchyma and may be the cause of her failure to improve on antibiotics.

➤ **Most likely diagnosis:** Parapneumonic effusion as a complication of pneumonia.

➤ **Next step:** Diagnostic thoracentesis to help diagnose the cause of the pleural effusion and to determine the necessity for fluid drainage.

ANALYSIS

Objectives

1. Understand the use of Light criteria to distinguish transudative effusions from exudative effusions, as a guide to the etiology of the effusion.
2. Learn what pleural fluid characteristics suggest a complicated parapneumonic effusion or empyema, and the need for drainage.
3. Know the treatment of a complicated parapneumonic effusion that does not improve after thoracentesis.

Considerations

In this patient, the effusion is large and if it is free-flowing, which would be evaluated with a lateral decubitus film, then diagnostic thoracentesis can easily be accomplished. It is important to determine if the effusion is, in fact, caused by the pneumonia, and, if so, whether it is likely to resolve with antibiotics alone or will require drainage with tube thoracostomy.

APPROACH TO
Pleural Effusion

DEFINITIONS

EXUDATE: Effusion caused by inflammatory or malignant causes, usually with high protein or high lactate dehydrogenase (LDH) levels.

PLEURAL EFFUSION: Accumulation of fluid in the pleural space.

TRANSUDATE: Effusion caused by alteration of oncotic forces, usually with low protein and low LDH levels.

CLINICAL APPROACH

Diagnostic thoracentesis should be considered for every patient who presents with a pleural effusion for which the cause is unknown. Possibly the only exception to this rule is if the patient is known to have congestive heart failure (CHF) with equal bilateral effusions or if the effusion is too small, that is, less than 10 mm on lateral decubitus film. If the pleural effusion of CHF does not significantly improve after a trial of diuresis, however, a diagnostic tap should be performed. Table 45–1 gives the correlations of pleural fluid appearance. Approximately 50 mL of fluid is needed in order to be visible on a lateral decubitus film (more reliable in detecting smaller effusions), and fluid volume more than 500 mL usually obscures the whole hemidiaphragm.

Table 45–1 PLEURAL FLUID APPEARANCE	
Clear yellow	Transudative, eg, secondary to CHF, cirrhosis, nephrotic syndrome
Frank pus	Infectious process, empyema
Bloody	If the hematocrit of the pleural fluid is: <1% : Blood caused by traumatic tap 1%-20%: Cancer, pulmonary embolus, tuberculosis >50%: Hemothorax, most commonly secondary to trauma but also seen in malignancy and pulmonary embolism
Milky, turbid	Chylothorax triglycerides >110 mg/dL resulting from disruption of thoracic duct, cholesterol effusion
Dark green	Biliothorax

Indications for thoracentesis:

- Uneven pleural effusion or unilateral pleural effusion
- Evidence of infection, for example, productive cough, fever, or pleurisy
- Normal cardiac silhouette (no heart failure)
- Alarming signs, for example, significant weight loss, hemoptysis, or hypoxia
- Need to evaluate underlying lung parenchyma

A simple "diagnostic" thoracentesis can be performed, but if the effusion is significant in size and the patient is dyspneic, especially at rest, a "therapeutic" thoracentesis may also be performed, with safe removal of up to 1500 mL. With removal of more fluid, the patient is at risk for developing reexpansion pulmonary edema.

Transudate Versus Exudate

To appreciate the pathophysiology of the formation of a transudate versus an exudate is to understand the differential under each category. Approximately 10 mL of pleural fluid is formed every day by the visceral pleura and absorbed by the parietal pleura (capillaries and lymphatics). Processes that disturb this "equilibrium" lead to fluid accumulation. Clinical settings in which the hydrostatic pressure is increased, for example, CHF and constrictive pericarditis; the oncotic pressure is decreased, for example, nephrotic syndrome and cirrhosis; or the intrapleural pressure is reduced, for example, atelectasis, lead to the formation of a "transudate." In contrast, "exudates" are more a result of local inflammation, for example, infection, malignancy, and connective tissue diseases, which cause a protein leak into the pleural space. Less commonly, impaired lymphatic drainage, as occurs in chylothorax, or lymphangitic spread of a malignancy may cause an exudative fluid. Pulmonary emboli can cause both exudative and transudative effusions. Tables 45–2 and 45–3 list the etiologies of transudative and exudative pleural effusions, respectively.

Table 45–2 CAUSES OF TRANSUDATIVE PLEURAL EFFUSIONS

TRANSUDATE	CLINICAL CORRELATES OR RADIOGRAPHIC FEATURES
Congestive heart failure	Most commonly bilateral and symmetric, at times isolated right-sided effusion
Nephrotic syndrome	Bilateral and subpulmonic effusion
Cirrhosis with ascites	Patients usually have significant ascites
Malignancy	Secondary to decreased drainage of daily fluid by obstructed lymphatics
Pulmonary embolism	May also be exudative or bloody; rarely large
Hypothyroidism	Seen in myxedema

Table 45–3 CAUSES OF EXUDATIVE PLEURAL EFFUSIONS

EXUDATE	COMMENT
Infection	Bacterial pneumonia, viral etiology, fungal infection, parasitic (eosinophilic) involvement; subdiaphragmatic abscesses
Tuberculosis	One-third have parenchymal involvement; lymphocytes >80%; adenosine deaminase >43 U/L; total protien >4.0 g/dL; diagnostic yield of fluid for acid-fast bacilli <10%; pleural biopsy increases yield to between 80% and 90%
Malignancy	Lymphocytic predominant and occasionally bloody; cytologic examination positive in >50% of cases; usually indicative of dismal prognosis
Connective tissue disease	Rheumatoid pleurisy: very low glucose, rheumatoid factor >1:320 and >serum titer and LDH >1000 IU/L; more common in men Lupus pleuritis: positive lupus erythematosus cells; pleural fluid/serum antinuclear antibody >1.0; usually responsive to steroid treatment
Pancreatitis	Elevated pancreatic amylase isoenzyme; salivary isoenzyme seen in esophageal rupture with associated low pH
Chylothorax	Triglycerides >110 mg/dL
Asbestos exposure	Spectrum of disease ranges from pleural plaques to effusion and malignancy; also usually eosinophilic

Pleural Fluid—Light Criteria: The most widely used criteria to distinguish between a transudative and exudative fluid are the Light criteria first described in 1997. For a fluid to be labeled an **exudate**, it must meet **at least one of the following criteria** (transudates meet none of these criteria):

1. Pleural fluid protein/serum protein ratio more than 0.5
2. Pleural fluid LDH/serum LDH ratio more than 0.6
3. Pleural fluid LDH greater than two-thirds the upper limit of normal for serum LDH

Pleural LDH correlates with the degree of **pleural inflammation** and along with **fluid protein** should always be sent in the initial evaluation.

Parapneumonic Effusions and Empyemas

Pleural effusions occur in 40% of patients with an underlying bacterial pneumonia. Most of these effusions should resolve with appropriate antibiotic treatment, but if the fluid characteristics predict a **"complicated" parapneumonic** effusion, urgent tube drainage is indicated to prevent formation of fibrous peels, which may need surgical decortication.

The following fluid characteristics suggest chest tube drainage is necessary:
- Empyema (frank pus in the pleural space)
- Positive Gram stain of fluid
- Presence of loculations
- pH less than 7.10
- Glucose less than 40 mg/dL
- LDH more than 1000 U/L

If the patient does not meet the criteria for immediate drainage, a 1-week trial of antibiotics is indicated, with close reevaluation of those patients who do not respond or who clinically deteriorate.

If tube thoracostomy drainage is required, a chest tube is placed until drainage rate has decreased to less than 50 mL/d. Postdrainage imaging must be obtained to confirm complete drainage of fluid and to assess the need for placement of a second tube if the fluid has not been adequately drained (as is often seen if the effusion is loculated). Complete sterilization of the cavity is desirable when treating an empyema with 4 to 6 weeks of antibiotics, as is complete obliteration of the space by lung expansion. Multiloculated empyemas are treated further by administering fibrinolytic agents such as streptokinase or urokinase through the chest tube. Video-assisted thorascopic surgery (VATS) is another option for trying to break up fibrinous adhesions.

Comprehension Questions

45.1 A 55-year-old man with congestive heart failure develops bilateral pleural effusions. Which of the following is the most likely pleural fluid characteristic if thoracentesis is performed?
A. Pleural fluid LDH 39, LDH ratio 0.2, protein ratio 0.7
B. Pleural fluid LDH 39, LDH ratio 0.2, protein ratio 0.1
C. Pleural fluid LDH 599, LDH ratio 0.9, protein ratio 0.1
D. Pleural fluid LDH 599, LDH ratio 0.9, protein ratio 0.7

45.2   A 39-year-old man develops a moderate free-flowing pleural effusion
        following a left lower lobe pneumonia. Thoracentesis reveals straw-
        colored fluid with gram-positive diplococci on Gram stain, pH 6.9,
        glucose 32 mg/dL, and LDH 1890. Which of the following is the best
        next step?
        A. Send the fluid for culture.
        B. Continue treatment with antibiotics for pneumococcal infection.
        C. Tube thoracostomy to drain the effusion.
        D. Schedule a follow-up chest X-ray in 2 weeks to document resolu-
           tion of the effusion.

45.3   A 69-year-old man complains of gradually worsening dyspnea and a
        nagging cough over the past 3 months but no fevers. He is found to
        have a right-sided pleural effusion, which is tapped and is grossly
        bloody. Which of the following is the most likely diagnosis?
        A. Parapneumonic effusion
        B. Malignancy in the pleural space
        C. Rupture of aortic dissection into the pleural space
        D. Pulmonary embolism with pulmonary infarction

ANSWERS

45.1   **B.** Congestive heart failure is commonly associated with bilateral
        pleural effusions, which are transudative, as a consequence of alter-
        ation of Starling forces. The effusions of heart failure are best man-
        aged by treating the heart failure, for example, with diuretics, and
        typically do not require thoracentesis.

45.2   **C.** The positive Gram stain, low pH, low glucose, and markedly elevated
        LDH all suggest that this parapneumonic effusion is "complicated," that
        is, it is unlikely to resolve with antibiotic therapy and is likely to produce
        loculated pockets of pus, which will require surgical intervention.
        Drainage by serial thoracentesis or tube thoracostomy is essential.

45.3   **B.** The most common causes of hemorrhagic pleural effusion are
        malignancy, pulmonary embolism, and tuberculosis. Pulmonary
        embolism would be suggested by acute onset of dyspnea and pleuritic
        chest pain rather than this subacute presentation. Similarly, aortic
        rupture can produce a hemothorax but would have an acute presen-
        tation with pain and hemodynamic compromise.

Clinical Pearls

➤ Transudative effusions meet *none* of the following criteria (exudative effusions meet at least one):
(a) Pleural fluid protein/serum protein ratio more than 0.5. (b) Pleural fluid LDH/serum LDH ratio more than 0.6. (c) Pleural fluid LDH greater than two-thirds normal serum LDH.

➤ Tube thoracostomy or more aggressive drainage of parapneumonic effusion usually is required with gross pus (empyema), positive Gram stain or culture, glucose less than 40 mg/dL, pH less than 7.10, and loculations.

➤ The most common cause of pleural effusion is congestive heart failure, which typically gives bilateral symmetric transudative effusions and is best treated with diuresis.

➤ The most common causes of bloody pleural effusion (in the absence of trauma) are malignancy, pulmonary embolism with infarction, and tuberculosis.

REFERENCES

Colice, GL, Curtis A, Deslauriers J, et al. Medical and surgical treatment of parapneumonic effusions: an evidence-based guideline. *Chest.* 2000;118:1158-1171.

Light RW. Disorders of the pleura and mediastinum. In: Kasper DL, Braunwald E, Fauci AS, et al, eds. *Harrison's Principles of Internal Medicine.* 17th ed. New York, NY: McGraw-Hill; 2008:1658-1661.

Light RW. Pleural effusion. *N Engl J Med.* 2002;346:1971-1977.

Case 46

A 25-year-old man presents to your clinic for a general checkup and cholesterol screening. He denies having medical problems and takes no medications on a regular basis. He works as a computer programmer, exercises regularly at a gym, and does not smoke or use illicit drugs. He drinks two to three beers on the weekend. His father suffered his first heart attack at age 36 years and eventually died of complications of heart disease at age 49 years. The patient's older brother recently was diagnosed with "high cholesterol."

The patient's blood pressure is 125/74 mm Hg and heart rate 72 bpm. He is 69 in tall and weighs 165 lb. His physical examination is unremarkable.

Fasting lipid levels are drawn. The next day, you receive the results: total cholesterol 362 mg/dL, triglycerides 300 mg/dL, high-density lipoprotein (HDL) 36 mg/dL, and low-density lipoprotein (LDL) 266 mg/dL.

➤ What is the most likely diagnosis?

➤ What is your next step?

➤ What are the possible complications if left untreated?

ANSWERS TO CASE 46:
Hypercholesterolemia

Summary: A healthy 25-year-old man presents for a physical examination and is found to have markedly elevated total and LDL cholesterol and triglycerides, and low HDL cholesterol. He has an unremarkable physical examination. He is normotensive and is a nonsmoker, but he has a strong family history of hypercholesterolemia and premature atherosclerotic coronary artery disease (CAD).

➤ **Diagnosis:** Familial hypercholesterolemia.

➤ **Next step:** Counsel regarding lifestyle modification with low-fat diet and exercise, and offer treatment with an HMG-CoA (β-hydroxy-β-methylglutaryl-coenzyme A) reductase inhibitor.

➤ **Complications if untreated:** Development of atherosclerotic vascular disease, including coronary heart disease (CHD).

ANALYSIS

Objectives

1. Know the risk factors for developing coronary artery disease and know how to estimate the risk for coronary events using the Framingham risk scoring system.
2. Be familiar with the recommendations for cholesterol screening and for the treatment of low-, intermediate-, and high-risk patients.
3. Understand how the different classes of lipid-lowering agents affect lipid levels and the potential side effects of those agents.
4. Know the secondary causes of hyperlipidemia.

Considerations

A young man presents to the clinic for a checkup and is found to have markedly elevated total cholesterol (normal <200 mg/dL) and LDL levels (normal <100 mg/dL), and low HDL levels (normal >45 mg/dL). He does not have any apparent secondary causes of dyslipidemia, and has no signs or symptoms of vascular disease. He does have a strong family history of hypercholesterolemia and premature death caused by myocardial infarction (MI). The decisions regarding the method and intensity of lipid-lowering therapy are based on one's **estimation of the patient's 10-year risk of major coronary events.** Because of his very high lipid levels and family history, he is a high-risk patient and, thus, should be counseled about lipid-lowering medical therapy. The very high cholesterol levels at a young age in the absence of secondary causes leads one to suspect familial hypercholesterolemia, a condition caused by defective or absent LDL surface receptors and subsequent inability to metabolize LDL particles. Meanwhile, the importance of lifestyle modification cannot be overemphasized.

APPROACH TO
Hyperlipidemia

DEFINITIONS

HYPERLIPIDEMIA: An excess of fats or lipids in the blood, principally due to either elevated cholesterol or triglycerides.

ATHEROSCLEROSIS: Deposition of atheromatous plaques containing cholesterol and lipids on the innermost layer of the walls of large and medium-sized arteries.

STATIN MEDICATIONS: A class of agents that lower cholesterol by inhibiting 3-Hydroxy-3-methylglutaryl-coenzyme (HMG-CoA) reductase, which is a key enzyme in cholesterol synthesis.

CLINICAL APPROACH

Atherosclerotic coronary artery disease is the **leading cause of death of both men and women** in the United States. Because of the association of hypercholesterolemia and development of atherosclerotic heart disease, most authorities recommend routine screening of average risk individuals at least every 5 years. Clinical laboratories usually measure total cholesterol, HDL, and triglycerides. The LDL cholesterol may be calculated by using the formula:

$$LDL = Total\ cholesterol - HDL - (Triglycerides/5)$$

A fasting sample should be measured, if possible, but the total cholesterol and HDL are still reliable in a nonfasting sample. The triglycerides and the calculated LDL levels are affected by recent dietary intake and should be drawn in the fasting state.

Approximately 25% of American adults have a total cholesterol level of more than 240 mg/dL, which is considered elevated according to the guidelines of the National Cholesterol Education Program (NCEP). Management of patients with hypercholesterolemia involves assessment of other atherosclerotic risks to estimate the 10-year risk of coronary events, such as fatal or nonfatal myocardial infarction. The LDL goal is set based on the estimated cardiovascular risk as described in the 2002 Adult Treatment Panel III (ATP III).

High-risk patients already have an **established CHD** or other **atherosclerotic vascular disease**: their 10-year risk for future coronary events is more than 20%. The presence of **diabetes now is considered a "CHD risk equivalent"** in patients because of their higher risk of vascular disease as well as higher mortality rate from myocardial infarction than is the case with nondiabetics. High-risk individuals have an **LDL goal** of less than **100 mg/dL** according to the ATP III. The intensity of lipid lowering for secondary prevention of CHD in patients with established atherosclerosis is controversial and is evolving. Based on additional studies published after the ATP III, some authors have proposed lower targets **(LDL <70 mg/dL)** for patients in the **"very high risk" category: those with established CHD PLUS multiple major risk factors such as diabetes OR severe and poorly controlled risk factors such as continued smoking, OR a recent acute coronary event.**

The LDL goal for individuals who do not have established CHD or CHD equivalents (diabetes or other vascular disease such as stroke, peripheral vascular disease, or abdominal aortic aneurysm) is based on a **risk stratification** process. First, the number of risk factors for CHD is counted (Table 46–1). The absolute 10-year risk for patients with two or more risk factors may be estimated using a scoring system based on data from the Framingham heart study (Figure 46–1). Patients with multiple risk factors then are assigned to high risk (>20%), intermediate risk (10%-20%), or low risk (<10%). Those in the intermediate-risk category should have an LDL goal of less than **130 mg/dL,** whereas the lowest-risk patients have an LDL goal of less than **160 mg/dL.**

One should exclude a secondary cause of lipid disorder, either by clinical or laboratory evaluation. Underlying disorders include diabetes, hypothyroidism, obstructive liver disease, chronic renal failure/nephrotic syndrome, and medication side effects (progestins, anabolic steroids, corticosteroids). High cholesterol levels in young patients in the absence of secondary causes suggest familial hypercholesterolemia, a condition caused by defective or absent LDL surface receptors and subsequent inability to metabolize LDL particles. Homozygotes for this condition may develop atherosclerotic disease in childhood and usually require intensive lipid-lowering drug therapy.

Table 46–1 CHD RISK FACTORS

Cigarette smoking
Hypertension (elevated blood pressure when seen, or patient on antihypertensives)
Low HDL cholesterol (<40 mg/dL)
Family history of premature coronary artery disease (in men <55 y or in women <65 y)
Age of the patient (men >45 y, women >55 y)

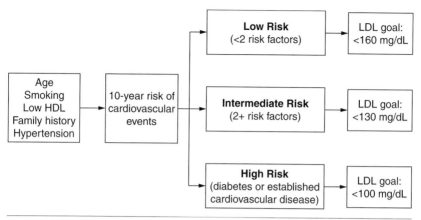

Figure 46–1.   Risk stratification for coronary heart disease and LDL goals based on CHD risk factors.

Lowering serum cholesterol levels decrease the risk of major coronary events and death in hypercholesterolemic patients without a prior history of CHD **(primary prevention)**, as well as reducing the overall mortality and coronary disease mortality in patients who have established cardiovascular disease **(secondary prevention).** All patients should first be educated regarding therapeutic lifestyle changes. These changes include a diet low in saturated fat (<7% of total daily calories) and low in cholesterol (<200 mg/d), as well as exercise, which can help to lower cholesterol.

When lifestyle modifications are not enough to reach the LDL goal, multiple lipid-lowering medications are available. Table 46–2 lists their effects on lipids and their potential side effects. **Side effects of statins** are uncommon but include **myopathy**, which may manifest as muscle tenderness with elevated creatine kinase (CK) levels and may progress to rhabdomyolysis. Less commonly, **elevated liver enzymes,** or even severe hepatitis, have been reported. When these drugs are used, routine clinical or laboratory monitoring for these effects is advisable.

Table 46–2 DRUGS FOR HYPERLIPIDEMIA

DRUG CLASS	THERAPEUTIC EFFECTS	SIDE EFFECTS	MONITORING
HMG-CoA reductase inhibitors ("statins")	Lower LDL 25%-55% Lower TG 10%-25% Raise HDL 5%-10%	Hepatic injury, myositis	Monitor LFTs and creatine kinase
Nicotinic acid (eg, niacin)	Lower TG 25%-35% Lower LDL 15%-25% Raise HDL 15%-30%	Flushing, tachycardia	Flushing may be relieved by aspirin
Bile acid resins (eg, cholestyramine)	Lower LDL 20%-30% Raise HDL 5%	Constipation, nausea, GI discomfort	Binds fat-soluble vitamins
Fibric acid derivatives (eg, gemfibrozil)	Lower TG 25%-40% Raise HDL 5%-15%	Gallstones, nausea, increased LFTs	Caution if used with statins

GI, gastrointestinal; HDL, high-density lipoprotein; LDL, low-density lipoprotein; LFT, liver function test; TG, triglycerides.
Data from Rader DJ, Hobbs HH. Disorders of lipoprotein metabolism. In: Braunwald E, Fauci AS, Kasper KL, et al, eds. Harrison's Principles of Internal Medicine. 17th ed. New York, NY: McGraw-Hill; 2008:2428.

Comprehension Questions

46.1   A 35-year-old man with no history of cardiac or other vascular disease asks how often he should have routine cholesterol screening. Which of the following is the best answer?
   A. Every 3 months
   B. Annually
   C. Every 5 years
   D. Every 7 to 10 years

46.2   A 38-year-old man presents to your office following a health fair screening of his cholesterol level because he was told that it is high. He watches his diet, plays tennis, exercises 3 to 5 times per week, and appears to be in good physical condition. He is a nonsmoker and has no family history of cardiovascular disease. His profile is total cholesterol 202 mg/dL, HDL 45 mg/dL, LDL 128 mg/dL, and triglycerides 145 mg/dL. Following a review of this patient's profile, which of the following would you recommend?

A. Administer gemfibrozil
B. Administer HMG-CoA reductase inhibitor
C. Administer low-dose niacin and slowly increase to achieve 3 g daily
D. Suggest he continue his current diet and exercise program

46.3   Which of the following patients is the best candidate for lifestyle modification alone rather than lipid-lowering medications?

A. A 60-year-old diabetic male smoker with a recent myocardial infarction: cholesterol 201 mg/dL, HDL 47 mg/dL, and LDL 138 mg/dL
B. A 62-year-old diabetic man: cholesterol 210 mg/dL, HDL 27 mg/dL, and LDL 146 mg/dL
C. A 57-year-old asymptomatic woman: cholesterol 235 mg/dL, HDL 92 mg/dL, and LDL 103 mg/dL
D. A 39-year-old man with nephrotic syndrome: cholesterol 285 mg/dL, HDL 48 mg/dL, LDL 195 mg/dL

ANSWERS

46.1   **C.** The recommended interval for cholesterol screening in this population of healthy adults is every 5 years. Cholesterol levels do not change rapidly over a person's lifetime. A rapid change should prompt investigation for an underlying secondary cause.

46.2   **D.** In this scenario, this 38-year-old man's only risk factor for CHD is male sex; thus, his 10-year risk is less than 10%. His total cholesterol is barely in the borderline high category, fairly near the desirable level, his LDL is less than 130 mg/dL, and his HDL is acceptable.

46.3   **C.** Patient A is at highest risk for future events because he has established CHD and diabetes, he smokes, and he recently had a myocardial infarction. His goal LDL is less than 70 mg/dL. Patient B has diabetes, a CHD equivalent. Besides lifestyle modifications, he should start drug therapy to lower his LDL and raise his HDL. Patient C has very high HDL, which is protective, and probably contributes to her elevated total cholesterol. Patient D has nephrotic syndrome causing hyperlipidemia, which may be treated by reduction of proteinuria using angiotensin-converting enzyme (ACE) inhibitors but often requires drug therapy such as statins.

Clinical Pearls

> ➤ The intensity of lipid-lowering therapy is based on the patient's estimated 10-year risk for coronary events: high-risk goal low-density lipoprotein (LDL) goal less than 100 mg/dL, intermediate-risk goal LDL less than 130 mg/dL, and low-risk goal LDL less than 160 mg/dL.
>
> ➤ The patients at highest risk are those with established coronary heart disease (CHD), and other atherosclerotic vascular disease, such as stroke or peripheral vascular disease, or diabetes, which is considered a "CHD equivalent." The low-density lipoprotein goal for very high-risk patients may be less than 70 mg/dL.
>
> ➤ Low-density lipoprotein is the primary target of lipid-lowering therapy; treatment reduces coronary events and death in patients with and without established coronary heart disease.
>
> ➤ The major side effects of statins are myopathy and hepatocellular injury.

REFERENCES

Expert Panel on Detection, Evaluation, and Treatment of High Blood Cholesterol in Adults. Executive summary of the third report of the National Cholesterol Education Program Expert Panel on Detection, Evaluation, and Treatment of High Blood Cholesterol in Adults (Adult Treatment Panel III). JAMA. 2001;285:2486-2497.

Grundy SM, Cleeman JI, Merz CN, et al. Implications of recent trials for the National Cholesterol Education Program Adult Treatment Panel III guidelines. *Circulation*. 2004;110:227-239.

Libby P. The pathogenesis, prevention, and treatment of atherosclerosis. In: Braunwald E, Fauci AS, Kasper KL, et al., eds. *Harrison's Principles of Internal Medicine*. 17th ed. New York, NY: McGraw-Hill; 2008:1501-1509.

Rader DJ, Hobbs HH. Disorders of lipoprotein metabolism. In: Braunwald E, Fauci AS, Kasper KL, et al., eds. *Harrison's Principles of Internal Medicine*. 17th ed. New York, NY: McGraw-Hill; 2008:2416-2429.

Case 47

A 72-year-old man is admitted to the hospital because of acute onset of a right facial droop, right arm weakness, and some difficulty speaking. These symptoms started 6 hours ago while he was sitting at the breakfast table. He had no headache, no diminishment of consciousness, and no abnormal involuntary movements. Two weeks ago, he had a transient painless loss of vision in his left eye, which resolved spontaneously within a few hours. His medical history is significant for long-standing hypertension and a myocardial infarction (MI) 4 years previously, which was treated with percutaneous angioplasty. His medications include a daily aspirin, metoprolol, and simvastatin. He does not smoke. When you see him in the emergency room, his symptoms have nearly resolved. He is afebrile, heart rate 62 bpm, and blood pressure 135/87 mm Hg. The corner of his mouth droops, with slight flattening of the right nasolabial fold, but he is able to fully elevate his eyebrows. His strength is 4/5 in his right arm and hand, and the rest of his neurologic examination is normal. He has no carotid bruits, his heart rhythm is regular with no murmur but with an S_4 gallop. The remainder of his physical examination is normal. Laboratory studies, including renal function, liver function, lipid profile, and complete blood count (CBC), all are normal. Within a few hours, all of the patient's symptoms have resolved.

➤ What is the most likely diagnosis?

➤ What is the next step?

ANSWERS TO CASE 47:

Transient Ischemic Attack

Summary: A 72-year-old man is admitted because of an acute onset of right facial droop and, right arm weakness, and some difficulty speaking, which resolves within hours. He denies headache, diminishment of consciousness, or abnormal involuntary movements. Two weeks ago, he had a transient painless loss of vision in his left eye, which resolved spontaneously within a few hours. He has no carotid bruits, but he does have a known atherosclerotic disease.

➤ **Most likely diagnosis:** Transient ischemic attack (TIA) caused by atheroembolism from the left internal carotid artery.

➤ **Next step:** Perform a noninvasive study, such as a high-resolution carotid ultrasonography or a magnetic resonance angiogram (MRA), to evaluate for carotid artery stenosis.

ANALYSIS

Objectives

1. Know the most common mechanisms for ischemic stroke: carotid stenosis, cardioembolism, lipohyalinosis, or other small-vessel disease.
2. Understand the evaluation of a stroke patient with the goal of secondary prevention.
3. Learn which patients are best managed with medical therapy and which patients benefit from carotid endarterectomy.

Considerations

Patients who present with acute focal neurologic deficits require rapid evaluation for suspected stroke. **Noncontrast computed tomography (CT) of the brain** is necessary to differentiate between ischemic stroke and hemorrhagic stroke, which cannot be definitively distinguished clinically. If CT shows no hemorrhage, or a very large stroke (>1/3 of the MCA territory), patients with the clinical diagnosis of acute ischemic may receive **thrombolytics** (IV recombinant tissue plasminogen activator) as long as it can be delivered **within 3 hours** of the onset of symptoms, with a reduction in mortality and disability.

This 72-year-old man presented more than 6 hours after the onset of symptoms and has had resolution of neurologic deficits, the hallmark of TIA. He has established atherosclerotic coronary disease but no known carotid artery disease. He denies headache, which is important because migraine headache may be associated with neurologic deficits; it would be rare for an elderly man to have the first presentation of migraine headache. Various neurologic diseases, such as multiple sclerosis, may be characterized by complete resolution of neurologic deficits, but the symptoms usually last longer than 24 hours. He does not have abnormal motor activity, which would suggest seizure disorder. His evaluation will be focused on secondary prevention of another, perhaps more devastating cerebrovascular event.

Initially, noninvasive imaging of the carotid arteries should be performed to determine the extent of stenosis. With these symptoms, if there is more than 70% stenosis of the left internal carotid artery, the possibility of left carotid endarterectomy should be discussed.

APPROACH TO
Transient Ischemic Attack/Stroke

DEFINITIONS

AMAUROSIS FUGAX: Transient monocular blindness that often is described as a gray shade being pulled down over the eye caused by ischemia to the retinal artery.

STROKE: Acute onset of a focal neurologic deficit due to a cerebral infarction or hemorrhage.

TRANSIENT ISCHEMIC ATTACK (TIA): Transient neurologic deficit secondary to ischemia in a defined vascular territory that lasts less than 24 hours (most commonly <1 hour).

CLINICAL APPROACH

Transient ischemic attacks, often called "mini-strokes," refer to the sudden onset of a focal neurologic deficit, with spontaneous resolution within 24 hours (usually within the first hour). Not all transient focal neurologic events actually represent ischemia, however. The differential diagnosis includes classic migraine, postictal paralysis, seizures, cerebral hemorrhage, or even slow-evolving intracranial processes such as subdural hematoma, abscess, or tumors, which can suddenly produce symptoms because of edema or hemorrhage or result in seizure activity. However, clinical evaluation and imaging studies of the brain should be sufficient to exclude most or all of these diagnoses.

The **focal neurologic symptoms** produced by ischemia depend on the **area of the cerebral circulation** involved and may include (a) amaurosis fugax, (b) hemiparesis, (c) hemianesthesia, (d) aphasia, or (e) dizziness/vertigo as a result of vertebrobasilar insufficiency. The significance of a TIA is not the symptoms it produces, because by definition it is self-resolved, but the risk for future events it portends. **The highest-risk patients for stroke are those with**

previous ischemic events such as TIA; that is, it can be looked upon as a warning sign of impending potential disaster.

TIAs are produced by temporary ischemia to a vascular territory, usually caused by thrombosis or embolism and less commonly by vasculitis, hematologic disorders such as sickle cell disease or vasospasm. By far, the most common causes of stroke or TIA are **carotid atherosclerosis** (large-vessel disease), **cardioembolism** usually to branches of the middle cerebral artery (medium-size vessel disease), or **lipohyalinosis** affecting small lenticulostriate arteries (small-vessel disease). Table 47–1 lists the etiologies of a TIA/stroke.

The workup for a TIA begins with a history and physical examination. Pertinent historical factors include onset, course, and duration of symptoms, atherosclerotic risk factors, and relevant medical history (ie, atrial fibrillation). Physical examination should begin with blood pressures in four extremities and should include a funduscopic examination. In this patient, the first symptom was amaurosis fugax due to cholesterol emboli, called **Hollenhorst plaques**, which often can be seen lodged in the retinal artery. Auscultation for carotid bruits, cardiac murmurs, assessment of cardiac rhythm, evidence of embolic events to other parts of the body, and a complete neurologic examination should also be assessed.

Laboratory data that should always be obtained include a complete blood count, fasting lipid profile, and serum glucose level. Other laboratory data, such as an erythrocyte sedimentation rate in elderly populations to evaluate for temporal arteritis, should be tailored to the demographic of the patient. Generally, a 12-lead electrocardiogram (ECG) must be obtained to evaluate for atrial fibrillation. An echocardiogram can be useful to evaluate for valvular or mural thrombi. **A noncontrast CT scan of the brain also must be performed initially.** Noncontrast CT scans of the brain are very sensitive in detecting acute cerebral hemorrhage but are relatively insensitive to acute ischemic strokes, particularly when the area of the stroke is less than 5 mm in diameter, are located in the region of the brainstem, or are less than 12 hours old. Further imaging with magnetic resonance may be considered.

Finally, imaging of the extracranial vasculature to detect severe **carotid artery stenosis is essential to guide further stroke prevention therapy.** Carotid Doppler ultrasound and magnetic resonance angiography are effective noninvasive imaging studies and are often used as first-line diagnostic tools.

Stroke prevention begins with **antiplatelet therapy**, and **aspirin** should be used in all cases unless there is a contraindication to its use. Use of **clopidogrel** or combination **aspirin and dipyridamole** may be slightly superior to aspirin for stroke prevention but at a substantially higher dollar cost. Combination therapy with aspirin and clopidogrel has not been shown to provide greater benefit in stroke prevention but does produce a higher rate of bleeding complications. For patients with TIA/stroke as a consequence of carotid atherosclerosis, medical management includes antiplatelet agents, blood pressure control, treatment of hyperlipidemia, and smoking cessation.

Table 47–1 ETIOLOGY OF TRANSIENT ISCHEMIC ATTACKS

Emboli of cardiac origin

Intracardiac thrombus or mass
- Myocardial infarction (anterior wall sputum, akinetic segment)
- Cardiomyopathy (infectious, idiopathic)
- Arrhythmia (atrial fibrillation)
- Cardiac myxoma

Valvular heart disease
- Rheumatic heart disease
- Bacterial endocarditis
- Nonbacterial endocarditis (carcinoma, Libman-Sacks disease)
- Mitral valve prolapse
- Prosthetic valve

Vasculitides

Primary central nervous system vasculitis
Systemic necrotizing vasculitis (polyarteritis nodosa, allergic angiitis)
Hypersensitivity vasculitis (serum sickness, drug-induced, cutaneous vasculitis)
Collagen vascular diseases (rheumatoid arthritis, scleroderma, Sjögren disease)
Giant cell (temporal arteritis, Takayasu arteritis)
Wegener granulomatosis
Lymphomatoid granulomatosis
Behçet disease
Infectious vasculitis (neurovascular syphilis, Lyme disease, bacterial and fungal meningitis, tuberculosis, acquired immunodeficiency syndrome, ophthalmic zoster, hepatitis B)

Hematologic disorders

Hemoglobinopathies (sickle cell, sickle cell hemoglobin C [HbSC])
Hyperviscosity syndromes (polycythemia, thrombocytosis, leukocytosis, macroglobulinemia, multiple myeloma)
Hypercoagulable states (carcinoma, pregnancy, puerperium)
Protein C or S deficiency
Antiphospholipid antibodies (lupus anticoagulant, anticardiolipin antibody)

Drug related

Street drugs (cocaine, crack, amphetamines, lysergic acid, phencyclidine, methylphenidate, sympathomimetics, heroin, pentazocine)
Alcohol
Oral contraceptives

Table 47–1 ETIOLOGY OF TRANSIENT ISCHEMIC ATTACKS (CONTINUED)
Other
Fibromuscular dysplasia
Arterial dissection (trauma, spontaneous, Marfan syndrome)
Homocystinuria
Migraine
Subarachnoid hemorrhage or vasospasm
Other emboli (fat, bone marrow, air)
Moyamoya

For patients with cardioembolic stroke as a result of atrial fibrillation, long-term anticoagulation with warfarin (Coumadin) is recommended. For patients with small-vessel disease producing lacunar infarctions, blood pressure control and antiplatelet agents are the mainstays of therapy.

Surgical endarterectomy for severe carotid artery stenosis has successfully reduced the long-term risk of stroke in both symptomatic and asymptomatic patients. The North American Symptomatic Carotid Endarterectomy Trial (NASCET) showed that in patients who had suffered a TIA or stroke and had an ipsilateral **carotid artery stenosis** greater than **70%**, endarterectomy reduced the rate of stroke from 26% to 9% over 2 years compared with standard medical management. The Asymptomatic Carotid Artery Stenosis (ACAS) trial also showed benefit from carotid endarterectomy in patients with **asymptomatic carotid artery stenoses** (those without prior TIA or stroke), **greater than 60%.** However, the risk reduction was smaller than in symptomatic patients, from 11% to 5% over 5 years compared to medical management. It should also be noted that the surgery is not without risk and can actually cause strokes. In both trials, the stipulation was made that in order to achieve the risk reduction benefit; **surgery should be performed in a center with very low surgical morbidity and mortality.** For asymptomatic patients, the benefits of the procedure do not begin to exceed the perioperative morbidity for at least 2 years, so it should be viewed as a "long-term investment" in patients with relatively low comorbidity and a long life expectancy.

Carotid angioplasty and stenting is another procedure available for patients with carotid stenosis but, like endarterectomy, also carries a risk of embolization and stroke. Angioplasty has not been proven to be superior to surgical endarterectomy, and its exact role is not yet defined. It may be considered as an alternative to surgery for symptomatic patients, those with previous TIA or stroke, whose surgical risk is believed to be too high or who are believed to have a high risk for restenosis.

Comprehension Questions

47.1   A healthy 55-year-old man without prior history of stroke or TIA is seen for his annual physical examination. He is found to have a right carotid bruit. On duplex ultrasound, he is found to have a 75% stenosis of the right carotid artery. Which of the following is the best therapy?

A. Aspirin
B. Warfarin (Coumadin)
C. Carotid endarterectomy
D. Observation and reassurance

47.2   One year ago, a 24-year-old woman had an episode of diplopia of 2 weeks' duration. The symptoms resolved completely. Currently, she complains of left arm weakness but no headache. Which of the following is the most likely diagnosis?

A. Recurrent transient ischemic attacks
B. Subarachnoid hemorrhage
C. Complicated migraine
D. Multiple sclerosis

47.3   A 67-year-old woman with extensive atherosclerotic cerebrovascular disease complains of dizziness and vertigo. Which of the following arteries is most likely to be affected?

A. Vertebrobasilar
B. Carotid
C. Aorta
D. Middle cerebral

ANSWERS

47.1   **C.** In this asymptomatic patient, carotid endarterectomy may be considered for severe stenosis, provided it can be performed in a center with very low surgical morbidity and mortality, and the patient has a life expectancy sufficient to justify the perioperative risk.

47.2   **D.** Multiple neurologic deficits separated in space and time in a young patient are suggestive of multiple sclerosis.

47.3   **A.** Vertigo and dizziness can be seen vertebrobasilar insufficiency.

Clinical Pearls

➤ The most common causes of cerebral infarction are carotid atherosclerotic stenosis, cardioembolism, and small-vessel disease such as lipohyalinosis.

➤ Cerebral infarction, transient ischemic attack, and amaurosis fugax all may be symptoms of carotid stenosis.

➤ In symptomatic patients with severe stenosis >70%, carotid endarterectomy is superior to medical therapy in stroke prevention provided the surgical risk is low (<3%).

➤ For other patients, stroke prevention consists mainly of antiplatelet agents (aspirin, clopidogrel) and risk factor modification, for example, lowering blood pressure, hypercholesterolemia, smoking cessation.

REFERENCES

Brott TG, Brown RD Jr, Meyer FB, et al. Carotid revascularization for prevention of stroke: carotid endarterectomy and carotid artery stenting. *Mayo Clin Proc.* 2004; 79:1197-1208.

Pulsinelli WA. Ischemic cerebrovascular disease. In: Goldman L, Bennett JC, eds. *Cecil's Textbook of Medicine*, 21st ed. Philadelphia: WB Saunders; 2000:2099-2109.

Sacco RL. Extracranial carotid stenosis. *N Engl J Med.* 2001;345:1113-1118.

Smith WS, English JD, Johnston SC. Cerebrovascular diseases. In: Fauci AS, Braunwald E, Kasper DL, eds. *Harrison's Principles of Internal Medicine*, 17th ed. New York, NY: McGraw-Hill; 2008:2513-2536.

Case 48

A 25-year-old man comes to an outpatient clinic complaining of low-grade fever and sore throat, and he receives an injection of intramuscular penicillin for presumed streptococcal pharyngitis. He is otherwise healthy and takes no regular medications. Within 20 minutes, he begins to complain of swelling of his face and difficulty breathing. He looks dyspneic and frightened. His heart rate is 130 bpm, blood pressure 90/47 mm Hg, and respiratory rate 28 breaths per minute and shallow. His face and lips are edematous, and he can barely open his eyes because of swelling. He is wheezing diffusely, and he has multiple raised urticarial lesions on his skin. An ambulance has been called.

➤ What is the most likely diagnosis?

➤ What is your next step?

ANSWERS TO CASE 48:
Anaphylaxis/Drug Reactions

Summary: A 25-year-old man develops facial edema and difficulty breathing minutes after receiving an injection of penicillin. He is tachypneic and tachycardic, with borderline hypotension. He is wheezing diffusely, his abdomen is nondistended with hyperactive bowel sounds, and his skin is warm with multiple raised urticarial lesions.

> **Most likely diagnosis:** Anaphylaxis as a result of penicillin hypersensitivity.

> **Next step:** Immediate administration of intramuscular epinephrine, along with corticosteroids and H_1 and H_2 blockers. Close observation of the patient's airway and oxygenation, with possible endotracheal intubation if he becomes compromised.

ANALYSIS

Objectives

1. Learn the clinical presentation and emergency management of anaphylaxis.
2. Understand the diagnosis and complications of serum sickness.
3. Be able to recognize and treat erythema multiforme minor and major.

Considerations

This young man developed manifestations of immediate hypersensitivity, with urticaria, facial angioedema, and bronchospasm. Penicillin is fairly allergenic and leads to an immunoglobulin (Ig)E–mediated release of histamines and other vasoactive chemicals. Epinephrine is the agent of choice in acute anaphylaxis. Antihistamines may also help. Because the airway is vulnerable to compromise as a result of severe edema, intubation to protect the airway is sometimes indicated.

APPROACH TO
Suspected Anaphylaxis

DEFINITIONS

ANGIOEDEMA: Swelling of the lips, periorbital region, face, hands, or feet.
ANAPHYLACTOID REACTIONS: Similar clinical picture to anaphylaxis but not caused by immunologic mechanisms.

ANAPHYLAXIS: Syndrome with varied mechanisms, clinical presentations, and severity that is an acute life-threatening reaction resulting from an immunologic IgE-mediated mechanism.

CLINICAL APPROACH

Common causes of anaphylaxis include drugs, hymenoptera stings, radiographic contrast media (anaphylactoid), blood products, latex in medical products, allergen immunotherapy injections, and foods. **The most common cause of drug-related anaphylaxis is a-lactam antibiotics such as penicillins.** The **most common cause of food-related anaphylaxis is peanuts,** partly because of the frequency with which peanut products are included in other types of foods. However, it is important to note that almost any agent that can activate mast cells or basophils can cause an anaphylactic reaction. Approximately, one-third of all cases of anaphylaxis are idiopathic.

The clinical presentation of anaphylactic reactions varies greatly, but the following guidelines are a good rule of thumb. Symptoms usually develop within 5 to 60 minutes following exposure, although a delayed reaction is possible. Symptoms and signs are variable and are listed in Table 48–1. The key fact to remember is that a **true anaphylactic reaction is life-threatening.** Angioedema may occur with or without urticaria but is not anaphylaxis unless the reaction is associated with other life-threatening processes, such as hypotension or laryngeal edema.

Treatment of anaphylaxis begins with first assessing the **ABCs** (airway, breathing, circulation). Intubation, if required, should not be delayed. Second, **epinephrine** should be administered to help control symptoms and blood pressure. Intramuscular epinephrine injected in the anterolateral thigh leads to more rapid and higher peak levels than does either subcutaneous or deltoid intramuscular injection. Additional treatment measures include placing the patient in a recumbent position, elevating the legs, administration of

---

Table 48–1 CLINICAL MANIFESTATIONS OF ANAPHYLAXIS

Pruritus
Flushing, urticaria, and angioedema
Diaphoresis
Sneezing, rhinorrhea, nasal congestion
Hoarseness, stridor, laryngeal edema
Dyspnea, tachypnea, wheezing, bronchorrhea, cyanosis
Tachycardia, bradycardia, hypotension, cardiac arrest, arrhythmias
Nausea/vomiting, diarrhea, abdominal cramping
Dizziness, weakness, syncope
Sense of impending doom
Seizures

oxygen as needed, normal saline (NL) volume replacement and/or pressors as required, and administration of diphenhydramine 50 mg orally or intravenously every 4 hours as needed (Table 48–2).

Other considerations in the differential diagnosis of anaphylaxis include erythema multiforme major and minor. **Erythema multiforme minor** often occurs after herpes simplex virus (HSV) or other infections. It manifests as urticarial or bullous skin lesions. The pathognomonic finding is a **target lesion**, described as a lesion that is centrally inflamed but is surrounded by an area of less inflamed skin. Treatment includes management of the underlying cause when known, withdrawal of suspected causative drugs, and acyclovir if HSV involvement is suspected. **Erythema multiforme major** (Stevens-Johnson syndrome [SJS]) is similar to erythema multiforme minor but is more severe and involves two or more mucosal surfaces. It is also more likely to be induced by drugs such as sulfonamides or nonsteroidal anti-inflammatory drugs (NSAIDs) than is erythema multiforme minor. Skin findings may include petechiae, vesicles, bullae, and some desquamation of the skin. If the epidermal detachment involves less than 10% of the skin, it is considered SJS. If the epidermal detachment involves more than 30% of the skin, it is considered **toxic epidermal necrolysis** (TEN). Other symptoms include fever, headache, malaise, arthralgias, corneal ulcerations, arrhythmia, pericarditis, electrolyte abnormalities, seizures, coma, and sepsis. Treatment involves withdrawal of the suspected offending agent, treatment of concurrent infections, aggressive fluid maintenance, and supportive treatment similar to burn care. Use of corticosteroids is controversial, but they are often prescribed.

Most drug rashes are maculopapular and occur several days after starting treatment with an offending drug. They usually are not associated with other signs and symptoms, and they resolve several days after removal of the offending agent. **Serum sickness**, on the other hand, is an allergic reaction that occurs

Table 48–2 SUGGESTED TREATMENT OF ANAPHYLAXIS

Address ABCs (airway, breathing, circulation); intubate, if needed
Epinephrine either as intravenous solution (1:1000 0.1-0.3 mL in 10 mL of normal saline over several minutes) or intramuscularly (1:1000 0.3-0.5 mL every 5 min as needed)
Oxygen as needed
Place the patient in a recumbent position, elevate the legs
Normal saline volume replacement and/or pressors as required
Diphenhydramine 50 mg orally or intravenously every 4 h as needed
Other measures
• Ranitidine or other H_2 blockers
• Albuterol or levalbuterol for bronchospasm
• Glucagon if the patient is taking beta-blockers
• Systemic steroids to prevent delayed reactions

7 to 10 days after primary administration or 2 to 4 days after secondary administration of a foreign serum or a drug (ie, a heterologous protein or a nonprotein drug). It is characterized by fever, polyarthralgia, urticaria, lymphadenopathy, and sometimes glomerulonephritis. It is caused by the formation of immune complexes of IgG and the offending antigen. Treatment is based on symptomatology, as the disease usually is self-limiting. Treatment may include administration of antihistamines, aspirin, or NSAIDs, and therapy for associated disease.

Finally, several other types of drug reactions do not fit into the categories discussed. Two of the most important types are iodine allergy and phenytoin (Dilantin) hypersensitivity. "Iodine allergy" is often associated with **radiologic contrast media**. Reactions to contrast media are the result of the hyperosmolar dye causing degranulation of mast cells and basophils rather than a true allergic reaction. These reactions can be prevented by pretreatment with diphenhydramine, H_2 blockers, and corticosteroids beginning 12 hours before the procedure. There is no evidence that a history of seafood allergy is related to adverse events from radiocontrast media. **Dilantin hypersensitivity** can manifest in a range from skin rash to TEN. It may be associated with a syndrome of "drug fever" that resembles infectious mononucleosis and includes fever and lymphadenopathy, with or without a rash. This is not IgE mediated, and the exact mechanism remains unclear. Treatment is withdrawal of the offending agent.

Comprehension Questions

48.1 A 55-year-old accountant complains of facial and tongue swelling. He recently started using a new bath soap. His medical problems include osteoarthritis and mild hypertension, for which he takes acetaminophen and captopril, respectively. Which of the following is the most likely etiology?

A. Captopril
B. Soap hypersensitivity
C. Hypothyroidism
D. Acetaminophen
E. Food-related allergy

48.2 An 18-year-old man with epilepsy controlled with medication develops fever, lymphadenopathy, a generalized maculopapular rash, and arthralgias. He notes having been bitten by ticks while working in the yard outside. Which of the following is the most likely etiology?

A. Severe poison ivy dermatitis
B. Reaction to epilepsy medication
C. Acute human immunodeficiency virus (HIV) infection
D. Lyme disease

48.3   A 34-year-old man is brought into the emergency room for a severe allergic reaction caused by fire ant bites. He is treated with intramuscular epinephrine and intravenous corticosteroids. His oxygen saturation falls to 80%, and he becomes apneic. Which of the following is the best next step?
        A. Intravenous diphenhydramine
        B. Intravenous epinephrine
        C. Oxygen by nasal cannula
        D. Endotracheal intubation
        E. Electrical cardioversion

48.4   A 57-year-old woman with congestive heart failure (CHF) has a positive cardiac stress test. Cardiac catheterization is required to evaluate for coronary bypass grafting. She states that she has an allergy to iodine. Which of the following is the best next step?
        A. Desensitization with increasing doses of oral iodine
        B. Infusion of diphenhydramine during the procedure
        C. Cancel the procedure and proceed to surgery
        D. Diphenhydramine and corticosteroids the night before the procedure

ANSWERS

48.1   **A.** Angiotensin-converting enzyme (ACE) inhibitors are often associated with angioedema.

48.2   **B.** This is a common presentation of phenytoin (Dilantin) hypersensitivity. Poison ivy is not associated with fever and lymphadenopathy.

48.3   **D.** He has developed airway obstruction due to an anaphylactic reaction. He requires intubation and positive-pressure ventilation to maintain oxygenation.

48.4   **D.** Pretreatment with diphenhydramine, H_2 blockers, and corticosteroids beginning 12 hours before the procedure greatly decreases the reaction to contrast dye.

Clinical Pearls

➤ Anaphylaxis is characterized by respiratory distress caused by bronchospasm, cutaneous manifestations such as urticaria or angioedema, and gastrointestinal hypermotility. Patients may die as a consequence of airway compromise or hypotension and vascular collapse caused by widespread vasodilation.

➤ Treatment of anaphylaxis is immediate epinephrine, antihistamines, airway protection, and blood pressure support as necessary. Corticosteroids may help prevent late recurrence of symptoms.

➤ Serum sickness is an immune complex–mediated disease that may include fever, cutaneous eruptions, lymphadenopathy, arthritis, and glomerulonephritis. It usually is self-limited, but treatment may be necessary for renal complications.

➤ Erythema multiforme minor is characterized by urticarial or bullous eruptions, often with target lesions, usually following herpes simplex virus infections. Erythema multiforme major (Stevens-Johnson syndrome) usually is caused by drugs and includes cutaneous and mucosal involvement.

REFERENCES

Austen KF. Allergies, anaphylaxis, and systemic mastocytosis. In: Fauci AS, Braunwald E, Kasper DL, eds. *Harrison's Principles of Internal Medicine*, 17th ed. New York, NY: McGraw-Hill; 2008:2061-2070.

Gruchalla RS, Pirmohamed M. Antibiotic allergy. *N Engl J Med*. 2006;354:601-609.

Roujeau JC, Stern RS, Wintroub BU. Cutaneous drug reactions. In: Kasper DL, Braunwald E, Fauci AS, et al., eds. *Harrison's Principles of Internal Medicine*, 17th ed. New York, NY: McGraw-Hill; 2008:343-349.

Sampson HA. Peanut allergy. *N Engl J Med*. 2002;346:1294-1299.

Vittorio CC, Muglia JJ. Anticonvulsant hypersensitivity syndrome. *Arch Intern Med*. 1995;155:2285-2290.

Case 49

A 68-year-old woman is noted to have memory loss and confusion. Her daughter relates a history of progressive decline in her mother's cognitive function over the last year. The mother has lived on her own for many years, but recently she has begun to become unable to take care of herself. The daughter states that her mother has become withdrawn and has lost interest in her usual activities, such as gardening and reading. The patient was always a fastidious housekeeper; however, recently she is noted to wear the same clothes for several days, and her house is unkempt and dirty. She seems anxious and confused, and she calls her daughter several times a day, worried that the neighbors, previously good friends, are spying on her. She denies bowel or urinary incontinence, and she has had no trouble with headaches or gait instability. Overall the patient has been very healthy, and she only receives treatment with hydrochlorothiazide for hypertension. She never smoked and drank alcohol only rarely. On examination, her blood pressure is 116/56 mm Hg, heart rate 78 bpm, temperature 98.7°F, and respiratory rate 18 breaths per minute. Her weight is 160 lb and her height is 5 ft 3 in. She is noted to be well developed, but her affect throughout the examination is rather flat. She is oriented to person and place, but she is a little confused as to the date. Head, neck, and cardiovascular examinations are unremarkable. Abdomen is benign. The extremities are without edema, cyanosis, or clubbing. Neurologic examination reveals that the cranial nerves are intact, and the motor and sensory examinations are within normal limits. Cerebellar examination is unremarkable, and the gait is normal. Mini-Mental State Examination (MMSE) reveals a score of 24 out of 30.

➤ What is the most likely diagnosis?

➤ What are the next diagnostic steps?

➤ What is the best treatment for this condition?

ANSWERS TO CASE 49:
Alzheimer Dementia

Summary: A 68-year-old woman has memory loss, confusion, and fatigue. She is more withdrawn and is noted to have a flat affect. She is oriented to person and place, but not to time. The remainder of the examination, including neurologic examination, is normal. Notable, however, is her low MMSE score.

➤ **Most likely diagnosis:** Alzheimer dementia.

➤ **Next diagnostic step:** Assess for depression and reversible causes of dementia.

➤ **Probable treatment:** Acetylcholinesterase inhibitor.

ANALYSIS

Objectives

1. Know some of the common causes and evaluation of dementia.
2. Understand the presentation and diagnosis of Alzheimer dementia.
3. Know acetylcholinesterase inhibitors may slow the progression of dementia.

Considerations

In this elderly patient with slowly progressive decline in memory and cognitive functioning, dementia due to Alzheimer disease is the most likely diagnosis. As in other cases of major organ system failure (heart and kidney failures), dementia (brain failure) deserves some investigation into treatable or reversible causes before assigning a diagnosis such as Alzheimer disease, which is incurable and progressive and for which no highly effective therapy exists (Table 49–1).

Table 49–1 ABBREVIATED WORKUP FOR DEMENTIA

Complete blood count (CBC) and consider erythrocyte sedimentation rate (ESR)
Chemistry panel
Thyroid-stimulating hormone (TSH) level
Venereal Disease Research Laboratory (VDRL)
Human immunodeficiency virus (HIV) assay
Urinalysis
Serum vitamin B_{12} and folate levels
Chest radiograph
Electrocardiogram (ECG)
Computed tomography (CT) or magnetic resonance imaging (MRI) of the head

APPROACH TO
Dementia

DEFINITIONS

DEMENTIA: Impairment of memory and at least one other cognitive function (eg, language, visuospatial orientation, judgment) without alteration in consciousness, representing a decline from previous level of ability and interfering with daily functioning and independent living.

ALZHEIMER DISEASE: Leading cause of dementia, accounting for half of the cases involving elderly individuals, correlating to diffuse cortical atrophy and hippocampal atrophy with ventricular enlargement. The pathologic changes in the brains of patients with Alzheimer disease include neurofibrillary tangles with deposition of abnormal amyloid in the brain.

MULTI-INFARCT DEMENTIA: Dementia in the setting of cerebrovascular disease, occurring after multiple cerebral infarctions, whether large or small (lacunar).

CLINICAL APPROACH

In assessing the patient with dementia, the clinician should strive to answer three questions: (1) What is the most likely diagnosis? (2) Is any treatable or reversible condition contributing to the patient's cognitive decline? (3) What interventions are available to preserve the patient's level of function and relieve the burden to caregivers?

To answer the first question, the most important investigation is the history of symptoms. If the patient has an acute or subacute onset of confusion or has a fluctuating level of consciousness, the most likely diagnosis is a **delirium** resulting from infection, intoxication, or adverse medication effects, or metabolic derangements such as hyponatremia, hypercalcemia, or hypoglycemia.

If cognitive decline occurs with prominent mood disturbance, then one consideration is **depression** or pseudodementia. Distinguishing which occurred first is often difficult because many elderly patients with cognitive decline and a declining level of independent functioning suffer from a reactive depression. History provided by involved family members regarding the onset of symptoms or history of prior depression or other psychiatric illness may help establish the diagnosis, and an empiric trial of antidepressants may be considered.

If the patient has a history of irregular stepwise decline in functioning, especially if the patient has had apparent stroke symptoms or transient ischemic events or has a known cardiovascular disease or atrial fibrillation, then **multi-infarct dementia** is the most likely diagnosis. This type of vascular dementia is the second most common cause of dementia in the United

States, composing 10% to 20% of dementias. Other patients with cerebrovascular disease, especially as a result of long-standing hypertension, may develop diffuse subcortical white matter changes seen on imaging and an insidious rather than sudden stepwise decline in cognitive function. This condition is often referred to as *Binswanger disease*.

Other common causes of dementia include cognitive decline as a result of long-standing **alcoholism** or dementia associated with **parkinsonism**. Both of these underlying conditions are readily discovered by the appropriate associated medical history.

Less common causes of dementia include medical conditions such as Wernicke encephalopathy resulting from thiamine (vitamin B_1) deficiency, vitamin B_{12} deficiency resulting from pernicious anemia, untreated **hypothyroidism**, or chronic infections such as **HIV** dementia or **neurosyphilis**. A variety of primary central nervous system (CNS) diseases can lead to dementia, including Huntington disease, multiple sclerosis, neoplastic diseases such as primary or metastatic brain tumors (although they are much more likely to produce seizures or focal deficits rather than dementia), or leptomeningeal spread of various cancers.

Normal pressure hydrocephalus is a potentially reversible form of dementia in which the cerebral ventricles slowly enlarge as a result of disturbances to cerebral spinal fluid resorption. The **classic triad is dementia, gait disturbance, and urinary or bowel incontinence**. Relief of hydrocephalus through placement of a ventriculoperitoneal shunt may reverse the cognitive decline. Descriptions of the primary neurologic diseases associated with cognitive dysfunction are listed in Table 49–2.

Once likely diagnoses have been established by history and physical examination, investigation should be undertaken to look for treatable or reversible causes. The choice of laboratory or imaging tests is not straightforward because of the numerous, yet uncommon, causes of reversible dementia, so testing is generally low yield. Tests that may be considered for the evaluation of dementia are listed in Table 49–1. The American Academy of Neurology recommends routine assessment of thyroid function tests, a vitamin B_{12} level, and a neuroimaging study (either CT or MRI of the brain).

For patients with Alzheimer disease, the average life expectancy after diagnosis is 7 to 10 years. The clinical course is characterized by progressive decline of cognitive functions (memory, orientation, attention, and concentration) and the development of psychological and behavioral symptoms (wandering, aggression, anxiety, depression, and psychosis; Table 49–3). The goals of treatment in Alzheimer disease are to (a) improve cognitive function, (b) reduce behavioral and psychological symptoms, and (c) improve the quality of life. Donepezil, rivastigmine, and galantamine are cholinesterase inhibitors that are effective in improving cognitive function and global clinical state. Antagonists to N-methyl-D-aspartate (NMDA) receptors, such as memantine, also seem to reduce the rate of decline in patients with Alzheimer dementia. Risperidone reduces psychotic symptoms and aggression in patients with dementia. Other

Table 49–2 NEUROLOGIC DISEASES IMPAIRING COGNITIVE ABILITY

DISEASE	CLINICAL FEATURES	TREATMENT
Alzheimer disease	Slow decline in cognitive and behavioral ability; pathology: neurofibrillary tangles, enlarged cerebral ventricles, atrophy	Cholinesterase inhibitors such as donepezil or rivastigmine
Normal-pressure hydrocephalus	Gait disturbance, dementia, incontinence; enlarged ventricles without atrophy	Ventricular shunting process
Multi-infarct dementia	Focal deficits, stepwise loss of function; multiple areas of infarct usually subcortical	Address atherosclerotic risk factors, identify and treat thrombus
Parkinson disease	Extrapyramidal signs (tremor, rigidity), slow onset	Dopaminergic agents
HIV infection	Systemic involvement; risk factors for acquisition; positive HIV serology	Treat specific infection
Neurosyphilis	Optic atrophy, Argyll Robertson pupils, gait disturbance; positive cerebrospinal fluid serology	High-dose intravenous penicillin
Multiple sclerosis	Brainstem signs, optic atrophy, long-standing disease with exacerbations and remissions; MRI showing white matter abnormalities	Recombinant interferon, corticosteroids
Intracranial tumor	Focal signs, papilledema, seizures	Corticosteroids to reduce intracranial pressure, treat the lesion

issues include wakefulness, nightwalking and wandering, aggression, incontinence, and depression. A structured environment, with predictability, and judicious use of pharmacotherapy, such as a selective serotonin reuptake inhibitor (SSRI) for depression or a short-acting benzodiazepine for insomnia, are helpful. The primary caregiver is often overwhelmed and needs support. The Alzheimer Association is a national organization developed to give support to family members and can be contacted through its Web site at *www.alz.org*.

Table 49–3 CLINICAL COURSE OF ALZHEIMER DISEASE

CLINICAL STAGE	MANIFESTATIONS
Early	Mild forgetfulness, poor concentration, fairly good function, denial, occasional disorientation
Intermediate	Drastic deficits of recent memory, can travel to familiar locations; suspicious, anxious, aware of confusion
Late	Cannot remember names of family members or close friends; may have delusions or hallucinations, agitation, aggression, wandering, disoriented to time and place; needs substantial care
Advanced	Totally incapacitated and disoriented, incontinent, personality and emotional changes; eventually all verbal and motor skills deteriorate, leading to need for total care

Comprehension Questions

49.1   A 78-year-old woman is diagnosed with Alzheimer disease. Which of the following agents is most likely to help with the cognitive function?
       A. Haloperidol
       B. Estrogen replacement therapy
       C. Donepezil
       D. High-dose vitamin B_{12} injections

49.2   A 74-year-old man was noted to have excellent cognitive and motor skill 12 months ago. His wife noted that 6 months ago his function deteriorated noticeably, and 2 months ago another level of deterioration was noted. Which of the following is most likely to reveal the etiology of his functional decline?
       A. HIV antibody test
       B. Magnetic resonance imaging of the brain
       C. Cerebrospinal fluid (CSF) Venereal Disease Research Laboratory (VDRL) test
       D. Serum thyroid-stimulating hormone

49.3   A 55-year-old man is noted by his family members to be forgetful and
        become disoriented. He has difficulty making it to the bathroom in
        time and complains of feeling as though "he is walking like he was
        drunk." Which of the following therapies is most likely to improve his
        condition?
        A. Intravenous penicillin for 21 days
        B. Rivastigmine
        C. Treatment with fluoxetine for 9 to 12 months
        D. Ventriculoperitoneal shunt
        E. Enrollment into alcoholic anonymous

49.4   Which of the following are commonly seen in brain imaging of
        patients with Alzheimer disease?
        A. Normal cerebral ventricles and atrophic brain tissue
        B. Enlarged cerebral ventricles and atrophic brain tissue
        C. Enlarged cerebral ventricles and no atrophy of brain tissue
        D. Normal cerebral ventricles and normal brain tissue, acetylcholine
           deficiency

ANSWERS

49.1   **C.** Cholinesterase inhibitors help with the cognitive function in
        Alzheimer disease and may slow the progression somewhat.

49.2   **B.** The stepwise decline in function is typical for multi-infarct dementia,
        diagnosed by viewing multiple areas of the brain infarct.

49.3   **D.** The classic triad for normal pressure hydrocephalus is dementia,
        incontinence, and gait disturbance; one treatment is shunting the
        cerebrospinal fluid.

49.4   **B.** Alzheimer disease typically has enlarged cerebral ventricles and
        brain atrophy, whereas normal pressure hydrocephalus has enlarged
        brain ventricles without brain atrophy.

Clinical Pearls

➤ Alzheimer disease is the most common type of dementia, followed by
  multi-infarct (vascular) dementia.

➤ Approximately 5% of people older than 65 years and 20% older than 80 years
  have some form of dementia.

➤ Depression and reversible causes of dementia should be considered in the
  evaluation of a patient with memory loss and functional decline.

➤ A cholinesterase inhibitor such as donepezil is effective in improving cognitive function and global clinical state in patients with Alzheimer disease.

REFERENCES

Bird TD, Miller BL. Dementia. In: Kasper DL, Braunwald E, Fauci AS, et al., eds. *Harrison's Principles of Internal Medicine*, 17th ed. New York, NY: McGraw-Hill; 2008:2536-2549.

Geldmacher DS, Whitehouse PJ. Evaluation of dementia. *N Engl J Med*. 1996; 335:330-336.

Knopman DS, DeKosky ST, Cummings JL, et al. Practice parameter: diagnosis of dementia (an evidence-based review). *Neurology*. 2001;56:1143-1153.

Case 50

A 59-year-old woman comes to your office because she is concerned that she might have a brain tumor. She has had a fairly severe headache for the last 3 weeks (she rates it as an 8 on a scale of 1-10). She describes the pain as constant, occasionally throbbing but mostly a dull ache, and localized to the right side of her head. She thinks the pain is worse at night, especially when she lies with that side of her head on the pillow. She has had no nausea, vomiting, photophobia, or other visual disturbances. She has had headaches before, but they were mostly occipital and frontal, which she attributed to "stress," and they were relieved with acetaminophen. Her medical history is significant for hypertension, which is controlled with hydrochlorothiazide, and "arthritis" of her neck, shoulders, and hips for which she takes ibuprofen when she feels stiff and achy. On physical examination, her temperature is 100.4°F, heart rate 88 bpm, blood pressure 126/75 mm Hg, and respiratory rate 12 breaths per minute. Her visual acuity is normal, visual fields are intact, and her funduscopic examination is significant for arteriolar narrowing but no papilledema or hemorrhage. She has moderate tenderness over the right side of her head but no obvious scalp lesions. Her chest is clear, her heart rhythm is regular, with normal S_1 and S_2 but an S_4 gallop. Abdominal examination is benign. She has no focal deficits on neurologic examination. She has no joint swelling or deformity but is tender to palpation over her shoulders, hips, and thighs.

➤ What is the most likely diagnosis?

➤ What is the best next step to confirm the diagnosis?

ANSWERS TO CASE 50:
Headache/Temporal Arteritis

Summary: A 59-year-old woman complains of a 3-week history of severe right-side headaches that are worse at night, when she lies with that side of her head on the pillow. Her medical history is significant for hypertension and "arthritis" of her neck, shoulders, and hips, for which she takes ibuprofen. She has a temperature 100.4°F and normal neurologic and eye examinations. She has moderate tenderness over the right side of her head but no obvious scalp lesions.

➤ **Most likely diagnosis:** Temporal arteritis (TA).

➤ **Best next step to confirm diagnosis:** Erythrocyte sedimentation rate (ESR).

ANALYSIS

Objectives

1. Be familiar with the clinical features that help to distinguish a benign headache from the one representing a serious underlying illness.
2. Know the clinical features and diagnostic tests for TA.
3. Know the clinical features of migraine and cluster headaches and of subarachnoid hemorrhage.

Considerations

Although headaches are a very common complaint, this patient has features that are of greater concern: older age of onset, abrupt onset and severe intensity, and dissimilarity to previous milder headaches. These are three of the nine factors of concern for significant underlying pathology outlined in Table 50–1. She is very concerned about the headaches and is worried that they indicate a brain tumor. She has no meningeal signs and her neurologic examination is

Table 50–1 RED FLAGS FOR SECONDARY HEADACHE DISORDERS

Fundamental change or progression in headache pattern
First severe and/or worst headache
Abrupt-onset attacks, including those awakening one from sleep
Abnormal physical examination findings (general or neurologic)
Neurologic symptoms lasting >1 h
New headache in individuals aged <5 y or >50 y
New headache in patients with cancer, immunosuppression, pregnancy
Headache associated with alteration in or loss of consciousness
Headache triggered by exertion, sexual activity, or Valsalva maneuver

nonfocal. She has stiffness and achiness of the shoulder and hip girdles. Together these factors make the diagnosis of TA a strong possibility. TA usually has its onset in patients aged 50 years or older (females more than males), and involves inflammation of the medium- or large-size vessels. Her low-grade fever and generalized body aches may represent polymyalgia rheumatica, which is closely associated with TA. The diagnosis would be suggested by an elevated ESR, and then confirmed by temporal artery biopsy. Although TA is not a common cause of headache, untreated patients often progress to permanent visual loss as a consequence of involvement of the ophthalmic artery, so a high index of suspicion is necessary to begin investigation. An elevated ESR necessitates further diagnostic testing, such as a temporal artery biopsy. In the meantime, empiric corticosteroids may help prevent complications.

APPROACH TO
Headaches

DEFINITIONS

TEMPORAL ARTERITIS (TA): Also known as giant cell arteritis (GCA), temporal arteritis is a common form of systemic vascular inflammation affecting patients older than 50 years. Medium- and large-sized vessels especially the superficial temporal artery are affected.

BERRY ANEURYSM: A small outpouching that looks like a berry and classically occurs at the point at which a cerebral artery departs from the circular artery (the circle of Willis) at the base of the brain. They can rupture causing subarachnoid hemorrhage.

CLINICAL APPROACH

Headache is one of the most common complaints of patients in the western world. It periodically afflicts 90% of adults, and almost 25% have recurrent severe headaches. As with many common symptoms, a broad range of conditions, from trivial to life-threatening, might be responsible. The **majority of patients** presenting with **headache** have **tension-type, migraine,** or **cluster**; however, fewer than 1 in 20 have significant underlying pathology. Because headache symptoms usually are accompanied by a paucity of associated findings, including those on laboratory examination, the clinician must depend largely upon a thorough history with a general and focused neurologic examination as the initial workup. Careful inquiry and meticulous physical examination, keeping in mind the "red flags" of headaches (Table 50–1), will serve the clinician well. Differentiating serious underlying causes of headache from more benign causes may be difficult. Table 50–2 lists some typical features of serious causes of headache.

Table 50–2 CAUSES OF PATHOLOGIC HEADACHES

DISEASE	CLINICAL FEATURES	DIAGNOSTIC FINDINGS
Meningitis	Nuchal rigidity, headache, photophobia, and prostration; may not be febrile	Lumbar puncture is diagnostic
Intracranial hemorrhage	Nuchal rigidity and headache; may not have clouded consciousness or seizures	Hemorrhage may not be seen on CT scan; lumbar puncture shows "bloody tap" that does not clear by the last tube; a fresh hemorrhage may not be xanthochromic
Brain tumor	May present with prostrating pounding headaches that are associated with nausea and vomiting; should be suspected in progressively severe new "migraine" that is invariably unilateral	CT or MRI
Temporal arteritis	May present with a unilateral pounding headache; onset generally in older patients ≤ 50 y) and frequently associated with visual changes	Erythrocyte sedimentation rate is the best screening test and usually is markedly elevated (ie, >50 mm/hr); definitive diagnosis can be made by arterial biopsy
Glaucoma	Usually consists of severe eye pain; may have nausea and vomiting; the eye usually is painful and red; the pupil may be partially dilated	Elevated intraocular pressure
Migraine headache	Unilateral throbbing headache with preceding aura, photophobia, and nausea, which is relieved with sleep	
Cluster headache	Male predominance; precipitated by alcohol; occurs with rhinorrhea and lacrimation	
Tension headache	Occipital-frontal headache; constant, "bandlike"; relieved with relaxation	

Adapted with permission, from Raskin NH. Headache. In: Braunwald E, Fauci AS, Kasper KL, et al., eds. Harrison's Principles of Internal Medicine, 16th ed. New York, NY: McGraw-Hill; 2005:86.

One of the most catastrophic secondary causes of headache is **subarachnoid hemorrhage**, usually secondary to a ruptured intracerebral (berry) aneurysm. Up to 4% of patients presenting to an emergency center with severe headache, or the classic "worst ever headache," have a subarachnoid bleed. The initial hemorrhage may be fatal, may result in severe neurologic impairment, or may produce only minor symptoms such as headache. A high index of suspicion is needed because no neurologic findings may be present initially, and the patient who will benefit the most from intervention will often have the mildest symptoms. The first diagnostic study should be a noncontrast CT scan with thin imaging cuts at the region of the brain base. This study will be positive in more than 90% of cases on the first day, with decreasing sensitivity over the next several days. If hemorrhage is suspected but the CT is negative, lumbar puncture should be performed as soon as possible to assess for the presence of red cells or xanthochromia (yellowish discoloration of cerebrospinal fluid [CSF]); this finding indicates presence of bilirubin and differentiates subarachnoid hemorrhage from a traumatic lumbar puncture.

Giant cell arteritis, or **temporal arteritis** (TA), is a chronic vasculitis of large- and medium-size vessels, usually involving the cranial branches of the arteries arising from the aortic arch. The clinical criteria for diagnosis include age of onset older than 50 years, new onset or type of headache pattern, tenderness or decreased pulsation of the temporal artery, elevated ESR, and abnormal findings on biopsy of the temporal artery. The presence of three or more criteria yields more than 90% sensitivity and specificity for the diagnosis. TA is closely related to **polymyalgia rheumatica** (PR), a condition associated with bilateral aching and stiffness of neck, torso, shoulders, or proximal parts of the arms and thighs, as well as an elevated ESR. Both conditions probably are polygenic diseases in which various environmental and genetic factors influence susceptibility and severity. Clinical symptoms may include jaw claudication, and the most worrisome complication is permanent or partial loss of vision in one or both eyes, which can occur as an early manifestation in up to 20% of patients. Temporal artery biopsy is recommended in all patients suspected of having TA, and long segments of the artery may require excision in order to find the typical areas of segmental inflammation. Corticosteroids are the drugs of choice to treat both polymyalgia rheumatica and TA, with daily doses of 10 to 20 mg of prednisone for polymyalgia rheumatica and 40 to 60 mg for TA. Steroids may prevent, but usually do not reverse, visual loss. Steroid dosage is gradually tapered, but relapse is common, as are complications of corticosteroid therapy.

Migraine headache is much more common than TA but is more variable in its presentation. It is the most common cause of initial office visits for headache because of its frequency, disabling qualities, and associated multiorgan symptoms. Migraine attacks are more common in women than in men. Migraine attacks may or may not have a preceding aura, may be unilateral or bilateral, and may have either throbbing or nonpulsatile pain, including the neck. They may have cranial autonomic features such as tearing or nasal congestion, leading to the misdiagnosis of sinus disease. A number of evidence-based guidelines are available for managing migraine headaches. In general, preventive therapies include tricyclic antidepressants and beta-blockers. Treatment of acute episodes involves the initial use of nonsteroidal anti-inflammatory drugs (NSAIDs), followed by dihydroergotamine or sumatriptan if symptoms persist.

Episodic **cluster headache** is much less common, but it is more easily diagnosed by its distinctive pattern of periodic attacks of intense, unilateral, periorbital pain with nasal or ocular watering lasting only minutes to hours but recurring daily over several weeks or months. Acute attacks can be treated with oxygen or subcutaneous sumatriptan.

Comprehension Questions

Match the headache type (A-E) to the clinical presentation described in Questions [50.1] to [50.3].

    A. Common migraine headache
    B. Classic migraine headache
    C. Cluster headache
    D. Subarachnoid hemorrhage
    E. Meningitis

50.1   A 42-year-old man with polycystic kidney disease who complained of a sudden onset of severe headache and then lost consciousness

50.2   A 22-year-old college student with fever, headache, photophobia, and 25 white blood cells per high-power field but no red blood cells or xanthochromia in CSF

50.3   A 31-year-old woman with a long history of intermittent severe unilateral headache lasting hours to days associated with nausea and photophobia, but no preceding symptoms and no visual disturbance

ANSWERS

50.1   **D.** The sudden onset of severe headache with diminution in level of consciousness is classic for subarachnoid hemorrhage. This patient likely had rupture of a cerebral artery aneurysm, which is associated with polycystic kidney disease.

50.2   **E.** The presence of white blood cells but no red blood cells in the CSF is indicative of meningeal inflammation, likely due to viral or bacterial infection.

50.3   **A.** The patient's history is strongly suggestive of migraine (common type), which is not associated with a preceding aura or visual symptoms as seen in classic-type migraine.

Clinical Pearls

➤ Temporal arteritis usually involves one or more branches of the carotid artery and almost always occurs in patients older than 50 years. Diagnosis is suggested by an elevated erythrocyte sedimentation rate and confirmed by temporal artery biopsy.

➤ Visual loss is a common complication of temporal arteritis and can be prevented by initiation of high-dose corticosteroids when the diagnosis is suspected.

➤ Subarachnoid hemorrhage typically presents as a sudden onset of severe headache and is diagnosed by visualization of blood on a computed tomographic (CT) scan or by finding red blood cells or xanthochromic fluid on a lumbar puncture.

➤ Migraine is the most common type of headache for which patients seek medical attention in an office setting. The classic variety has a preceding aura, whereas the common type does not.

REFERENCES

Edlow J, Caplan L. Avoiding pitfalls in the diagnosis of subarachnoid hemorrhage. *N Engl J Med.* 2000;342:29-36.

Goadsby PJ, Raskin NH. Headache. In: Kasper DL, Braunwald E, Fauci AS, et al., eds. *Harrison's Principles of Internal Medicine*, 17th ed. New York, NY: McGraw-Hill; 2008:95-107.

Kaniecki R. Headache assessment and management. *JAMA.* 2003;289:1430-1433.

Salvarani C, Cantini F, Boiardi L, et al. Polymyalgia rheumatica and giant cell arteritis. *N Engl J Med.* 2002;347:261-278.

Snow V, Weiss K, Wall E, et al. Pharmacologic management of acute attacks of migraine and prevention of migraine headache. *Ann Intern Med.* 2002;137: 840-852.

Case 51

A 75-year-old white woman presents to the emergency room with right wrist pain after a fall at home. She tripped and fell while preparing dinner, and she says that she tried to stop her fall with her outstretched right hand. She heard a "snap" and felt immediate pain. Her medical history is remarkable only for three normal pregnancies, menopause at age 50 years, and hypertension that is well controlled with diuretics. She has a 50-pack per year history of smoking. Her weight is 100 lb and her height is 5 ft 6 in. Her examination is remarkable for normal vital signs; a swollen, deformed right distal forearm and wrist, with limited mobility because of pain; and good radial pulses and capillary refill in the right fingernail beds. An X-ray confirms a fracture of the right radial head, and the radiologist notes osteopenia.

➤ What risk factor for fracture is this woman likely to have?

➤ What are the causes of this condition?

➤ What can her physician offer her to prevent future fractures?

ANSWERS TO CASE 51:

Osteoporosis

Summary: A 75-year-old white woman tried to stop her fall using her outstretched right hand, heard a "snap," and felt immediate pain. Her medical history is remarkable only for menopause at age 50 years and hypertension that is well controlled with diuretics. She does have a 50-pack per year history of smoking. She has a swollen, deformed, right distal forearm and wrist, with limited mobility because of pain, and good radial pulses and capillary refill in the right fingernail beds. An X-ray confirms a fracture of the right radial head, and the radiologist notes osteopenia.

➤ **Risk factor for fracture:** Osteoporosis.

➤ **Causes of this condition:** Decreased bone strength as a consequence of demineralization and increased bone turnover as a result of decreased levels of sex steroids (estrogen and testosterone), medications, other hormonal conditions, or diseases of decreased calcium absorption.

➤ **Preventive measures:** Several medications are available to increase bone density, which may decrease the risk of future fractures. Also, her physician would want to work with her to prevent future falls by limiting unnecessary medications that may cause instability, making changes in the home environment, and evaluating her gait, visual acuity, and peripheral sensory system. The patient should be advised to quit smoking.

ANALYSIS

Objectives

1. Understand the pathophysiology of osteoporosis.
2. Learn the risk factors that predispose both men and women to osteoporosis.
3. Be familiar with the tests used to evaluate bone density.
4. Know the treatment options for osteoporosis.

Considerations

This 75-year-old woman with a fracture after a fall likely sustained the fracture because of osteoporosis. Her risk factors for osteoporosis are her race, smoking history, postmenopausal state without hormone replacement therapy, and thin physique. Osteoporosis puts her at risk for future fractures with substantial morbidity, such as painful vertebral compression fractures or incapacitating hip fractures. She requires intervention to reduce her risk of fractures as well as her risk of falls.

APPROACH TO
Osteoporosis

DEFINITIONS

BISPHOSPHONATES: Synthetic carbon phosphate compounds (alendronate, risedronate, ibandronate) that build bone mass by binding to pyrophosphatase in bone and by inhibiting osteoclast bone resorption.

OSTEOPENIA: T score between −1.0 and −2.5 standard deviations (SD) below the mean.

OSTEOPOROSIS: Decrease in bone mass leading to increased bone fragility and predisposing to fracture of the hip, vertebrae, and long bones, with a defined bone mineral density (BMD) less than 2.5 SD below the mean of young healthy adults.

T SCORE: BMD comparison against young healthy adults (in standard deviations from the mean).

CLINICAL APPROACH

Osteoporosis is an important health issue because the resultant bone fractures cause a great deal of morbidity in chronic pain, loss of independence, and loss of function, as well as mortality. Risk factors for the development of osteoporosis include a low peak skeletal density reached in young adulthood, increasing age, loss of steroid hormone production (menopause or hypogonadism), smoking, nutritional deficiencies, and genetically low bone density. Approximately 14% of white women and 3% to 5% of white men will develop osteoporosis in their lifetime. The prevalence is lower in other ethnic groups.

Osteoporosis can be either idiopathic or a manifestation of another underlying disease process. Probably the most common form of **secondary osteoporosis** is caused by **glucocorticoid excess**, usually iatrogenic steroid use for an inflammatory disease such as rheumatoid arthritis. Patients, both men and women, with rheumatoid arthritis are susceptible to accelerated bone loss with even low doses of glucocorticoids. **Gonadal deficiency** is another common cause, which is seen physiologically in menopausal women but is seen pathologically in women who are amenorrheic (eg, female athletes such as gymnasts or marathon runners) or as a result of hyperprolactinemia. Men with gonadal failure for whatever reason also are prone to develop osteoporosis.

Osteoporosis is a common feature of several endocrinopathies. Patients with **hyperparathyroidism** will develop osteoporosis because of increased calcium mobilization from bone. Long-standing **hyperthyroidism**, either naturally occurring, as in Graves disease, or as a result of excessive replacement of levothyroxine in patients with hypothyroidism, will also lead to accelerated bone loss. Malnutrition and nutritional deficiencies are causative and are often seen in patients with malabsorption; for example, most patients, both men and women, with **celiac sprue** have osteoporosis. Certain medications, such as cyclosporine, antiepileptics, heparin, and gonadotropin-releasing hormone (GnRH) inhibitors, among others, may accelerate bone loss.

Peak bone density occurs in young adulthood under the influence of sex steroid hormone production. Other influential factors include genetics, which may account for 80% of total bone density, adequate calcium intake, and level of physical activity, especially **weight-bearing activity.** The type of bone growth at this stage is called *modeling.* After skeletal maturation is reached, the bone growth enters a new phase, termed *remodeling,* in which repairs are made to damaged bone, existing bone is strengthened, and calcium is released to maintain serum levels under the influence of estrogens, androgens, parathyroid hormone, vitamin D, and various cytokines and other hormones. The activity of the osteoclasts approximates the activity of the osteoblasts in that overall bone density remains stable. However, after age 35 years, bone breakdown begins to exceed bone replacement, and this increases **markedly after menopause** as a consequence of **increased osteoclast activity.**

Diagnostic Approach

The benefits and costs of universal screening for osteoporosis are unclear. Rather, a targeted approach is advocated. Those with a family history or other risk factors should be offered screening, as well as patients undergoing a chronic drug (steroid) therapy that may lead to osteoporosis. **Currently, all women older than 65 years or those who have sustained a fracture before age 65 years are recommended to undergo BMD testing.** Dual-energy X-ray absorptiometry (DEXA scan) is the technique used to define diagnostic thresholds; however, whether the hip, spine, or forearm is the best site for screening is not clearly established. DEXA scan results can be expressed as a Z score, which compares BMD to that in persons of the same age, and a T score, which compares to the young adult normal range. **T scores are more useful for predicting fracture risk.** Every 1 SD decrease in BMD below the mean doubles the fracture risk. As mentioned, osteoporosis is defined as a T score of −2.5 SD.

Other laboratory evaluations should routinely be considered in patients with osteoporosis. The **serum levels of calcium, phosphorus, and alkaline phosphatase should be normal** in patients with osteoporosis, although the alkaline phosphatase level sometimes is mildly elevated in the presence of a healing fracture. Laboratory abnormalities should prompt consideration of alternative diagnoses for the bone disease: hypercalcemia in hyperparathyroidism or hypocalcemia in osteomalacia.

If a patient suffers a pathologic fracture, that is, one with minimal trauma, other diagnoses must be excluded. **Osteomalacia** is defective mineralization of bone matrix with accumulation of unmineralized osteoid and is most often caused by vitamin D deficiency or phosphate deficiency.

Patients with osteomalacia frequently have diffuse bone pain and tenderness, proximal muscle weakness, and laboratory abnormalities such as elevated alkaline phosphatase level and low or low to normal calcium level. In the absence of fractures, patients with osteoporosis should have no bone pain or laboratory abnormalities. Both of these disease processes can coexist. A less common bone disease is **Paget disease**, which is characterized by disorganized bone remodeling with a high alkaline phosphatase level causing weakened and enlarged bones with skeletal deformities. Other important causes of pathologic fracture that must be considered include **malignancy**, such as multiple myeloma or metastatic disease, and vertebral osteomyelitis.

Treatment

Treatment takes a multifaceted approach. Adequate **calcium intake**, 1000 to 1200 mg/d for premenopausal women and adult men to prevent bone loss and 1500 mg with 400 to 800 IU of **vitamin D** per day for postmenopausal women, leads to decreased fractures. Estrogen replacement can increase bone density and reduce fracture, as can the use of bisphosphonates, both in combination with calcium and vitamin D. **Bisphosphonates** can lead to **severe esophagitis** and must be used with caution in individuals with gastric reflux disease. Bisphosphonates should be taken on an empty stomach, with a large quantity of water, and the patient should remain in the upright position for at least 30 minutes. Selective estrogen receptor modifiers are used for treatment of osteoporosis as well.

    Weight-bearing physical activity decreases bone loss and improves coordination and muscle strength, which may prevent falls. Ensuring that patients can see adequately, that they use a cane or walker if needed, that throw rugs are removed, that patients have railings to hold on to in the shower or bath, or that they wear hip protectors can further decrease the risk of life-altering bone fractures.

Comprehension Questions

51.1   Which of the following patients is most likely to be a candidate for bone mineral density screening?

    A. A 65-year-old, thin, white woman who smokes and is 15 years postmenopausal

    B. A 40-year-old white woman who exercises daily and still menstruates

    C. A healthy 75-year-old white man who is sedentary

    D. A 60-year-old overweight African American woman

    E. A 35-year-old asthmatic woman who took prednisone 40 mg/d for a 2-week course 1 week ago

51.2   During which of the following periods in a woman's life is the most bone mass accumulated?
    A. Ages 15 to 25
    B. Ages 25 to 35
    C. Ages 35 to 45
    D. Ages 45 to 55

51.3   A 60-year-old woman presents with the results of her DEXA scan. She has a T score of −1.5 SD at the hip and −2.5 at the spine. Which of the following is the most accurate interpretation of these results?
    A. She has osteoporosis at the spine and osteopenia at the hip.
    B. She has osteoporosis in both areas.
    C. This is a normal examination.
    D. She has osteoporosis of the hip and osteopenia at the spine.
    E. You need to know the Z score.

51.4   You see a 70-year-old woman in your office for a routine checkup, and you order a DEXA scan for bone mineral density screening. The T score returns as −2.5 standard deviations SD in the spine and −2.6 in the hip. Which of the following statements is most accurate?
    A. This patient has osteopenia.
    B. Estrogen replacement therapy should be started with an anticipated rebuilding of bone mass to near-normal within 1 year.
    C. Swimming will help build bone mass.
    D. Bisphosphonates would reduce the risk of hip fracture by 50%.

ANSWERS

51.1   **A.** Of the choices, this woman is the only individual with risk factors. Risk factors include white race, age, postmenopausal status, smoking, positive family history, poor nutritional status, and chronic treatment with a drug known to predispose to bone loss.

51.2   **A.** The time of greatest accumulation of bone mass in women is during adolescence.

51.3   **A.** The T score is the number of standard deviations of a patient's bone mineral density from the mean of young, adult, white women. It is the standard measurement of bone mineral density used by the World Health Organization. A score of −2.5 SD is the definition of osteoporosis. A Z score is the number of standard deviations from the mean bone mineral density of women in the same age group as the patient.

51.4   **D.** Estrogen primarily inhibits loss of bone mass, although it can help to build a modest amount of bone mass. Weight-bearing exercise, and not swimming, is important in preventing osteoporosis. Bisphosphonates decrease the incidence of hip fractures by 30% to 50%.

Clinical Pearls

➤ Bone mineral density screening should be offered to patients with risk factors for osteoporosis and to all women older than 65 years.

➤ Every 1 standard deviation (SD) decrease in bone mineral density below the mean of young adults doubles the fracture risk. Osteoporosis is defined as a T score of −2.5 SD.

➤ Patients with osteoporosis should have normal serum calcium, phosphorus, and alkaline phosphatase levels. Laboratory abnormalities should prompt a search for an alternative diagnosis.

➤ Fractures can have a devastating effect upon a patient's quality of life, and a multifaceted approach through nutritional counseling, home improvements, gait stabilization through exercise and with canes or walkers, and medical interventions to improve eyesight or with medications to improve bone density should be offered to patients at risk.

➤ In patients with a pathologic fracture, osteoporosis is a diagnosis of exclusion; osteomalacia, Paget disease, and metastatic malignancies also must be considered.

REFERENCES

Lindsay R, Cosman F. Osteoporosis. In: Kasper DL, Braunwald E, Fauci AS, et al, eds. *Harrison's Principles of Internal Medicine*. 17th ed. New York, NY: McGraw-Hill; 2008:2397-2408.

Mauck KF, Clarke BL. Diagnosis, screening, prevention, and treatment of osteoporosis. *Mayo Clin Proc*. 2006;81:662-672.

Rosen CJ. Clinical practice: postmenopausal osteoporosis. *N Engl J Med*. 2005;353: 595-603.

Case 52

A 57-year-old man was admitted to the hospital 2 days ago following a motor vehicle accident. He suffered multiple contusions and a femur fracture that was surgically repaired 24 hours ago. He also had a laceration on his forehead but had a CT scan of his head on admission that showed no intracranial bleeding. His hospital course has been uncomplicated, and the only medications he currently is taking are morphine as needed for pain and subcutaneous enoxaparin for prophylaxis of deep venous thrombosis. This evening he has been agitated and combative, having pulled out his intravenous (IV) line. He is cursing at the nurses and is trying to get out of bed to leave the hospital. When you see him, he is febrile with a temperature of 100.8°F, heart rate 122 bpm, blood pressure 168/110 mm Hg, respiratory rate 28 breaths per minute, and oxygen saturations 98% on room air. He is awake and fidgety, staring around the room nervously. He is disoriented to place and time; he seems to be having auditory hallucinations and is brushing off unseen objects from his arms. On examination, his forehead wound is bandaged, his pupils are dilated but reactive, and he is mildly diaphoretic. Auscultation of the chest reveals few inspiratory crackles in the left base, his heart rhythm is tachycardic but regular, his abdomen is benign, and he is tremulous. You are able to contact family members by phone. They confirm that prior to his car accident, the patient had no medical problems, had no dementia or psychiatric illness, and was employed as an attorney. They report that he took no medications at home, did not smoke or use illicit drugs, and drank three to four mixed drinks every day after work.

➤ What is your most likely diagnosis?

➤ What should be your next step?

ANSWERS TO CASE 52:
Delirium/Alcohol Withdrawal

Summary: A 57-year-old man has been hospitalized for 2 days for multiple contusions and surgery performed 24 hours ago for a femur fracture sustained in a motor vehicle accident. Computed tomographic (CT) scan of his head is normal. His only medications are morphine and subcutaneous enoxaparin. This evening he is agitated and combative, and he is trying to leave the hospital. His temperature is 100.8°F, heart rate 122 bpm, blood pressure 168/110 mm Hg, respiratory rate 28 breaths per minute, and oxygen saturations 98% on room air. He is awake, fidgety, and disoriented, and he seems to be having auditory and tactile hallucinations. His pupils are dilated, and he is mildly diaphoretic and tremulous. Family members confirm that the patient had no medical problems and no dementia or psychiatric illness. He took no medications, did not smoke or use illicit drugs, and drank three to four mixed drinks every day after work.

➤ **Most likely diagnosis:** Delirium as a result of an acute medical illness or possibly alcohol withdrawal.

➤ **Next step:** Look for serious or reversible underlying medical causes for the delirium. If no other medical problems are identified, based on the patient's daily alcohol use, a possible diagnosis is alcohol withdrawal syndrome.

ANALYSIS

Objectives

1. Be able to recognize delirium in a hospitalized patient.
2. Know the most common causes of delirium.
3. Understand the management of an agitated, delirious patient.
4. Know the special considerations applicable to an elderly demented patient with delirium.
5. Learn the stages, treatment, and complications of alcohol withdrawal syndrome.

Considerations

This 57-year-old man had been in a normal physical and mental state prior to hospitalization. He then developed an acute change in mental status, with fluctuating consciousness and orientation, the hallmark of delirium. There are many possible causes for his delirium: pulmonary embolism, acute electrolyte disturbances, occult infection, central nervous system (CNS) hemorrhage or infection, or drug intoxication or withdrawal. These conditions require investigation before ascribing the symptoms to alcohol withdrawal because they are potentially very serious or even fatal. In addition, further investigation to quantify his alcohol intake is necessary. Although the patient in the clinical scenario has all the features of alcohol withdrawal—agitation, hyperalert, confusion, possible hallucinations, and the gamut of signs of adrenergic stimulation (dilated pupils, fever, tachycardia, tachypnea, hypertension, tremor, peripheral vasodilation)—so many possibilities exist that approaching his care with awareness of the many etiologies of delirium is mandatory.

APPROACH TO
Delirium

DEFINITIONS

DELIRIUM: An acute confusional state that is one of the most common mental disorders encountered in hospitalized or otherwise medically ill patients.

DEMENTIA: Significant loss of intellectual abilities such as memory capacity, severe enough to interfere with social or occupational functioning, usually over a long period of time.

CLINICAL APPROACH

The *Diagnostic and Statistical Manual of Mental Disorders, Fourth Edition (DSM-IV)* defines delirium as having the following features:

- Disturbance of consciousness with impairment of attention
- Change in cognition or the development of perceptual disturbances, for example, hallucinations
- Symptoms developing over a short period
- Evidence that the above features are caused by a medical condition, medications, or intoxicants

One of the earliest signs of a disturbance of consciousness is an inability to focus or sustain attention, which may be evident as distractibility in conversation. Usually there also is disturbance of the sleep–wake cycle. As symptoms progress, patients may become lethargic or even stuporous (arousable only to painful stimuli). In alcohol withdrawal, signs of autonomic hyperactivity predominate, and patients may go to the opposite extreme, becoming hypervigilant and agitated.

Regarding changes in cognition or perception, patients may have difficulty with memory, orientation, or speech. It is important to ascertain from family members whether these impairments were chronic, as in dementia, or developed acutely. Delirious patients may have hallucinations or vague delusions of harm, but hallucinations are not a mandatory feature of the condition. Delirium is an acute process, with **symptoms developing over a period of hours to days**. Additionally, the patient's mental status fluctuates, with symptoms often becoming most severe in the evening and at night. Not uncommonly, hospitalized patients appear relatively lucid on morning rounds, especially if mental status is only superficially assessed, but then the night staff reports severe confusion and agitation.

Finally, delirium is a manifestation of an underlying medical disorder. Sometimes, the underlying condition is apparent. At other times, especially in elderly demented patients, delirium may be the first or the only sign of an acute illness, or it may be a serious decompensation or complication of a stable medical condition. Table 52–1 lists conditions that should be considered as causes of delirium. Of these conditions, the most common are drug toxicity (especially anticholinergics, sedatives, or narcotics in elderly patients), infection, electrolyte disturbances (most commonly hyponatremia or hypoglycemia), and withdrawal from alcohol or other sedatives.

Regardless of etiology, delirium produces a profound disturbance of brain function, and all etiologies are serious and potentially fatal illnesses. **Delirium must be approached as an acute medical emergency.** A detailed history, aggressively pursued, is mandatory, and because the responses from these patients cannot be relied upon, information from family, friends, or other caregivers is essential. A thorough physical examination with emphasis on neurologic status, clarity of speech, level of awareness, attention span, facial droop, and weakness

Table 52–1 MEDICAL CAUSES OF DELIRIUM

Discrete CNS lesion present

Head injury; stroke or intracranial bleed
Infection: meningitis, meningoencephalitis, brain abscess
Mass lesion: hematoma, tumor
Seizure, postictal

No discrete CNS lesion

Metabolic encephalopathy
- Anoxia: any cause, heart or respiratory failure, pulmonary embolus, sleep apnea, etc
- Hepatic encephalopathy
- Uremic encephalopathy
- Hypo-, hyperglycemia
- Hyponatremia/hypercalcemia
- Hypo-, hyperthermia
Toxic encephalopathy
- Drug withdrawal, especially alcohol and benzodiazepines, and also meperidine (Demerol) and many others
- Drug toxicity, eg, dilantin
- Substance abuse
- Infections, especially pneumonia, urinary tract infections, intra-abdominal infection, bacteremia; all more frequent in the elderly

of an extremity must be established because such changes must be carefully and frequently assessed. Basic laboratory studies should focus on chemical abnormalities (glucose, creatinine, bilirubin, serum sodium levels) and evidence of hypoxia. The two threatening and potentially easily reversible conditions—hypoxia and hypoglycemia—should be immediately investigated and treated.

Delirium develops more commonly in those with an underdeveloped brain (eg, the febrile delirium of young children) and in those with involuting or diseased brains (many of the elderly). Delirium in the geriatric population can be the presenting manifestation of any acute illness, with an incidence of up to 10% on admission and up to 30% during an acute hospitalization. Causes of delirium in the elderly include pneumonia, urinary tract infection, myocardial infarction, gastrointestinal hemorrhage, traumatic injury, or virtually anything else that precipitates an acute hospitalization. This is even more of a problem after major surgery; nearly half of individuals (usually elderly) who suffer hip fractures develop delirium postoperatively.

Persons at any stage of dementia may develop delirium with any superimposed acute illness or injury or with additional pharmaceutical agent(s). Dementia is a chronic illness with no impairment of awareness in its earlier stages, whereas delirium is an acute event with alteration of consciousness. Additionally, an acute delirium may "unmask" an early underlying, undetected dementia. The confused and disoriented geriatric patient cannot be dismissed as having one or the other, and the history on which this differential diagnosis is dependent should concentrate on any changes in the behavioral status of the patient since the acute event.

The management of delirium is first and foremost the identification and treatment of the acute underlying illness. Adequate hydration, oxygenation, good nursing care, and round the clock careful supervision are always the initial measures. Management of agitation and disruptive behavior is the most challenging aspect of care of the delirious patient. If no specific treatable problem is identified, physical restraint should be used as a last resort. Frequent reassurance and orientation from familiar persons or constant supervision from a nurse or hospital aide are preferable. **Agitation with psychotic symptoms (hallucinations and delusions) can be treated with a neuroleptic such as low-dose haloperidol.** Older patients are more likely to experience extrapyramidal side effects; however, so newer atypical antipsychotics such as **risperidone** may be used. Benzodiazepines have a rapid onset of action but may worsen confusion and sedation.

Alcohol Withdrawal

Alcohol withdrawal manifests as a spectrum of symptoms, ranging from minor tremulousness and insomnia to the most severe form, **delirium tremens (DT)**, characterized by delirium, tremor, and autonomic hyperactivitiy. The severity of withdrawal can be assessed using a validated assessment tool, the Clinical Institute Withdrawal Assessment (CIWA) scale. Risk factors for the development of **delirium tremens** include a history of sustained drinking, prior withdrawal symptoms, age older than 30 years, and a concurrent medical illness. Withdrawal can coexist with or mimic other conditions, such as infection, intracranial bleeding, hepatic failure, gastrointestinal bleeding, or other drug overdose. DT is a diagnosis of exclusion; other serious diagnoses must be excluded before the patient's mental status and autonomic signs are attributed to withdrawal. There should be a search for infection (blood cultures), pneumonia (chest radiograph), and hypoxia (blood gases or oximetry), and, although it is early in the patient's course, the possibility of pulmonary embolus must be kept in mind. It is important to understand the temporal course of the spectrum of alcohol withdrawal syndromes (Table 52–2).

Table 52–2 ALCOHOL WITHDRAWAL SYMPTOMS

STAGE	SYMPTOMS
Tremulousness	Earliest symptom occurring within 6 hours of abstinence, caused by CNS and sympathetic hyperactivity, often referred to as the "shakes" or "jitters," and can occur even when patients still have a significant blood alcohol level. In addition to the typical 6- to 8-Hz tremor, which can be violent or subtle, insomnia, anxiety, gastrointestinal upset, diaphoresis, and palpitations can occur. Tremor typically diminishes over 48-72 h, but anxiety, easy startling, and other symptoms can persist for 2 weeks.
Withdrawal seizures	Also called "rum fits" and typically generalized tonic–clonic seizures, often occurring in clusters of two to six episodes, and almost always within 6-48 h of abstinence. Typically seen in patients with a long history of chronic alcoholism.
Alcoholic hallucinosis	Typically develops within 12 h of abstinence and resolves within 48 h. Hallucinations are most often visual (eg, bugs, pink elephants) but can be auditory or tactile. When auditory, they are often maligning or reproachful human voices. Despite the hallucinations, patients maintain a relatively intact sensorium.
Delirium tremens (DT)	Most dramatic and serious form of alcohol withdrawal, but occurs in only 5% of patients with withdrawal symptoms. DT typically begins within 48-72 h after the last drink and can last several days, often with a resolution as abrupt as its onset. Characterized by hallucinations, agitation, tremor, and sleeplessness, as well as signs of sympathetic hyperactivity: dilated pupils, low-grade fever, tachycardia, hypertension, diaphoresis, and hyperventilation. Delirium tremens is a serious condition with an in-hospital mortality of 5%-10%, usually from arrhythmias or infection, which is often unsuspected.

In contrast to other causes of delirium, **benzodiazepines are the drugs of choice in alcohol withdrawal**. They can be given on a fixed schedule in high-risk patients (previous history of DT or withdrawal seizures) to prevent withdrawal symptoms. If symptoms have already developed, benzodiazepines can be given according to one of two strategies. Long-acting benzodiazepines such as diazepam can be given in high doses until withdrawal symptoms cease and then the slow clearance of the drug allowed to prevent further withdrawal symptoms. Alternatively, shorter acting agents such as lorazepam can be given as needed only when the patient has symptoms. Both strategies are effective. In either case, the key to successful management is initially aggressive upward titration of dosage until the patient is heavily sedated but responsive, followed by rapid downward titration as agitation decreases, usually over 48 to 72 hours. Supportive measures are also important, such as adequate hydration, replacement of electrolytes, and supplementation with thiamine and other B vitamins in malnourished, chronic alcoholics to prevent the development of Wernicke encephalopathy.

Comprehension Questions

52.1 Which of the following agents most closely resembles the action of alcohol in the brain?
A. Amphetamines
B. Marijuana
C. Cocaine
D. Benzodiazepine
E. Acetaminophen

52.2 Compared with dementia, which of the following is a characteristic of delirium?
A. A fluctuating level of consciousness
B. Slow onset
C. Can be due to deficiencies of thiamine or cyanocobalamin
D. Decreased memory ability

52.3 A 34-year-old man is brought to the emergency room for extreme tremors and auditory hallucinations. Which of the following statements is most likely to be correct?
A. Auditory hallucinations are unique to alcohol withdrawal and cannot be caused by a brain tumor.
B. If the serum blood alcohol level is higher than the legal limits of intoxication, these symptoms cannot be alcohol withdrawal.
C. This patient should receive glucose intravenously for possible hypoglycemia.
D. If the patient also has hypertension, fever, and tachycardia, he has a 5% to 15% chance of mortality.

ANSWERS

52.1   **D.** Alcohol and benzodiazepines both interact with the γ-aminobutyric acid (GABA) system; thus, benzodiazepines are the drugs of choice for treatment of acute alcohol withdrawal.

52.2   **A.** Fluctuating levels of alertness and consciousness are typical of delirium.

52.3   **D.** DT with autonomic instability and sympathetic overactivity is associated with a 5% to 15% mortality. Auditory hallucinations can occur from a number of illicit agents or even brain tumors. The fall in serum blood alcohol level and not the absolute level may induce symptoms of withdrawal. An individual who abuses alcohol should first be given thiamine, before glucose is administered, to prevent acute Wernicke encephalopathy.

Clinical Pearls

➤ Delirium is characterized by acute onset of impaired attention and cognition, and fluctuating levels of consciousness, often with psychomotor and autonomic hyperactivity.

➤ Delirium requires urgent investigation to search for serious underlying systemic or metabolic causes.

➤ Frequent reassurance and orientation, and constant observation are useful in managing the agitated delirious patient. Low-dose haloperidol can be used to control agitation or psychotic symptoms. Physical restraint is used as a last resort.

➤ Delirium tremens is the most severe and dramatic form of alcohol withdrawal, with abrupt onset from 2 to 4 days after cessation of drinking and sudden resolution several days later, and is associated with a mortality rate of 5%.

➤ Therapy for alcohol withdrawal syndromes includes benzodiazepines, hydration, electrolyte replacement, and B vitamins to prevent Wernicke encephalopathy.

REFERENCES

Inouye SK. Delirium in older persons. *N Engl J Med.* 2006;354:1157-1165.

Josephson SA, Miller BL. Confusion and delirium. In: Fauci AS, Braunwald E, Kasper DL, eds. *Harrison's Principles of Internal Medicine.* 17th ed. New York, NY: McGraw-Hill; 2008:158-162.

Kosten TR, O'Connor PG. Management of drug and alcohol withdrawal. *N Engl J Med.* 2003;348:1786-1795.

Shuckit MA. Alcohol and alcoholism. In: Kasper DL, Braunwald E, Fauci AS, et al, eds. *Harrison's Principles of Internal Medicine.* 17th ed. New York, NY: McGraw-Hill; 2008:2274-2729.

Case 53

A 66-year-old woman comes in for a routine physical examination. She volunteers that her menopause occurred at age 51 years, and that she is currently taking an estrogen pill along with a progestin pill each day. The medical history is unremarkable. Her family history includes one maternal cousin with ovarian cancer. On examination, she is found to have blood pressure 120/70 mm Hg, heart rate 70 bpm, and temperature 98°F. Her weight is 140 lb and her height is 5 ft 4 in. The thyroid is normal to palpation. Breast examination reveals no masses or discharge. Abdominal, cardiac, and lung evaluations are within normal limits. Pelvic examination shows a normal multiparous cervix, a normal-size uterus, and no adnexal masses. She had undergone a mammogram 3 months previously. The patient states that she has regular Papanicolaou (Pap) smears, and that the last one performed 1 year ago was normal.

➤ What is your next step?

➤ What would be the most common cause of mortality for this patient?

ANSWERS TO CASE 53:
Health Maintenance

Summary: A 66-year-old woman presents for health maintenance. A mammogram had been performed 3 months previously.

➤ **Next step:** Each of the following should be performed: stool for occult blood, colonoscopy or barium enema, pneumococcal vaccine, influenza vaccine, tetanus vaccine (if not within 10 years), cholesterol screening, fasting blood glucose, and urinalysis.

➤ **Most common cause of mortality:** Cardiovascular disease.

ANALYSIS

Objectives

1. Understand which health maintenance studies should be performed for a 66-year-old patient.
2. Know the most common cause of mortality in a woman in this age group.
3. Understand that preventive maintenance consists of immunizations, cancer screening, and screening for common diseases.

Considerations

The approach to health maintenance consists of three parts: (a) cancer screening, (b) immunizations, and (c) addressing common diseases for the particular patient group. For a 66-year-old woman, this includes annual mammography for breast cancer screening, colon cancer (annual stool for occult blood and either periodic colonoscopy or barium enema), tetanus booster every 10 years, pneumococcal vaccine, and yearly influenza immunization. Screening for hypercholesterolemia every 5 years up to age 75 years and fasting blood glucose levels every 3 years also are recommended. Finally, the most common cause of mortality is cardiovascular disease. Cervical cancer screening can be stopped at age 65 or 70 years if all previous Pap smears have been normal.

APPROACH TO
Health Maintenance

DEFINITIONS

COST-EFFECTIVENESS: Comparison of resources expended (dollars) in an intervention versus the benefit, which may be measured in life-years or quality-adjusted life-years.

PRIMARY PREVENTION: Identifying and modifying risk factors in subjects who have never had the disease of concern.

SCREENING TEST: Device used to identify asymptomatic disease in the hope that early detection will lead to an improved outcome. An optimal screening test has high sensitivity and specificity, is inexpensive, and is easy to perform.

SECONDARY PREVENTION: Actions taken to reduce the morbidity or mortality once a disease has been diagnosed.

CLINICAL APPROACH

When the patient does not have an apparent disease or complaint, the goal of medical intervention is prevention of disease. One method of targeting diseases is according to the patient's age. For example, the most common cause of death in a 16-year-old is motor vehicle accidents; hence, the teenage patient is well served by the physician encouraging her to wear seat belts and to avoid alcohol intoxication when driving. In contrast, a 56-year-old woman is most likely to die of cardiovascular disease, so the physician might focus on exercise and weight loss, and screen for hyperlipidemia.

Additionally, physicians should seek to identify high-risk behaviors in a nonjudgmental fashion, and promote lifestyle modification: Patients should be screened for tobacco, alcohol, and illicit drug use. They should be advised to quit smoking and limit alcohol consumption to one drink per day for women and two drinks per day for men. Adjuvant pharmacological agents are more successful in tobacco cessation than quitting abruptly. Patients with a history of intravenous (IV) drug use should be offered testing for human immunodeficiency virus (HIV) and hepatitis C. Screening for sexually transmitted diseases (STDs) should be offered to patients based on their risk factors. Annual screening for gonorrhea and chlamydia is recommended for all sexually active women 25 years and younger. Overweight (BMI >25) and obese (BMI >30) patients should be advised to lose weight through diet modification and exercise. Obesity can lead to numerous complications including diabetes, hypertension, heart disease, menstrual irregularities, osteoarthritis, sleep apnea and respiratory difficulties, and hyperlipidemia.

In each age group, particular screening tests are recommended (Table 53–1).

Table 53–1 SCREENING BASED ON AGE

	13-18 YEARS	19-39 YEARS	40-64 YEARS	65+ YEARS
Cancer screening	Pap smear 3 y after initiation of intercourse	Annual Pap smear	Annual Pap smear Age 50: stool for occult blood, barium enema + flexible sigmoidoscopy every 5 y or colonoscopy every 10 y, Age 40: annual clinical breast exam and mammography	Annual stool for occult blood; barium enema + flexible sigmoidoscopy every 5 y, or colonoscopy every 10 y; annual clinical breast exam and mammography
Immunizations	Tetanus booster once between ages 11 and 16 y HPV vaccine up to age 26	Tetanus every 10 y	Tetanus every 10 y Age 50: annual influenza vaccine	Tetanus every 10 y; pneumococcal vaccine; annual influenza vaccine
Other diseases	Depression; firearms	Cardiovascular diseases; cholesterol screening every 5 y beginning at age 20 y	Cholesterol screening every 5 y	Osteoporosis
Most common causes of mortality	1. Motor vehicle accidents 2. Homicide 3. Suicide	1. Motor vehicle accidents 2. Cardiovascular disease 3. AIDS	1. Cardiovascular disease 2. Cancer	1. Heart disease 2. Cancer 3. Cerebrovascular disease

Data from: The US Preventive Services Task Force Guide to Clinical Preventive Services 2007, American Cancer Society Screening Guidelines, 2008.

Comprehension Questions

53.1   A 59-year-old woman is being seen for a health maintenance appoint-
        ment. She has not seen a doctor for over 10 years. She had undergone
        a total hysterectomy for uterine fibroids 12 years ago. The patient
        takes supplemental calcium. The physician orders a fasting glucose
        level, lipid panel, mammogram, colonoscopy, and a pap smear of the
        vaginal cuff. Which of the following statements is most accurate
        regarding the screening for this patient?
        A. The Pap smear of the vaginal cuff is unnecessary.
        B. In general, colon cancer screening should be initiated at age 60 but
           this patient has very sporadic care, therefore colonoscopy is
           reasonable.
        C. Because the patient takes supplemental calcium, a DEXA scan is
           not needed.
        D. Pneumococcal vaccination should be recommended.

53.2   A 63-year-old male has had annual health maintenance appointments
        and has followed all the recommendations offered by his physician.
        The physician counsels him about varicella zoster vaccine. Which of
        the following is the most accurate statement about this vaccine?
        A. This vaccine is recommended for patients who are aged 65 and
           older.
        B. This vaccine is not recommended if a patient has already devel-
           oped the shingles
        C. This vaccine is a live attenuated immunization.
        D. This vaccine has some cross-reactivity with herpes simplex virus
           and offers some protection against HSV.

53.3   An 18-year-old female is being seen for a health maintenance appoint-
        ment. She has not had a pap smear previously. She currently takes oral
        contraceptive pills. She began sexual intercourse 1 year previously.
        Which of the following statements is most accurate regarding health
        maintenance for this individual?
        A. A pap smear should not be performed in this patient at this time.
        B. The HPV vaccine should be administered only if she has a history
           of genital warts.
        C. The most common cause of mortality for this patient would be
           suicide.
        D. Hepatitis C vaccination should be offered to this patient.

ANSWERS

53.1   **A.** Cervical cytology of the vaginal cuff is unnecessary when the hysterectomy was for benign indications (not cervical dysplasia or cervical cancer), and when there is no history of abnormal pap smears. Colon cancer screening is generally started at age 50. DEXA scan for osteoporosis screening should be considered in any postmenopausal woman at risk, such as having an osteoporosis-related fracture, a family history, or being thin and Caucasian. Pneumococcal vaccine is generally given at age 65.

53.2   **C.** The varicella zoster vaccine is a live attenuated vaccine, recommended for individuals aged 60 and above, and has been shown to greatly reduce the incidence of herpes zoster (shingles), and the severity and likelihood of post-herpetic neuralgia. It has no efficacy in preventing HSV.

53.3   **A.** Cervical cytology should be deferred until age 21 or 3 years after iniatiation of sexual intercourse. This is due to the fact that adolescents many times will clear the HPV infection, and cause an abnormal pap smear to normalized. The HPV vaccine should be recommended to all females between the age of 9 and 26, regardless of exposures. The most common cause of mortality for adolescent females is motor vehicle accidents. The hepatitis C vaccine is currently not available, but hopefully in several years, it may be developed.

Clinical Pearls

➤ The basic approach to health maintenance is age-appropriate immunizations, cancer screening, and screening for common diseases.

➤ The most common cause of mortality in a woman younger than 20 years is motor vehicle accidents.

➤ The most common cause of mortality in men or women age 40 years or older is cardiovascular disease.

➤ Major conditions in women 65 years and older include osteoporosis, heart disease, breast cancer, and depression.

➤ Obesity is a major concern and has numerous complications including diabetes, hyperlipidemia, heart disease, sleep apnea, and respiratory difficulties.

➤ Tobacco use should be queried at each visit and patients should be counseled actively about cessation; pharmacological therapy is associated with a higher success rate.

REFERENCES

American College of Obstetricians and Gynecologists. Osteoporosis. ACOG Practice Bulletin 50. Washington, DC: American College of Obstetricians and Gynecologists, 2004.

American College of Obstetricians and Gynecologists. Primary and preventive care: Periodic assessments. ACOG Committee Opinion 292. Washington, DC: American College of Obstetricians and Gynecologists, 2003.

Martin GJ. Screening and prevention of disease. In: Fauci AS, Braunwald E, Kasper DL. *Harrison's Principles of Internal Medicine*, 17th ed. New York, NY: McGraw-Hill; 2008: 24-27.

U.S. Preventive Services Task Force, 2005. Guide to Clinical Prevention Services, 3rd ed. *http://www.ahrq.gov/clinic/uspstfix.htm*. Accessed 7-1-2008.

Case 54

You are the intern on call in the hospital, when the emergency room resident calls up a new admission. She describes an 84-year-old Alzheimer patient who was brought to the emergency room by ambulance from her long-term care facility for increased confusion, combativeness, and fever. Her medical history is significant for Alzheimer disease and well-controlled hypertension; otherwise she has been very healthy. The resident states that the patient is "confused" and combative with staff, which, per her family, is not her baseline mental status. Her temperature is 100.5°F, heart rate 130 bpm, blood pressure 76/32 mm Hg, respiratory rate 24 breaths per minute, and oxygen saturations 95% on room air. On examination, she is lethargic but agitated when disturbed, her neck veins are flat, her lung fields are clear, and her heart rhythm is tachycardic but regular with no murmur or gallops. Abdominal examination is unremarkable and her extremities are warm and pink.

After administration of 2 L of normal saline over 30 minutes, her blood pressure is now 95/58 mm Hg, and the initial laboratory work returns. Her white blood cell count (WBC) is 14,000/mm³, with 67% neutrophils, 3% bands, and 24% lymphocytes. No other abnormalities are noted. Chest X-rays obtained in the emergency room are normal. Urinalysis shows 2+ leukocyte esterase, negative nitrite, and trace blood. Microscopy shows 20 to 50 white blood cells per high-power field, 0 to 3 red blood cells (RBCs), and many bacteria.

➤ What is your diagnosis?

➤ What is your next step?

ANSWERS TO CASE 54:

Urosepsis in the Elderly

Summary: An 84-year-old woman, a nursing home resident with Alzheimer disease, is brought to the emergency room for agitation and confusion. She is found to be febrile, tachycardic, and hypotensive. Examination shows flat neck veins, clear lung fields, and no cardiac murmur or gallops; her extremities are warm and well perfused. Her hemodynamic status has improved with a fluid bolus. Laboratory examination shows evidence of a urinary tract infection (UTI).

➤ **Most likely diagnosis:** Shock, most likely as a consequence of urosepsis.

➤ **Next step:** Continued administration of blood pressure support with intravenous (IV) fluids or vasopressors as necessary. Broad-spectrum antibiotics should be started as soon as possible.

ANALYSIS

Objectives

1. Know how to diagnose a UTI.
2. Know effective treatments for UTI.
3. Recognize and know how to manage asymptomatic bacteriuria.
4. Know how to recognize and treat septic shock.

Considerations

In this patient presenting with shock, that is, hypotension leading to inadequate tissue perfusion, it is essential to try to determine the underlying cause and, thus, appropriate treatment. She has no history of hemorrhage or extreme volume losses, so hypovolemic shock is unlikely. She has flat neck veins and clear lung fields, suggesting she does not have right- or left-heart failure, respectively, so cardiogenic shock (eg, after a myocardial infarction) seems unlikely. Additionally, both hypovolemic and cardiogenic shock typically cause profound peripheral vasoconstriction, resulting in cold clammy extremities. This patient's extremities are warm and well perfused (inappropriately so) despite serious hypotension, suggesting a distributive form of shock. With the elevated white blood cell count with immature forms as well as the urine findings, septic shock as a consequence of UTI seems most likely.

APPROACH TO
Suspected Urosepsis

DEFINITIONS

ASYMPTOMATIC BACTERIURIA: Condition in which urine Gram stain or culture is positive, but no clinical signs or symptoms of infection are present.

LEUKOCYTE ESTERASE: Neutrophils within the urine release this enzyme, which can be detected by urinalysis.

NITRITE: Nitrites are converted from nitrates by some bacteria, particularly gram-negative organisms, and can be detected by urinalysis.

CLINICAL APPROACH

UTIs are a common affliction of the elderly, affecting both debilitated and healthy adults. UTIs are second only to respiratory infections as the most common infections in patients older than 65 years. Risk factors that contribute to the high incidence of UTIs in the elderly as well as in institutionalized patients include incontinence, a history of prior UTIs, neurologic impairment, polypharmacy (namely anticholinergics), immunosuppression, poor nutrition, and comorbid disease states. These conditions may confer functional abnormalities within the urinary tract or altered defenses against infection. Furthermore, frequent hospitalizations expose these patients to nosocomial pathogens and invasive instrumentation such as indwelling catheters.

UTIs typically are diagnosed based on a combination of symptoms and urinary findings. In symptomatic patients, bacteria typically are found in high concentrations in the urine, and **10^5 colony-forming units (CFU)/mL typically are recovered from a clean-catch** specimen. If the specimen is obtained by **catheterization, finding** more than 10^2 **CFU/mL** is considered significant. In **women with symptoms of acute cystitis**, urine cultures are often not obtained, but empiric treatment can be initiated based on the **dipstick findings of leukocyte esterase** (used as a marker for pyuria) **or nitrites** (used as a marker for bacteriuria).

Most UTIs can be described as one of three clinical syndromes: **acute uncomplicated cystitis** (lower tract infection), **acute uncomplicated pyelonephritis** (upper tract infection), or **complicated UTI** (associated with urinary catheterization or instrumentation, or anatomic or functional abnormalities). Symptoms of cystitis reflect bladder irritation and generally include dysuria, frequency, urgency, or hematuria. **Pyelonephritis** typically presents with **systemic symptoms such as fever, chills, or nausea**, with or without symptoms of cystitis. Another clinical finding that deserves mention is **asymptomatic bacteriuria**. Asymptomatic bacteriuria is characterized by positive urine cultures without clinical symptoms. Outside of pregnancy or immunocompromised patients such as transplant recipients, no adverse outcomes have been reported as a result of asymptomatic bacteriuria, and no benefits of treatment have been demonstrated. Up to 50% of women and 30% of men older than 65 years are reported to have asymptomatic bacteriuria. Although in younger patients fever, dysuria, urgency, or flank pain may be presenting symptoms for a UTI, elderly and institutionalized patients often present with less obvious symptoms. These patients may be febrile or hypothermic. Common manifestations include confusion or combativeness. **Mental status or behavioral changes in the elderly** should be considered **strong indicators for serious illness**, and a thorough workup should consider etiologies beyond infections. Even with localizing symptoms suggestive of a UTI, other sources of infection should still be investigated. Both urine and blood cultures should be sent in addition to a urinalysis and complete blood count. The results of the urine and blood cultures may take 2 to 3 days to yield an organism. If the clinical picture suggests a UTI, antibiotic treatment should not await these results and should be initiated immediately.

Antimicrobial therapy should not be directed solely at gram-negative organisms as in younger patients. The elderly and institutionalized patients commonly acquire gram-positive and mixed infections, so broad-spectrum antibiotics pending culture results are recommended. For uncomplicated UTIs, fluoroquinolones such as ciprofloxacin and gatifloxacin are considered first-line therapy. Treatment can range from 3 days in uncomplicated cystitis to 10 days in pyelonephritis. In patients presenting with a clinical picture of sepsis, broad-spectrum antibiotic coverage against enterococci and *Pseudomonas* is recommended until cultures are available to guide therapy. Suggested regimens include ampicillin with gentamicin, imipenem, or piperacillin with tazobactam. The duration of therapy should be dictated by the patient's clinical status. In cases where UTIs have progressed to bacteremia, aggressive and prompt treatment is necessary to prevent the onset of septic shock. This life-threatening state may develop with little warning in elderly and institutionalized patients with multiple comorbidities, as it did in the patient in the scenario, who presents with hypotension and altered mental status because of infection, that is, in septic shock.

Shock is the clinical syndrome that results from inadequate tissue perfusion. It can be classified in a variety of ways, but one useful schema divides the causes into hypovolemic shock, cardiogenic shock, or distributive shock, usually caused by sepsis. **Hypovolemic shock** is the most common form. It results from either hemorrhage or profound vomiting or diarrhea, resulting in loss of 20% to 40% of blood volume. **Cardiogenic shock** results from a primary cardiac insult, such as a myocardial infarction, arrhythmias, or end-stage heart failure such that the heart no longer pumps effectively. Both hypovolemic and cardiogenic shocks cause a marked fall in cardiac output and may appear clinically similar with tachycardia, hypotension, and with cold clammy extremities. It is essential to differentiate between the two, however, because the treatments are markedly different. Patients with **hypovolemic shock** should have **flat neck veins** and **clear lung fields**; those with **cardiogenic shock** are more likely to have markedly **elevated jugular venous pressure** and **pulmonary edema.** Treatment of hypovolemic shock is aggressive volume resuscitation, either with crystalloid solution or with blood products as necessary. Treatment of cardiogenic shock focuses on maintaining blood pressure with dopamine or norepinephrine infusions, relief of pulmonary edema with diuretics, and reducing cardiac afterload, for example, with an intraaortic balloon pump.

Distributive shock, in contrast, is characterized by an **increase in cardiac output** but an inability to maintain systemic vascular resistance, that is, there is **inappropriate vasodilation.** Clinically, it appears different than the other forms of shock in that, despite the hypotension, the **extremities are warm and well perfused,** at least initially. If septic shock continues, cardiac output falls as a consequence of myocardial depression, multiorgan dysfunction ensues, and **intense vasoconstriction** occurs in an attempt to maintain blood pressure, the so-called **"cold phase."** These findings portend a poor prognosis; hence, prompt recognition of septic shock in the early (warm) phase is paramount.

Although distributive shock may occur in neurogenic shock as a consequence of spinal cord injury or adrenal crisis, the most common cause is **septic shock,** most commonly from **gram-negative sepsis.** Gram-negative organisms may release **endotoxins,** which cause a decrease in systemic vascular resistance and cardiac contractility. The primary treatment is isotonic fluid replacement to maintain blood pressure. Other cornerstones of therapy include broad-spectrum antibiotics to attack the underlying infection and removal of the infection source. Patients often require vasopressor support (dopamine is the most commonly used agent) and mechanical ventilation to optimize tissue oxygenation. All types of shock are associated with high mortality rates exceeding 50%. Early diagnosis and prompt treatment are imperative because untreated shock progresses to an irreversible point that is refractory to volume expansion and other medical therapies.

Comprehension Questions

54.1   Which of the following asymptomatic patients would most benefit from treatment of the finding of more than 10^5 CFU/mL of *Escherichia coli* on urine culture?

   A. A 23-year-old asymptomatic sexually active woman
   B. A 33-year-old asymptomatic pregnant woman
   C. A 53-year-old asymptomatic diabetic woman
   D. A 73-year-old asymptomatic woman in a nursing home

54.2   Which of the following is the best treatment for a 39-year-old woman
        with fever 103°F, nausea, flank pain, and more than 10^5 CFU/mL of
        E coli in a urine culture?
        A. Oral trimethoprim-sulfamethoxazole for 3 days
        B. Single-dose ciprofloxacin
        C. Intravenous and then oral gatifloxacin for 14 days
        D. Oral ampicillin for 21 to 28 days

54.3   A 57-year-old man is noted to have a blood pressure 68/50 mm Hg,
        heart rate 140 bpm, elevated jugular venous pressure, inspiratory
        crackles on examination, and cold clammy extremities. Which of the
        following is the most likely etiology?
        A. Septic shock
        B. Adrenal crisis
        C. Cardiogenic shock
        D. Hypovolemic shock

54.4   A 45-year-old man is noted to have a blood pressure of 80/40 mm Hg,
        heart rate 142 bpm, and fever of 102°F. His abdomen is tender, particu-
        larly in the right lower quadrant, and acute appendicitis is diagnosed.
        Three liters of 0.9% saline is infused and intravenous antibiotics are
        administered as he is prepared for surgery. His blood pressure falls to
        70/42 mm Hg. Which of the following is the most appropriate next step?
        A. Administer a beta-blocker to control his heart rate.
        B. Check a cortisol level and administer corticosteroids.
        C. Infuse fresh-frozen plasma (FFP).
        D. Initiate dopamine intravenous infusion.
        E. IV Morphine for pain control.

ANSWERS

54.1   **B.** All of these patients are asymptomatic, and no benefit from treat-
        ment in terms of reduction in symptomatic UTIs or hospitalization
        has been shown for any of the other cases mentioned, except for
        pregnancy. Treatment is undertaken to prevent upper tract infection,
        preterm delivery, and possible fetal loss.

54.2   **C.** The patient in this scenario has symptoms of upper tract infec-
        tion, for example, pyelonephritis, and is moderately ill with nausea.
        She will need a 14-day course of treatment and may not be able to
        take oral antibiotics initially, so hospitalization and treatment with
        intravenous antibiotics likely will be necessary. Single-dose and 3-day
        regimens are useful only for acute uncomplicated cystitis in women.
        E coli are frequently resistant to ampicillin.

54.3 **C.** The patient is hypotensive with signs of left- and right-heart failure, that is, probably cardiogenic shock. Septic shock and adrenal crisis both are forms of distributive shock that would produce warm extremities. Hypovolemic shock should have flat neck veins and no pulmonary edema.

54.4 **D.** When septic shock is refractory to volume resuscitation, then vasopressors such as dopamine or norepinephrine are generally the next step. Corticosteroids can be administered empirically if hypotension is refractory to pressors. Intravenous morphine might lower his blood pressure further. FFP is used when the patient shows evidence of coagulopathy such as disseminated intravascular coagulation.

Clinical Pearls

➤ Urinary tract infections and pneumonia are the most common causes of sepsis in older patients.

➤ Urinary tract infections can be diagnosed by the presence of urinary symptoms and by more than 10^5 colony-forming units (CFU)/mL in a clean-catch specimen and more than 10^2 (CFU)/mL in a catheterized specimen.

➤ In healthy women with symptoms of acute uncomplicated cystitis, cultures are not routinely sent, and treatment can be initiated based on symptoms and on a urine dipstick finding of leukocyte esterase or nitrites.

➤ Asymptomatic bacteriuria is a common finding among elderly patients and requires no treatment; it is only routinely treated in pregnancy and in transplant recipients.

➤ With early septic shock, the patient has inappropriate vasodilation (feels warm) in the face of hypotension and tachycardia.

REFERENCES

Fihn SD. Acute uncomplicated urinary tract infection in women. *N Engl J Med.* 2003; 349:259-266.

Hotchkiss RS, Karl IE. The pathophysiology and treatment of sepsis. *N Engl J Med.* 2003;348:138-150.

Maier RV. Approach to the patient with shock. In: Fauci AS, Braunwald E, Kasper DL, eds. *Harrison's Principles of Internal Medicine,* 17th ed. New York, NY: McGraw-Hill; 2008:1689-1695.

Sessler CN, Perry JC, Varney KL. Management of severe sepsis and septic shock. *Curr Opin Crit Care.* 2004;10:354-363.

Shortliffe LMD, McCue JD. Urinary tract infection at the age extremes: pediatrics and geriatrics. *Am J Med.* 2002;113:55S-66S.

Case 55

A 28-year-old man is brought to the emergency room by Emergency Medical Services (EMS) after being found sitting at the side of the road, incoherent and disoriented. In the emergency room, he is uncooperative and combative. He is not oriented to self, place, or time. Security is called to help restrain him, and he is placed in five-point leather restraints for his own and the staff's protection. No specific complaints can be elicited from the patient; he continues to yell at the staff and seems to be having auditory and visual hallucinations. His temperature is 100.5°F, heart rate 120 bpm, and blood pressure 150/100 mm Hg. A Foley catheter is placed, and the urine is noted to be tea-colored. Urine dipstick reads 4+ for blood, but no red blood cells (RBCs) are seen on the microscopic examination. Urine drug screen is positive for cocaine and phencyclidine (PCP).

➤ What is your most likely diagnosis?

➤ What is your next step?

ANSWERS TO CASE 55:
Rhabdomyolysis, Cocaine-Induced

Summary: An uncooperative, disoriented, and combative 28-year-old man is brought to the emergency room and placed in five-point leather restraints. He seems to be having auditory and visual hallucinations. His temperature is 100.5°F, heart rate 120 bpm, and blood pressure 150/100 mm Hg. A Foley catheter is placed; the urine is noted to be tea-colored, with 4+ for blood, but no red blood cells on microscopy. Urine drug screen is positive for cocaine and PCP.

> **Most likely diagnosis:** Rhabdomyolysis secondary to cocaine and PCP (or angel dust) intoxication.

> **Next step:** Aggressive intravenous (IV) hydration with normal saline. To prevent further damage to muscle, chemical restraint of the patient, rather than physical restraint alone, may be advised.

Considerations

Rhabdomyolysis is muscle breakdown, which can occur due to severe exertion particularly in the face of dehydration, status epilepticus, or heat stroke. Malignant hyperthermia can also be associated with rhabdomyolysis. This 28 year old man has drug-induced hallucinations and severe muscular activity. Intravenous fluids are critical to prevent renal damage. Elevated CPK and SGOT enzymes would confirm the diagnosis.

ANALYSIS

Objectives

1. Know the clinically important toxic syndromes associated with cocaine and other drugs of abuse.
2. Learn the causes and natural history of untreated rhabdomyolysis.
3. Recognize the signs of myoglobinemia and myoglobinuria.
4. Learn the treatment of rhabdomyolysis.

APPROACH TO
Illicit Drug Effects

DEFINITIONS

OPIATE INTOXICATION: Physiological effect of miosis with depressed consciousness and respiratory rate due to substances related to heroin.

PHENCYCLIDINE (PCP): A piperidine derivative used chiefly in the form of its hydrochloride $C_{17}H_{25}N \cdot HCl$ especially as a veterinary anesthetic and sometimes illicitly as a psychedelic drug to induce vivid mental imagery, agitation, and convulsions.

CLINICAL APPROACH

Drug abuse is common and pervasive in our society. Contrary to popular belief, many highly educated and socioeconomically advantaged persons are involved in the illicit use of street drugs, legal drugs, or prescribed medications. The physician must have a high index of suspicion to be able to offer appropriate therapy and to prevent the disastrous consequences of such use. Alcohol and tobacco are the most commonly abused drugs; however, this discussion focuses on common "street" drugs that are known to have serious medical consequences with both acute and chronic use.

Heroin, or opiate, addiction, although less popular now than in the past, has seen something of a resurgence recently in some areas of the country. Acute intoxication causes hypotension, sedation or coma, nausea, and vomiting. The severity of the symptoms is dose-dependent. Long-term secondary effects include infections such as human immunodeficiency virus (HIV) or hepatitis through sharing of contaminated needles and infectious endocarditis. **Benzodiazepine** or **barbiturate** intoxication can cause a similar presentation of respiratory, cardiovascular, and central nervous system (CNS) depression. **PCP**, also called "angel dust," is a veterinary anesthetic that can be smoked or taken orally or intravenously. In a dose-dependent manner, people will develop agitation, excitability, acute psychosis, and convulsions when intoxicated with this drug.

Cocaine is a stimulant, vasoconstrictor, and local anesthetic derived from the leaves of the coca plant. The drug can be snorted, administered intravenously, or smoked. It blocks the reuptake of norepinephrine, serotonin, and dopamine at the receptor, which leads to elevated mood, heart rate, blood pressure, and temperature. Cocaine has a short half-life of approximately 1 hour, and its metabolites are detectable in the urine for approximately 3 to 5 days following use. Chronic use leads to tolerance of the effects, but high doses can be fatal. The resultant tachycardia, hypertension, and peripheral vasoconstriction may lead to ischemic stroke, subarachnoid hemorrhage, and hepatic or intestinal ischemia. Inhaling the cocaine or the chemicals used for purification can cause pneumonitis or adult respiratory distress syndrome. A common clinical problem is patients who present with **chest pain** after cocaine usage. Such patients may have undifferentiated chest pain, or they may have myocardial ischemia or infarction related to the tachycardia and vasoconstriction (mainly alpha-adrenergic mediated) of the drug. Of patients in whom myocardial infarction actually is precipitated, many have no cardiac risk factors other than smoking and they have normal coronary arteries. Patients with cocaine-associated chest pain generally undergo a period of observation and evaluation for ischemia. Most authorities recommend treatment with aspirin, benzodiazepines for anxiety, and nitrates for vasodilation. Beta-blockers are generally avoided because they may exacerbate the alpha-mediated vasoconstriction. Rhabdomyolysis, the breakdown of striated muscle, can also be caused by cocaine effect, through direct myotoxicity or vasoconstrictive ischemia. Other chemicals used to "cut" the cocaine may also be myotoxic. PCP can cause myoglobinemia because of muscle breakdown from the overexertion caused by the drug. Together, these effects may be additive and more toxic to the patient. Table 55–1 lists multiple other causes of rhabdomyolysis, ranging from injury to infection to genetic diseases.

Whatever the cause, the breakdown of muscle tissue leads to release of myoglobin into the blood, which then is bound up by the serum haptoglobin. This system, however, saturates at low levels of myoglobinemia. The **free myoglobin** is then filtered by the kidneys, where it can **precipitate in the tubules and cause obstruction and acute renal failure**. The damaged muscle itself can also sequester liters of fluid, leading to intravascular depletion and hypovolemia, poor renal perfusion, and further renal damage. Finally, the free iron released from the myoglobin also has some renal tubule toxicity.

Often patients with rhabdomyolysis are asymptomatic early in the course of the illness. Patients may complain of muscle pain and discolored urine. Many

Table 55–1 ETIOLOGIES OF RHABDOMYOLYSIS

Alcohol abuse

Drug abuse (cocaine, amphetamines, lysergic acid diethylamide [LSD], heroin, phencyclidine)

Medications (diuretics, narcotics, theophylline, corticosteroids, benzodiazepines, phenothiazines, tricyclic antidepressants)

Trauma

High temperatures

Heat stroke

Strenuous exercise

Seizures

Toxin ingestion

Infection

patients with rhabdomyolysis are acutely ill and unable to communicate. Therefore, in relevant clinical situations, the clinician needs to maintain a high index of suspicion to make the diagnosis, because early intervention can avert renal failure and possible multiorgan failure. One key finding is **urine dipstick showing blood but no red blood cells seen on microscopy**, suggesting hemoglobinuria or **myoglobinuria**. Serum markers, such as creatinine kinase (CK), then can be measured. The level of creatinine kinase elevation directly correlates with the risk of renal failure. Left untreated, early complications include hyperkalemia, hypocalcemia, possible cardiac arrest, and arrhythmia. Approximately 15% of patients later develop acute renal failure, which carries a high risk of future morbidity and mortality. **Early institution of aggressive IV hydration** with normal saline can reverse the hypovolemia and prevent precipitation of the myoglobin within the tubules. Some experts advocate the addition of **IV sodium bicarbonate to alkalinize the urine**, which may further decrease the toxicity and precipitation of myoglobin to the tubules. Others advocate the use of mannitol, an osmotic agent. Some patients may require hemodialysis. Diuretics, however, may worsen the situation and are not indicated.

Comprehension Questions

55.1   A 22-year-old man presents to the emergency room 30 minutes after smoking crack cocaine with the complaint of crushing substernal chest pain. His electrocardiogram (ECG) shows early repolarization with a heart rate of 116 bpm but no other changes, and his cardiac troponin levels are negative. His urine drug screen is positive for cocaine. Which of the following is the best next step?

A. Give the patient acetaminophen for pain and discharge home.
B. Treat with IV metoprolol to reduce the heart rate to less than 60 bpm.
C. Administer aspirin, sedation, and nitrates.
D. Administer thrombolytics and admit to the coronary care unit.
E. Give flumazenil to reverse the action of the cocaine.

55.2   A 35-year-old marathon runner has been training for his next run and is brought to the emergency room after collapsing on the road. His temperature is 108°F, and he is tachypneic and lethargic. Urine dipstick shows large blood, but no red blood cells are seen on microscopy. Which of the following interventions would be most useful in his management?

A. Immediate aggressive IV hydration with normal saline.
B. Use warm packs to prevent shivering.
C. Obtain blood culture and immediately start IV antibiotics.
D. Administer hypertonic glucose solution.
E. Administer sodium bicarbonate.

ANSWERS

55.1   **C.** The patient should be given oxygen, aspirin, sedation, and nitrates
        for vasodilation and will require some evaluation for an acute coro-
        nary syndrome. Beta-blockers are relatively contraindicated because
        they can worsen vasoconstriction. There is no indication for throm-
        bolytics. Flumazenil is the antagonist for benzodiazepines and would
        have no effect on cocaine.

55.2   **A.** The patient is likely suffering from exertional heat stroke and
        resulting rhabdomyolysis. Intravenous saline is critical, and also cool-
        ing. Antibiotics are not likely to help because the hyperthermia likely
        does not represent infection. Sodium bicarbonate is rarely helpful.

Clinical Pearls

➤ Cocaine intoxication causes hypertension, tachycardia, agitation, excita-
  tion, and vasoconstriction. These effects can cause organ ischemia that
  manifests as myocardial infarction, stroke, hepatic or intestinal necrosis, or
  subarachnoid hemorrhage.

➤ Rhabdomyolysis is the breakdown and necrosis of striated (skeletal)
  muscle.

➤ Positive urine dipstick for blood in the absence of red blood cells by
  microscopy on a spun fresh urine sample should raise suspicion of
  rhabdomyolysis.

➤ Rhabdomyolysis can cause acute renal failure, possible permanent renal
  damage, and hypovolemia as a result of fluid sequestration in the necrotic
  muscle tissue.

➤ Treatment of rhabdomyolysis is aggressive administration of intravenous
  normal saline to prevent renal failure.

REFERENCES

Bouchama A, Knochel JP. Heat stroke. *N Engl J Med.* 2002;346:1978-1988.

Hollander JE. The management of cocaine-induced myocardial ischemia. *N Engl J Med.* 1995;333:1267-1272.

Mendelson JH, Mello NK. Cocaine and other commonly abused drugs. In: Kasper DL, Braunwald E, Fauci AS, et al, eds. *Harrison's Principles of Internal Medicine*, 17th ed. New York, NY: McGraw-Hill; 2008:2733-2736.

Sauret JM, Marinides G, Wang G. Rhabdomyolysis. *Am Fam Physician.* 2002;65:907-912.

Case 56

A 56-year-old woman presents to her doctor's office complaining of gradually progressive, nonpainful enlargement of the terminal joint on her left hand over a 9-month period. She has some stiffness with typing but not first thing in the morning. She also reports pain in her right knee, which occasionally "locks up." The right knee also hurts after long walks. On examination, her blood pressure is 130/85 mm Hg, heart rate 80 bpm, and weight 285 lb. Examination reveals only a nontender enlargement of her left distal interphalangeal (DIP) joint, and the right knee is noted to have crepitus and slightly decreased range of motion. There is no redness or swelling.

➤ What is your next step?

➤ What is the most likely diagnosis?

➤ What is the best initial treatment?

ANSWERS TO CASE 56:
Osteoarthritis/Degenerative Joint Disease

Summary: The patient is a 56-year-old obese woman with complaints of activity-related joint disease in the left DIP and right knee. There is no evidence of synovitis on examination.

➤ **Next step:** Obtain erythrocyte sedimentation rate (ESR) and plain X-rays of the hand and knee.

➤ **Most likely diagnosis:** Osteoarthritis (OA).

➤ **Best initial treatment:** Acetaminophen up to 4 g qd.

ANALYSIS

Objectives

1. Know the major clinical characteristics of OA.
2. Be familiar with management approaches to OA.
3. Understand the major classes of medications used for OA.
4. Know how to differentiate OA from inflammatory arthritis.

Considerations

This patient's history and examination are characteristic of OA. Laboratory work, typically negative for inflammatory arthritis, and X-rays will confirm the diagnosis. The most important features are the gradual onset, the lack of active synovitis, and the fact that her symptoms worsen with activity. If there were evidence of inflammation or joint effusion, then the best next step would be to aspirate the fluid from the joint and send it for various studies, including Gram stain and culture to assess for infection, crystal analysis to assess for gout or pseudogout, and cell count to assess for inflammation.

APPROACH TO
Osteoarthritis

DEFINITIONS

BOUCHARD NODES: Bony enlargement of proximal interphalangeal (PIP) joints, often asymptomatic.

CREPITUS: A creaking or hook and loop (Velcro)-like sound made by a joint in motion. Typically not painful.

HEBERDEN NODES: Bony enlargement of DIP joints, often asymptomatic.

SYNOVITIS: Inflammation of the joint space characterized by redness, swelling, and tenderness to touch.

CLINICAL APPROACH

OA is the most common joint disease in adults. The disease affects women more often than men. The incidence increases sharply in the fifth and sixth decades of life. OA begins insidiously, progresses slowly, and eventually may lead to disability, recurrent falls, inability to live independently, and significant morbidity.

Patients with OA often experience joint stiffness, which occurs with activity or after inactivity ("gel phenomena") and lasts for less than 15 to 30 minutes. This is in contrast to the morning stiffness of patients with an inflammatory arthritis (eg, rheumatoid arthritis [RA]), which often lasts for 1 to 2 hours and often requires warming, such as soaking in a hot tub, to improve. Early in the disease, there are no obvious findings. There may be some crepitus (creaking sound) in the joint, and, unlike inflammatory arthritis, there is often no or minimal tissue swelling (except in the most advanced disease). Bony prominences, especially in the DIP/PIP joints, can occur later. Figure 22–1 shows a typical joint involvement in OA versus RA. Pain seen in OA typically can be reproduced with passive motion of the joint. Table 56–1 lists the patterns of typical joint involvement.

Laboratory examination typically is unremarkable; inflammatory markers such as ESR, creatinine phosphokinase (CPK), and white blood cells (WBCs) all are normal. Likewise, autoimmune studies such as antinuclear antibody (ANA), rheumatoid factor, and complement levels also are normal. If the joint is aspirated, then examination of the synovial fluid also reflects a lack of inflammation: WBCs less than 2000/mm^3, protein less than 45 mg/dL without

Table 56–1 JOINT INVOLVEMENT IN OSTEOARTHRITIS	
JOINTS AFFECTED IN OA (IN ORDER OF INVOLVEMENT/FREQUENCY)	**JOINTS SPARED**
Hands (often asymmetric)	Hands (all except DIP/PIP/CMP)
• DIP (Heberden nodes)	Wrist
• PIP (Bouchard nodes)	Elbow
• Carpal metacarpophalangeal (CMP) of thumb	Shoulder
Knee	Spine
Hip	
Feet (usually first toe metatarsophalangeal joint)	

crystals, and glucose equal to serum. X-ray evaluation in OA may show osteophytes that are the most specific finding in the disease but might not be found early. Other characteristics seen on X-rays include joint space narrowing, subchondral sclerosis, and subchondral cysts.

It is critical to differentiate OA from other conditions that may present similarly. Periarticular pain that is not reproduced with passive motion suggests bursitis or tendonitis. Prolonged pain lasting for more than 1 hour points toward an inflammatory arthritis. Intense inflammation suggests one of the microcrystalline diseases (gout/pseudogout) or infectious arthritis. Systemic constitutional symptoms, such as weight loss, fatigue, fever, anorexia, and malaise, indicate an underlying inflammatory condition, such as polymyalgia rheumatic, rheumatoid arthritis, systemic lupus erythematosus, or a malignancy, and generally demands aggressive evaluation.

Management

Education is critical. Encourage the patient to stay active, because not using the joint can cause further immobility. Multiple short periods of rest throughout the day are better than one large period.

Equipment such as canes and/or walkers are helpful for patients with advanced disease because these patients are less stable and, as a result, have frequent falls. Physical therapy in the form of heat applied to the affected joints in early disease often is helpful. Perhaps the most important intervention is having the patient maintain full/near-full range of motion with regular exercise.

Pharmacotherapy early in the course of the disease consists primarily of acetaminophen, the mainstay of therapy. It is well tolerated and as effective as nonsteroidal anti-inflammatory drugs (NSAIDs; both nonprescription and prescription strength). The nutraceutical agents glucosamine and chondroitin are as effective as the NSAIDs, but their onset of action is a bit slower. NSAIDs inhibit the enzyme cyclooxygenase (COX) in the prostaglandin catabolism pathway and work as either COX-1 or COX-2 inhibitors. For a long time, COX-1–type NSAIDs were the most commonly prescribed drug for OA. However, COX-1 NSAIDs have well-documented side effects of gastrointestinal irritation and bleeding and renal damage. The COX-2 inhibitor class has the same anti-inflammatory potential, with fewer gastrointestinal side effects. Recent evidence about increased risk of cardiovascular (CV) events in patients using COX-2 inhibitors have led to the withdrawal of rofecoxib and valdecoxib from the market, however, and the remaining members of the class should not be used in patients with known CV disease or multiple CV risk factors. Oral steroids are generally not used to treat OA. Intra-articular steroids may be rarely useful for long-term treatment and can be helpful for the rare inflammation of a loose cartilage fragment, which may cause the joint to "lock up."

Surgery is reserved for only the most severe cases, which include patients who have major instability, a loose body in the joint, intractable pain of advanced disease, or severe functional limitation. Joint replacement is the typical procedure.

Comprehension Questions

56.1 Which of the following is most likely to be associated with advanced OA?

A. Disability with recurrent falls and inability to live alone
B. Joints with redness and effusion
C. Best treated with oral steroids
D. Improvement throughout the day after approximately 1 to 2 hours of "unfreezing the joint"

Match the following disease processes (A-F) to the clinical setting described in Questions 56.2 to 56.5.

A. Gonococcal arthritis
B. Gout
C. Pseudogout
D. Osteoarthritis
E. Rheumatoid arthritis
F. Systemic lupus erythematosus

56.2 Symmetric bilateral ulnar deviation of both hands in a 42-year-old woman

56.3 Painful, swollen metatarsophalangeal great toe (unilateral) with redness and warmth after eating steak and shrimp dinner in a 45-year-old man

56.4 Acute onset of unilateral elbow swelling, warmth, and tenderness and cervical discharge in a 25-year-old woman

56.5 Unilateral nontender bony enlargement of the first DIP and activity-related right hip pain in a 68-year-old woman

56.6 A 72-year-old man complains of painful joints in his hips and knees, which you have diagnosed as osteoarthritis. Which of the following is the best agent to prescribe for this patient?

A. Naproxen sodium
B. Celecoxib
C. Oral prednisone
D. Intra-articular prednisone
E. Acetaminophen

ANSWERS

56.1 **A.** Degenerative joint disease is a major cause of decreased functional status in elderly patients and requires ongoing treatment and evaluation by the physician to try to improve symptoms and to promote mobility. Oral steroids are not helpful in this condition.

56.2   **E.** Rheumatoid arthritis gives the ulnar deviation of the fingers.

56.3   **B.** Gouty arthritis often affects the first metatarsophalangeal joint
        and can be precipitated by various foods or alcohol.

56.4   **A.** Cervical discharge and inflammatory joint are consistent with
        gonococcal arthritis, which can also present as a migratory arthritis.

56.5   **D.** The location and asymmetry of joint involvement, lack of inflam-
        matory signs, and worsening with exertion all are characteristic of OA.

56.6   **E.** Acetaminophen is the first agent of choice in the treatment of
        early osteoarthritis.

Clinical Pearls

> ➤ Osteoarthritis is the most common articular disease of adults, most often
>   affecting the distal interphalangeal joints > proximal interphalangeal joints
>   > knees > hip joints.
> ➤ Pain in osteoarthritis is worsened with activity and is not associated with
>   morning stiffness.
> ➤ No pharmacologic agents that modify or stop disease progression are
>   available. Treatment is aimed at symptom relief.
> ➤ Initial pharmacologic therapy should be acetaminophen. Joint replace-
>   ment for severe osteoarthritis is reserved for patients with intractable pain
>   despite medical therapy and for those with severe functional limitations.

REFERENCES

Felson DT. Osteoarthritis. In: Kasper DL, Braunwald E, Fauci AS, et al, eds. *Harrison's Principles of Internal Medicine*. 17th ed. New York, NY: McGraw-Hill; 2008:2158-2165.
Felson DT. Osteoarthritis of the knee. *N Engl J Med.* 2006;354:841-848.
Zhang W, Jones A, Doherty M. Does paracetamol (acetaminophen) reduce the pain of osteoarthritis? A meta-analysis of randomized controlled trials. *Ann Rheum Dis.* 2004;63:901-907.

Case 57

A 62-year-old man presents to the emergency room with sudden onset of abdominal discomfort and passage of several large, black, tarry stools. He became diaphoretic and began to experience chest pain, similar to that of his recent myocardial infarction. Three weeks ago, he suffered an uncomplicated non–ST-elevation myocardial infarction. A submaximal exercise treadmill test performed prior to discharge revealed no ischemia. He was discharged home with aspirin, clopidogrel, and metoprolol. On examination, his heart rate is 104 bpm. His blood pressure is 124/92 mm Hg while lying down but drops to 95/70 mm Hg upon standing. He appears pale and uncomfortable, and he is covered with a fine layer of sweat. His neck veins are flat, his chest is clear to auscultation, and his heart rhythm is tachycardic but regular, with a soft systolic murmur at the right sternal border and an S_4 gallop. His apical impulse is focal and nondisplaced. His abdomen is soft with active bowel sounds and mild epigastric tenderness, but no guarding or rebound tenderness, and no masses or organomegaly are appreciated. Rectal examination shows black, sticky stool, which is strongly positive for occult blood. His hemoglobin level is 5.9 g/dL, prothrombin time (PT) and partial thromboplastin time (PTT) both are normal, and he has normal renal function and liver function tests. Electrocardiogram (ECG) reveals sinus tachycardia with no ST-segment changes, but T-wave inversion in the anterior precordial leads and no ventricular ectopy. Creatine kinase (CK) is 127 U/L (units/liter) with a normal CK-MB (myocardial) fraction, and troponin I and serum myoglobin levels are normal.

➤ What is the most likely diagnosis?

➤ What is your next step?

ANSWERS TO CASE 57:
Transfusion Medicine

Summary: A man with a recent myocardial infarction but a negative postinfarction stress test, signifying no critical coronary artery stenosis, is admitted with angina pectoris at rest and ECG changes consistent with recurrent cardiac ischemia. In addition, he has melena and epigastric tenderness, indicating an upper gastrointestinal (GI) hemorrhage, likely caused by his use of aspirin. He is tachycardic and has orthostatic hypotension, indicating significant hypovolemia as a result of blood loss.

➤ **Most likely diagnosis:** Unstable angina, which has been precipitated by anemia because of acute GI blood loss.

➤ **Next step:** Transfusion with packed red blood cells (PRBCs).

ANALYSIS

Objectives

1. Understand the indications for transfusion of red blood cells.
2. Know the complications of transfusions.
3. Be aware of alternatives to transfusion.
4. Know the indications for transfusion of platelets and of fresh-frozen plasma (FFP).

Considerations

This patient has two urgent problems. He has suffered an upper GI hemorrhage, with enough blood loss to cause hemodynamic compromise. In addition, he has unstable angina, given his severe prolonged chest pain at rest but lack of definitive ECG or cardiac enzyme evidence of myocardial infarction. Rather than being a primary problem with his coronary arteries, such as thrombosis or vasospasm, the cardiac ischemia is secondary to his acute blood loss and consequent tachycardia and loss of hemoglobin and its oxygen-carrying capacity. He should be treated with urgent replacement of blood volume.

APPROACH TO
Symptomatic Anemia

DEFINITIONS

TRALI: Transfusion related acute lung injury, due to an immune mediated lung injury.

ACUTE HEMOLYTIC REACTION: Transfusion reaction due to antibody lysis of transfused red blood cells.

CLINICAL APPROACH

Symptoms attributable to anemia are manifold and depend primarily on the patient's underlying cardiopulmonary status and the chronicity with which the anemia developed. For a slowly developing, chronic anemia in patients with good cardiopulmonary reserve, symptoms may not be noted until the hemoglobin level falls very low, for example, from 3 to 4 g/dL. For patients with serious underlying cardiopulmonary disease who depend on adequate oxygen-carrying capacity, falls in hemoglobin level can be devastating. Such is the case with the man in this clinical scenario, who is suffering a cardiac complication as a consequence of his anemia, in this case, unstable angina. **Unstable angina** is defined as **ischemic chest pain at rest,** of **new onset,** or **occurring at a lower level of activity.** Unstable angina does not cause elevated levels of cardiac markers or a myocardial infarction tracing on ECG. The Braunwald classification defines patients into both class and clinical circumstance (Table 57–1).

Table 57–1 UNSTABLE ANGINA CLASSIFICATION

Class
  I. New or worsened angina not at rest
 II. Angina at rest, last occurred more than 48 h ago
III. Angina at rest within the last 48 h

and

Clinical circumstance
• Secondary angina—noncoronary precipitant (eg, anemia, thyrotoxicosis, infection)
• Primary angina—in the absence of an extracardiac condition
• Postinfarction angina—within 2 wk after a myocardial infarction, with those in class IIIC having the worst prognosis

Data from: Braunwald E. Unstable angina: a classification. Circulation. 1989; 80:410-414.

In this case of secondary angina, the anemia must be corrected, which requires an understanding of transfusion medicine. Anemia is generally considered to be a hemoglobin level <12 g/dL in women or less than 13 g/dL in men. Although lower values often can be tolerated or underlying etiologies treated, blood transfusions have been both necessary and lifesaving at times. In addition to PRBCs, there are other components of whole blood, including platelets, FFP, cryoprecipitate, and intravenous immunoglobulin (IVIg).

The indications for transfusion of PRBCs are acute surgical or nonsurgical blood loss, anemia with end-organ effects (eg, syncope, angina pectoris) or hemodynamic compromise, and in critical illness to improve oxygen-carrying capacity or delivery to tissues. However, there are no absolute guidelines or thresholds for transfusion. Many believe that a hemoglobin level of 7 g/dL is adequate in the absence of a clearly defined increased need, such as cardiac ischemia, for which a hematocrit level of at least 30% may be desired. In the absence of ongoing bleeding or destruction of red cells, we typically expect that each unit of PRBC will result in an increase of 1 g/dL in the hemoglobin level or 3% in the hematocrit level.

Transfusion carries a small but definite risk, including transmission of infection, reactions, and consequences. Viruses that are screened for but which can be passed include hepatitis C virus (1 in 103,000 units), human T-cell lymphocyte virus types I and II, human immunodeficiency virus (1 in 700,000), hepatitis B virus (1 in 66,000), and parvovirus B19. Rarely, bacterial contamination (eg, *Yersinia enterocolitica*) causes fevers, sepsis, and even death during or soon after transfusion. Parasites (eg, malaria) are screened for by questioning a donor's medical and travel history.

There are also noninfectious concerns, both immune and nonimmune mediated. With respect to immune mechanisms, it is possible that a recipient has preformed natural antibodies that lyse foreign donor erythrocytes, which can be associated with the major A and/or B or O blood types or with other antigens (eg, D, Duffy, Kidd). Because hemolysis can ensue, a "type and cross" is first performed, in which blood samples are tested for compatibility prior to transfusion. The most common cause of this reaction actually is clerical (ie, mislabeling). **Acute hemolytic reactions** may present with **hypotension, fever, chills, hemoglobinuria,** and **flank pain.** The transfusion must be halted immediately, and fluid and diuretics (or even dialysis) should be given to protect the kidney from failure via immune-complex deposits. Laboratory work for intravascular hemolysis should be checked (lactate dehydrogenase [LDH], indirect bilirubin, haptoglobin), as well as coagulation tests for disseminated intravascular coagulopathy (DIC). Less predictably, milder, delayed hemolytic reactions involving amnestic responses from the recipient can occur. Febrile nonhemolytic transfusion reactions can occur and may be helped by antipyretics. Reactions range from urticaria treated with diphenhydramine and transfusion interruption to anaphylaxis, in which case the transfusion must be stopped, and epinephrine and steroids are needed. Sometimes seen is transfusion-related acute lung injury (TRALI), in which the appearance of bilateral interstitial infiltrates in the lung represents noncardiogenic pulmonary edema.

Considering nonimmune consequences, the transfusion itself supplies 300 mL per unit of PRBC intravascularly, so patients can easily become volume overloaded. Adjusting the volume and rate and using diuretics will prevent this complication. Each unit of blood also provides 250 mg of iron. Multiple and frequent transfusions can cause iron overload and deposition, leading to cirrhosis, cardiac problems (eg, arrhythmia, heart failure), or diabetes. Finally, a transfusion confers a mild immunosuppression to patients, which is potentially important in already compromised populations, such as patients with cancer or AIDS.

Alternatives to transfusion have shown a role for **erythropoietin**, a hormone that promotes red cell production. It is often used in the treatment of patients with **renal failure**–related anemia. It also can be used in patients who are banking a presurgical autologous transfusion to encourage quicker recovery of their hemoglobin levels prior to surgery. Cell savers salvage some intraoperative blood losses, which are then transfused back into the patient. A Jehovah's Witness often does not wish to have foreign blood products transfused based on religious convictions. In some cases we can increase the baseline hemoglobin level by using erythropoietin and iron before planned surgery, minimize laboratory testing, and use cell savers. Ultimately, however, a competent patient's wishes are to be respected.

Thrombocytopenia can frequently be treated with platelet transfusion. When a patient has a platelet count of less than 50,000/mm^3 and is bleeding, or when a patient is at risk for spontaneous bleeding at a level of less than 10,000/mm^3, platelets can be transfused. Each unit increases the platelet count from 5000 to 10,000/mm^3. In cases such as immune thrombocytopenic purpura (ITP), in which platelets are being destroyed, however, transfusion is generally not helpful unless active bleeding is occurring.

FFP replaces clotting factors and is often given to reverse **warfarin (Coumadin) anticoagulation**. Cryoprecipitate from FFP replaces fibrinogen and some clotting factors, making it useful in patients with hemophilia A and von Willebrand disease (vMD).

IVIg is administered in patients with immune thrombocytopenia to temporarily block the reticuloendothelial system and thus elevate platelets counts quickly, albeit temporarily. One caution is that in patients with IgA deficiency (1 in 600 individuals of European origin), transfusion with IVIg or FFP can cause anaphylaxis because of the presence of anti-IgA antibodies.

Comprehension Questions

57.1 A 32-year-old man is brought into the emergency room after a motor vehicle accident. He is noted to be in hypovolemic shock with a blood pressure of 60/40 mm Hg. He is actively bleeding from a femur fracture. The patient's hemoglobin level is 7 g/dL. His wife is positive that the patient's blood type is A-positive. Which of the following is the most appropriate type of blood to be transfused?
   A. Give AB-positive blood, uncross-matched.
   B. Await cross-matched A-positive blood.
   C. Give type-specific A-positive blood, uncross-matched.
   D. Give O-negative blood, uncross-matched.

57.2 A 45-year-old woman is noted to have severe menorrhagia over 6 months and a hemoglobin level of 6 g/dL. She feels dizzy, weak, and fatigued. She receives three units of packed erythrocytes intravenously. Two hours into the transfusion, she develops fever to 103°F and shaking chills. Which of the following laboratory tests would most likely confirm an acute transfusion reaction?
   A. Lactate dehydrogenase (LDH) level
   B. Leukocyte count
   C. Direct bilirubin level
   D. Glucose level

57.3 A 57-year-old man has a prosthetic aortic valve for which he takes warfarin (Coumadin) 10 mg/d. He is noted to have an international normalized ratio (INR) of 7.0 and is actively bleeding large clots from his gums, rectum, and when urinating. Which of the following is the best management for this patient?
   A. Administer vitamin D.
   B. Transfuse with fresh-frozen plasma.
   C. Administer intravenous immunoglobulin (IVIg).
   D. Discontinue the warfarin (Coumadin) and observe.

ANSWERS

57.1 **D.** This patient needs a blood transfusion immediately, as evidenced by his dangerously low blood pressure. He does not have the 45 minutes required for cross-matching his blood. Even though the patient's wife is "absolutely sure" about the blood type, history is not completely reliable, and in an emergent situation such that uncross-matched blood must be given, O-negative blood (universal donor) usually is administered.

57.2   **A.** Elevated LDH and indirect bilirubin levels or decreased hapto-globin levels would be consistent with hemolysis.

57.3   **B.** When life-threatening acute bleeding occurs in the face of coag-ulopathy due to warfarin (Coumadin) use, the treatment is fresh-frozen plasma. The INR is extremely high, consistent with a severe coagulopathy. Sometimes vitamin K administration can be helpful if the bleeding is not severe.

Clinical Pearls

➤ The symptoms of anemia are related to the rapidity or chronicity with which the anemia developed as well as the patients' underlying cardiopulmonary status.

➤ Myocardial ischemia or infarction may be precipitated by factors not related to the coronary arteries, such as tachycardia or severe anemia, with loss of oxygen-carrying capacity.

➤ Transfusion of blood carries certain risks, such as hemolytic reaction, infection (eg, human immunodeficiency virus [HIV] or hepatitis C), and transfusion-related lung injury.

➤ Platelet transfusions are indicated for severe thrombocytopenia with bleeding symptoms, but they frequently are not useful for immune-mediated immune thrombocytopenic purpura and are definitely contraindicated in thrombotic thrombocytopenic purpura.

➤ Fresh-frozen plasma is used to correct coagulopathy by providing clotting factors.

REFERENCES

Cannon CP, Braunwald E. Unstable angina and non-ST-elevation myocardial infarction. In: Fauci AS, Braunwald E, Kasper DL, eds. *Harrison's Principles of Internal Medicine*. 17th ed. New York, NY: McGraw-Hill; 2008: 1527-1532

Dzieczkowski JS, Anderson KC. Transfusion biology and therapy. In: Kasper DL, Braunwald E, Fauci AS, et al, eds. *Harrison's Principles of Internal Medicine*. 17th ed. New York, NY: McGraw-Hill; 2008:707-713.

Goodnough LT, Brecher ME, Kanter MH, et al. Transfusion medicine (part 1). *N Engl J Med*. 1999;340:438-447.

Case 58

A 26-year-old woman presents to the emergency room on a Saturday afternoon with complaints of bleeding from her nose and mouth since the previous night. She also noticed small, reddish spots on her lower extremities when she got out of the bed in the morning. She denies fever, chills, nausea, vomiting, abdominal pain, or joint pain. The patient reports she had developed an upper respiratory infection 2 weeks prior to the emergency room visit, but the infection has now resolved. She denies significant medical problems. Her menses have been normal, and her last menstrual period was approximately 2 weeks ago. She denies excessive bleeding in the past, even after delivering her baby. Prior to this episode, she never had epistaxis, easy bruisability, or bleeding into her joints. There is no family history of abnormal bleeding. The patient does not take any medications.

On examination she is alert, oriented, and somewhat anxious. Her blood pressure is 110/70 mm Hg, her heart rate is 90 bpm, and she is afebrile. No pallor or jaundice is noted. There is bright red oozing from the nose and the gingiva. Skin examination reveals multiple 1-mm flat reddish spots on her lower extremities. The rest of the examination is normal. There is no lymphadenopathy or hepatosplenomegaly. Her complete blood cell count (CBC) is normal except for a platelet count of 18,000/mm^3. Prothrombin time (PT) and partial thromboplastin time (PTT) are normal.

➤ What is your most likely diagnosis?

➤ What is the best initial treatment?

ANSWERS TO CASE 58:
Immune Thrombocytopenic Purpura

Summary: A 26-year-old woman is seen in the emergency room because of persistent epistaxis. She denies excessive bleeding with menses or childbirth, easy bruisability, or bleeding into her joints. There is no family history of abnormal bleeding. The patient does not take any medications. Physical examination is significant only for the blood oozing from her nose and for the petechiae on her legs. There is no lymphadenopathy or hepatosplenomegaly. Her CBC shows thrombocytopenia, but the other cell lines are normal.

➤ **Most likely diagnosis:** Immune thrombocytopenia purpura (ITP).

➤ **Best initial treatment:** Oral corticosteroids.

ANALYSIS

Objectives

1. Learn the clinical approach to bleeding disorders, specifically platelets disorders versus coagulation disorders.
2. Learn about the differential diagnosis of thrombocytopenia, specifically thrombocytopenic purpura versus other platelet disorders, such as thrombotic thrombocytopenic purpura (TTP), hemolytic uremic syndrome (HUS), and disseminated intravascular coagulation (DIC).
3. Learn about the treatment of ITP.

Considerations

This patient presents with mucosal bleeding, petechiae, and thrombocytopenia. She has no other history, symptoms, or physical examination findings of any systemic disease, so her problem appears to an isolated hematologic problem. Review of her CBC is important to ensure that other cell lines (white blood cell count [WBC] and red blood cell count [RBC]) are normal – if they are abnormal, processes, such as acute leukemia or a bone marrow infiltrative process must be considered. Her coagulation studies (PT and PTT) are also normal – if they were deranged, we would suspect a consumptive coagulopathy causing the thrombocytopenia and a serious underlying disorder. Her current level of thrombocytopenia does not place her at risk for spontaneous hemorrhage, but at platelet counts less than between 5000 and 10,000/mm^3, she is risk for life-threatening bleeding.

APPROACH TO
The Patient with Abnormal Bleeding

DEFINITIONS

IMMUNE THROMBOCYTOPENIA PURPURA: A hematological disorder characterized by the destruction of blood platelets due to the presence of antiplatelet autoantibodies.

THROMBOTIC THROMBOCYTOPENIA PURPURA: A life-threatening syndrome of uncertain etiology characterized by a pentad of microangiopathic hemolytic anemia, thrombocytopenia, neurologic abnormalities, fever, and renal dysfunction.

HEMOLYTIC UREMIC SYNDROME: A clinical complex consisting of progressive renal failure that is associated with microangiopathic hemolytic anemia and thrombocytopenia

CLINICAL APPROACH

A careful history is the most effective way to determine the presence and significance of a bleeding disorder. For a patient with abnormal bleeding, the most important history relates to any prior history of bleeding. One should inquire about history of abnormal bleeding, epistaxis, menorrhagia, excessive prolonged bleeding from minor cuts, bruising, prolonged or profuse bleeding after dental extraction, excessive bleeding after major surgery or obstetric delivery, or trauma. Excessive mucosal bleeding (eg, gum and nose bleedings) and petechiae are suggestive of thrombocytopenia, or abnormal platelet function such as von Willebrand disease (vMD). On the other hand, hemarthrosis, deep hematomas, and retroperitoneal bleeding more likely reflect a severe coagulation abnormality, such as hemophilia, deficiencies of factors VIII or IX. The causes of thrombocytopenia can be divided into (a) decreased platelet production, (b) decreased platelet survival, (c) sequestration (hypersplenism), and (d) dilutional. **Impaired platelet production** is caused by a bone marrow abnormality, such as infiltration caused by malignancy or myelofibrosis, marrow suppression as a result of chemicals, drugs, or radiation, and viruses. In these cases, a deficit of platelet production is rarely seen without abnormalities in the production of white and red cells. Therefore, when impaired platelet production is the result of a bone marrow abnormality, we also expect abnormalities in the number of leukocytes and red cells. **Decreased platelet survival** is another cause of thrombocytopenia. Thrombocytopenia is defined as a platelet count of less than 150,000/mm^3, although spontaneous bleeding usually occurs at much lower levels. Mild thrombocytopenia may be seen in pregnancy and much more significant thrombocytopenia with HELLP (hemolysis, elevated liver enzymes, low platelets) syndrome. Decreased platelet survival can be a result of increased destruction of platelets, such as immune-mediated destruction triggered by medications, various infections, autoimmune diseases like systemic lupus erythematosus (SLE) or for uncertain causes as in idiopathic thrombocytopenic purpura (ITP). Decreased platelet survival can also be due to sequestration in an abnormally enlarged spleen.

ITP: Acute ITP is most common in early childhood, often following an antecedent upper respiratory infection, and usually is self-limiting. In children, ITP usually resolves spontaneously within 3 to 6 months. **ITP in adults** is more likely to have an insidious or subacute presentation, is most likely to occur in women ages 20 to 40 years old, and is more likely to persist for months to years, with **uncommon spontaneous remission.** The patient will present with the clinical manifestations of thrombocytopenia, such as petechiae and mucosal bleeding, but with no systemic toxicity, no enlargement of nodes or abdominal organs, and a normal blood count and normal peripheral blood smear except for thrombocytopenia. Laboratory testing is usually focused on a search for secondary causes of thrombocytopenia such as HIV, hepatitis C, ANA (for SLE), and a direct Coombs test to evaluate for autoimmune hemolytic anemia with ITP (Evans syndrome). Bone marrow examination is generally performed on older patients to exclude myelodysplasia, and often reveals increased megakaryocytes but otherwise normal findings.

In 80% of children affected with ITP, spontaneous remission occurs within 6 weeks, but spontaneous recovery in adults is less common. Many physicians elect to treat affected patients, especially adults, with **oral steroids**, such as prednisone 1 to 2 mg/kg of body weight. Platelet transfusions usually are unnecessary and should be reserved for rare life-threatening situations because survival of transfused platelets in ITP may be as short as a few minutes. **Intravenous immunoglobulin (IVIg)** is often used when platelet counts are less than 10,000/mm^3 and is used concurrently with steroids. Because the spleen removes the antibody-bound platelets, patients who do not respond to steroids may be candidates for **splenectomy.**

Drug-induced thrombocytopenia: When a patient presents with thrombocytopenia, any drug that the patient is using should be considered a possible cause. Common drugs known to cause thrombocytopenia, include H$_2$ blockers, quinine, and sulfonamides. In general, the diagnosis is made by clinical observation of the response to drug withdrawal. Discontinuation of the offending medication should lead to improvement in the platelet count within a time frame consistent with the drug's metabolism, almost always within 7 to 10 days.

Heparin-induced thrombocytopenia (HIT): There are two types of HIT: HIT-1 which is non-immune mediated usually occurring shortly after initiation of heparin (<48 hours), and caused by platelet clumping. Usually the patient is not clinically affected. HIT-2 is caused by platelet-activating antibodies and occurs 3 or more days after heparin is begun, and sooner if the patient had been sensitized by prior heparin use. HIT-2 can cause serious

consequences. HIT differs from other drug-induced causes of thrombocytopenia in that it is not associated with bleeding, but rather with increased risk of thrombosis. HIT typically develops 5-10 days after exposure to either unfractionated heparin (UFH) or low-molecular-weight heparins (LMWH), when an antibody forms against the complex of heparin and platelet factor IV. Typically, UFH puts the patient at increased risk for HIT. These HIT antibodies activate platelets and endothelial cells, and can cause thrombosis. Up to half of patients with HIT will develop clinically evident thrombosis. Diagnosis depends on clinical suspicion, and utilization of an enzyme-linked immunosorbent assay (ELISA) for the HIT antibodies. Treatment includes discontinuation of the heparin (one cannot switch from UFH to LMWH because HIT antibodies will cross-react), and instead use a direct thrombin inhibitor such as argatroban or lepirudin to treat thrombosis.

Thrombocytopenia may also be caused by consumptive coagulopathy, the most common of which is **disseminated intravascular coagulation (DIC).** DIC usually is triggered by serious underlying conditions such as bacterial sepsis, malignancy such as acute promyelotic leukemia, or with obstetric catastrophes such as abruptio placentae. Any of these disease processes can produce blood exposure to pathologic levels of tissue factor, triggering uncontrolled thrombin generation with systemic fibrin deposition in the microcirculation. This uncontrolled activation of coagulation results in consumption of platelets and clotting factors, leading secondarily to bleeding. Laboratory findings include thrombocytopenia and elevated PT and PTT (reflecting the consumptive coagulopathy), and decreased fibrinogen and elevated fibrin-split products and D-dimer (reflecting uncontrolled fibrin deposition). Usually, the cause of DIC is obvious, and treatment should be directed toward correcting the underlying cause, as well as replacement of platelets and coagulation factors if there is clinically significant bleeding.

A less common disease process which may be confused with DIC is **Thrombotic Thrombocytopenic Purpura (TTP).** TTP may be triggered by infection such as HIV, or medications such as clopidogrel, or it may be idiopathic. As originally described, TTP has a pentad of findings : **(a) thrombocytopenia; (b) microangiopathic hemolytic** anemia with elevated lactate dehydrogenase (LDH) level and schistocytosis in the peripheral blood smear; **(c) fever; (d) fluctuating central nervous system (CNS) deficits with altered mental status; and (e) renal failure.** Patients may be acutely ill, and differentiation from DIC may be challenging, except that the PT and PTT are typically normal in TTP, but elevated in DIC. Plasma exchange is the standard treatment and has reduced the mortality of this condition greatly. Table 58–1 compares DIC, TTP, and ITP.

von Willebrand disease patients, who appear to have impaired primary hemostasis (ie, petechiae, easy bruising, mucosal bleeding, menorrhagia) yet have normal platelet counts, should be suspected of having impaired platelet function, as in **vWD.** vWD is the **most common inherited bleeding disorder.**

Table 58–1 COMPARISON OF DIC, TTP, AND ITP

	ETIOLOGY	CLINICAL COURSE	TREATMENT
Disseminated intravascular coagulopathy (DIC)	Secondary to some other process: sepsis, trauma, metastatic malignancy, obstetric causes	Can be relatively mild indolent course or severe life-threatening process; ongoing coagulation and fibrinolysis can cause thrombosis or hemorrhage; consumption of coagulation factors is seen as prolonged PT and PTT.	Treatment aimed at underlying cause. No proven specific treatment for the coagulation problem: if bleeding, replace factors and fibrinogen with fresh-frozen plasma (FFP) or cryoprecipitate; if clotting, consider anticoagulate with heparin.
Thrombo cytopenic thrombotic purpura (TTP)	Multiple causes, many seemingly trivial: drugs/infection lead to endothelial injury and release of von Willebrand factor (vMF), triggering formation of microvascular thrombi	May present as septic-appearing patient with fever, altered mental status, thrombocytopenia, microangiopathic hemolytic anemia, and renal failure. Previously a very high mortality, mainly because of CNS involvement. Normal PT and PTT.	Plasmapheresis (removal of the excess/abnormal vWF), most patients recover. Corticosteroids.
Immune throm-bocytopenic purpura (ITP)	Antiplatelet antibody leading to platelet destruction	Children: following a viral illness with resolution; in adults, a more indolent course with progression and rarely spontaneous resolution. Isolated thrombocytopenia, normal PT, PTT. Increased megakaryocytes on bone marrow aspiration.	Oral corticosteroids; splenectomy if resistant to steroids. Intravenous immunoglobulin (IVIg).

It may occur as often as 1 in 1000 individuals. It is an **autosomal dominant disorder** but often is not recognized because of relatively mild bleeding symptoms or because of excessive bleeding attributed to other causes, for example, menorrhagia attributed to uterine fibroids. von Willebrand factor (vWF) is a large complex multimeric protein that has two major functions: it allows for platelet adhesion to endothelium at sites of vascular injury, and it is the carrier protein for coagulation factor VIII, which stabilizes the molecule. vWD is a heterogenous group of disorders, but a common feature is **deficiency in the amount** or **function of vWF**. Clinical features are those of primary hemostasis as discussed. Typical laboratory features are reduced levels of vWF, reduced vWF activity as measured by ristocetin cofactor assay, and reduced factor VIII activity. The platelet count is usually normal, bleeding time is increased, and pTT may or may not be prolonged. Treatment is **desmopressin acetate (DDAVP)**, which causes release of vWF from endothelial stores, or use of factor VIII concentrate, which contains large amount of vWF.

Comprehension Questions

58.1 A 28-year-old woman complains of excessive bleeding from her gums and has petechiae. Here CBC shows a platelet count of 22,000/mm^3 with a hemoglobin of 8.9 g/dL and a WBC count of 87,000/mm^3. Which of the following is the most likely etiology of her low platelet count?

A. Immune thrombocytopenia purpura
B. Systemic lupus erythematosus
C. Drug-induced thrombocytopenia
D. Acute leukemia

58.2 A 50-year-old man has been treated for rheumatoid arthritis for many years. He currently is taking corticosteroids for the disease. On examination, he has stigmata of rheumatoid arthritis and some fullness on his left upper abdomen. His platelet count is slightly low at 105,000/mm^3. His white blood cell count is 3100/mm^3 and hemoglobin level 9.0 g/dL. Which of the following is the most likely etiology of the thrombocytopenia?

A. Steroid induced
B. Splenic sequestration
C. Rheumatoid arthritis autoimmune induced
D. Prior gold therapy

58.3   A 30-year-old woman with ITP has been taking maximum corticos-
        teroid doses and still has a platelet count of 20,000/mm³ and frequent
        bleeding episodes. Which of the following should she receive before
        her splenectomy?
        A. Washed leukocyte transfusion
        B. Intravenous interferon therapy
        C. Pneumococcal vaccine
        D. Bone marrow radiotherapy

58.4   A 65-year-old man who has a prosthetic heart valve is hospitalized for a
        knee replacement surgery, and placed on IV heparin for anticoagulation
        before the procedure. He drinks one glass of wine each weekend and has
        been diagnosed with osteoarthritis for which he takes acetaminophen.
        His platelet count was normal, but now is 32,000/mm³. Which of the
        following is the most likely cause of the thrombocytopenia?
        A. Prosthetic heart valve
        B. Alcohol intake
        C. Acetaminophen
        D. Heparin

ANSWERS

58.1   **D.** The thrombocytopenia is seen with other hematologic abnormalities,
        the most abnormal of which is a markedly elevated WBC count, sug-
        gesting acute leukemia.

58.2   **B.** This patient with rheumatoid arthritis likely has splenomegaly,
        also known as Felty syndrome. Splenomegaly from any etiology may
        cause sequestration of platelets, leading to thrombocytopenia.

58.3   **C.** Patients who undergo splenectomy are at risk for infections of
        encapsulated organisms such as *Streptococcus pneumoniae* and thus
        should receive the pneumococcal vaccine. It usually is given 2 weeks
        prior to splenectomy so that the spleen can help in forming a better
        immune response.

58.4   **D.** The patient likely has heparin-induced thrombocytopenia, which
        may be confirmed by assay for HIT antibodies. Treatment consists of
        stopping the heparin.

Clinical Pearls

➤ Disorders of primary hemostasis (thrombocytopenia or von Willebrand disease) are characterized by mucosal bleeding and the appearance of petechiae or superficial ecchymoses.

➤ Disorders of secondary hemostasis (coagulation factor deficiencies such as hemophilia) usually are characterized by the development of superficial ecchymoses as well as deep hematomas and hemarthroses.

➤ Immune thrombocytopenic purpura is a diagnosis of exclusion. Patients have isolated thrombocytopenia (ie, no red or white blood cell abnormalities), no apparent secondary causes such as systemic lupus erythematosus, human immunodeficiency virus (HIV), or medication-induced thrombocytopenia, and normal to increased numbers of megakaryocytes in the bone marrow.

➤ Spontaneous hemorrhage may occur with platelet counts of less than 10,000/mm^3.

➤ Platelet transfusion in immune thrombocytopenic purpura is generally ineffective and is used only when there is severe life-threatening bleeding.

➤ Corticosteroids are the initial treatment of immune thrombocytopenic purpura. Patients with more severe disease can be treated with intravenous immunoglobulin; chronic refractory cases are treated with splenectomy.

REFERENCES

Cines DB, Blanchette VS. Immune thrombocytopenic purpura. *N Engl J Med*. 2002; 346:995-1008.

George JN, Raskob GE, Shah SR, et al. Drug-induced thrombocytopenia: a systematic review of published case reports. *Ann Intern Med*. 1998;129:886-890.

Konkle BA. Bleeding and thrombosis. In: Fauci AS, Braunwald E, Kasper DL, eds. *Harrison's Principles of Internal Medicine*, 17th ed. New York, NY: McGraw-Hill; 2008:363-369.

Konkle BA. Disorders of platelets and vessel wall. In: Fauci AS, Braunwald E, Kasper DL, eds. *Harrison's Principles of Internal Medicine*, 17th ed. New York, NY: McGraw-Hill; 2008:718-725

Case 59

A 45-year-old woman returns today to your outpatient clinic for follow-up. You have seen her frequently over the last 3 months for various complaints. Over the past 2 to 3 weeks, however, she says that she has just felt terrible. Her symptoms include intermittent headaches, bilateral shoulder and neck pain, overwhelming fatigue, and difficulty sleeping. She cries easily, and she is irritable with her children. She feels unable to keep up with the demands of her work and family, and she feels her life is meaningless. The patient smokes half a pack of cigarettes per day and drinks an occasional glass of wine on weekends. She otherwise has no significant medical or family history, except for a maternal aunt with migraine headaches. The patient states that she has regular menses. She works as a waitress, and she is married with three teenage children. Physical examination reveals blood pressure 110/70 mm Hg, heart rate 80 bpm, and temperature 98°F. Her thyroid is normal to palpation. Her heart has a normal rate and rhythm without murmurs. Abdominal examination reveals no masses or hepatosplenomegaly. Neurologic examination reveals no deficits.

➤ What is your diagnosis?

➤ What is the best next step?

ANSWERS TO CASE 59:

Depression

Summary: A 45-year-old woman is seen in follow-up for various complaints. She has a 2- to 3-week history of intermittent headaches, bilateral shoulder and neck pain, overwhelming fatigue, insomnia, crying easily, irritability with her children, feeling unable to keep up with work and family demands, and feeling that her life is meaningless. She has a maternal aunt with migraine headaches. The patient states that she has regular menses. She is normotensive, and her thyroid is normal to palpation. Physical examination, including neurologic examination, reveals no deficits.

➤ **Most likely diagnosis:** Depression, perhaps major depression.

➤ **Next step:** Ascertain whether she has suicidal or homicidal ideation, or if hallucinations or psychosis are present, and investigate for medical causes of depression (hypothyroidism, substance abuse, physical or sexual abuse).

ANALYSIS

Objectives

1. Know the features of major depression.
2. Be able to distinguish depression from uncomplicated bereavement and from medical conditions that may mimic depression.
3. Know how to assess suicide risk and when to seek psychiatric evaluation.
4. Know the principles of treating depression.

Considerations

This 45-year-old woman has many of the criteria for major depression (Table 59–1). The first priority in the evaluation of this patient is to ensure her and others' safety; thus, assessing whether she has suicidal or homicidal ideation, has had "unusual thoughts," or has "seen or heard things that no one else does." This is best approached directly by asking, "Are you thinking about killing yourself?" The presence of suicidal ideation or psychosis generally requires psychiatric hospitalization. Other common illnesses and conditions can present with similar symptoms, such as hypothyroidism, abuse, anemia, and perimenopause, and should be considered in this middle-age female patient. The hypermetabolic condition of some cancers, renal failure, and other metabolic abnormalities can cause weight loss and fatigue that could be confused with depression. After ensuring that there is no underlying medical cause of the depressive symptoms, a selective serotonin reuptake inhibitor (SSRI), brief in-office counseling, or referral to a psychologist for more intensive counseling are reasonable treatment options.

Table 59–1 SYMPTOMS OF MAJOR DEPRESSION

SIG: E(nergy) **CAPS**. Each letter stands for a criterion (except for depressed mood) used in diagnosing a major depressive episode. Five or more of the following criteria are needed for at least 2 weeks:

S—sleep changes
I—(decreased) interest
G—(excessive) guilt
E—(decreased) energy
C—(decreased) concentration
A—appetite changes
P—psychomotor agitation or retardation
S—suicidal ideation

APPROACH TO
Depressive Disorder

DEFINITIONS

ATYPICAL DEPRESSION: Depressed mood with increased sleeping, increased eating, weight gain, and increased sensitivity to rejection.

DYSTHYMIA: Fewer, milder, but persistent depressive symptoms with low mood for more than 2 years.

MAJOR DEPRESSION: Depressed mood or loss of interest in activities for 2 weeks plus three or four of the other symptoms for a total of five (Table 59–1).

SOMATIZATION: Conversion of a mental or psychological disorder into a physical symptom.

CLINICAL APPROACH

Depression is highly prevalent in medical outpatients, thought to be second only to hypertension in general practice. It is estimated that 15% of the general population will experience a major depressive episode at some point in their life. Between 6% and 8% of outpatients in a primary care setting are estimated to satisfy diagnostic criteria for depression, although many seek care for other complaints. Consequently, a depressive condition may not be recognized or properly treated. Because of the high frequency of the disorder and the good outcomes with appropriate treatment, the United States Preventive Services Task Force recommends screening for depression, which may be as simple as asking questions about depressed mood or anhedonia.

When a patient presents with features of depression, the clinician must try to distinguish a depressive disorder from a transient situational disturbance or a more chronic personality problem, as well as considering medical illness that may mimic depression. One of the most common situational disturbances a primary care physician must assess and treat is an uncomplicated grief reaction. Patients experiencing **uncomplicated bereavement** after a significant loss, such as the death of a loved one, may have depressive symptoms for a period of time sufficient to qualify as major depression. However, these symptoms usually are self-limited, begin to resolve spontaneously in less than 6 months, and do not respond well to antidepressant medications. Treatment may include supportive counseling and medications to alleviate symptoms, such as sleep aids for insomnia. More extreme symptoms, such as **anhedonia, suicidal ideation,** or **persistent depressive** symptoms, may signify a more **complicated grief reaction** and may require psychiatric evaluation.

Depression shares several symptoms with other common medical disorders. A careful history with a thorough review of systems and physical examination may be all a physician must perform to exclude some diseases, such as some cancers, but others may require laboratory testing. When the suspicion of depression is high, the clinician should explain this to the patient at the beginning of the evaluation. Otherwise, when everything is normal and the patient is told all the symptoms are just a result of depression, sometimes this is interpreted as meaning, "It's all in your head."

Hypothyroidism often causes fatigue and mental slowing. Patients and physicians may interpret this as depression; however, the patient's mood usually is not altered. Nor should patients be experiencing the guilty feelings and poor self-esteem of depression. Anemia, especially the macrocytic anemia of vitamin B_{12} **deficiency,** often presents with neuropsychiatric changes early in the course of disease, especially in the elderly. Folate deficiency can produce similar symptoms, although they usually are less profound. **Metabolic disorders,** such as **renal failure, hyperglycemia, hyponatremia,** and **hypercalcemia,** can present with fatigue and mental confusion that may be mistaken for depression or dementia, especially in the elderly. However, these patients often have other symptoms, such as polyuria and polydipsia, or are taking medications that have such side effects. Other conditions that should be considered in evaluating a patient with depressive symptoms is substance abuse, although the two often coexist, organic brain disease in a patient with a history of brain injury and dementia in elderly patients.

When depressive symptoms are discovered, it is essential to assess the patient's suicide risk. Suicide is the most serious outcome of a depressive episode: **approximately 15% of patients requiring hospitalization for depression die by suicide.** Asking questions about suicidal or homicidal ideation does not "put the idea into the patient's head"; rather, it lets the patient know that you are willing to help. Patients who are an immediate threat to themselves or others require emergent admission to a psychiatric facility. Risk factors for suicide include male gender, older age, living alone, history of suicide attempt, or current suicidal ideation (especially when a specific plan has been formulated).

High-risk patients require immediate psychiatric evaluation and possible inpatient care.

Most patients, however, can be treated on an outpatient basis with medications and perhaps psychotherapy. In general, 60% to 70% of depressed patients will respond to any antidepressant, regardless of the drug class used. If a patient has taken an antidepressant previously and has had a good response, that drug should be the first choice for treatment. Conversely, if a patient has discontinued a medication because of unacceptable side effects, that is important information in choosing an agent or class of drugs. Overall, antidepressants are chosen based on side effect profile, patient preference, and medical considerations such as drug interactions. **SSRIs** have low side effect profiles, primarily gastrointestinal complaints which usually are short lived, and **sexual dysfunction** in approximately 30% of patients. They are considered safer than the older tricyclic antidepressants (TCAs) because of the risk for cardiac arrhythmias caused by TCA overdose, a particular concern in patients with suicidal ideation. Most SSRIs do have a number of drug interactions with medications metabolized through the cytochrome P-450 system. Some SSRIs have specific indications for anxiety as well as depression.

Other agents include trazodone, which is highly sedating and may be a good choice in patients with insomnia, and bupropion, which is nonsedating (in fact, may cause insomnia) and has a low incidence of sexual dysfunction but lowers seizure threshold in patients with epilepsy. TCAs are efficacious and useful in patients without active suicidal ideation, especially if cost is a factor, because TCAs are available in generic form.

Comprehension Questions

59.1 A 23-year-old woman is brought to the emergency room by ambulance for chest pain. She is frantic, crying, hyperventilating, and holding her chest. She says that she feels like she is about to die and that her heart is pounding out of her chest. Her blood pressure is 120/74 mm Hg, heart rate 118 bpm, respiratory rate 30 breaths per minute, and oxygen saturation 100% on room air. Her electrocardiogram (ECG), except for a sinus tachycardia, is completely normal. After a few minutes she begins to calm down, and she explains that she has these episodes about once per week. She suddenly feels like she can't breathe, that she's going to die, and that her heart is pounding. She's been to the emergency room four times with similar episodes, and nothing abnormal has been found. Which of the following is the most likely diagnosis?

A. Wolff-Parkinson-White syndrome
B. Myocardial ischemia
C. Panic disorder
D. Depression with anxious mood
E. Pheochromocytoma

59.2   A 73-year-old woman, whose health has always been perfect, is
        brought to your office by her family for worsening forgetfulness and
        personality changes. Until 6 months ago, she was active in her church
        and with her family. Now the family states that she rarely leaves her
        bed unless she is coerced, and she is sloppy in her personal appearance
        and in her housekeeping. The patient denies being sad, but says she doesn't
        have the energy she used to have. Mental status testing demonstrates
        poor short-term memory and concentration. Which of the following
        should be your next step?
        A. Prescribe a serotonin selective reuptake inhibitor
        B. Prescribe a tricyclic antidepressant
        C. Assess thyroid-stimulating hormone (TSH) level
        D. Referral to psychiatrist

59.3   A 35-year-old woman presents to your office for a second opinion. She
        believes that she has fibromyalgia and has suffered for years with daily
        generalized muscle pain that worsens with activity and responds only
        minimally to over-the-counter analgesics. Testing for rheumatologic
        and other medical disorders has been repeatedly negative. Following
        an exhaustive workup, her last doctor tried to start her on antidepres-
        sants. Although she is fatigued, lacks energy, has trouble concentrat-
        ing, and feels sad, she believes these symptoms are caused by her
        disease and so she never filled the prescription. Which of the follow-
        ing would be your advice?
        A. Repeat laboratory testing for rheumatologic disorders.
        B. Continue with over-the-counter analgesics and follow the response.
        C. Recommend trial of antidepressant medication.
        D. Recommend computed tomography (CT) of chest, abdomen, and
           pelvis to look for occult malignancy.
        E. Start empiric levothyroxine for subclinical hypothyroidism.

ANSWERS

59.1   **C.** This young woman is most likely suffering from panic disorder.
        The other diagnoses are unlikely given her normal blood pressure,
        ECG, and age. Panic disorder is the unexplained occurrence of sudden
        episodes of intense fear, often associated with palpitations, sweating,
        dizziness, difficulty breathing, and chest pain. These episodes are recur-
        rent and unpredictable. The first episode often occurs outside the
        home, and the unpredictable nature may lead to fear of leaving the
        house (agoraphobia). Depression is frequently a concomitant diagnosis.
        Illicit drug use also must be considered.

59.2   **C.** In this otherwise healthy, elderly woman, a sudden change in her behavior is concerning for a metabolic problem. Depression is a possibility, even though this patient denies feeling sad, as depression often is "masked" by symptoms of dementia in the elderly. Tests to consider in addition to assessment of TSH level are complete blood count, electrolytes, liver and renal function tests, and calcium level.

59.3   **C.** In many disorders, such as fibromyalgia, chronic fatigue syndrome, and chronic pain, which physicians poorly understand and for which we have few therapeutic options, depression may be present. It often is difficult to determine whether the depression preceded the illness or is a result of the illness. However, some patients with fibromyalgia or chronic pain do seem to benefit from the administration of antidepressant medications.

Clinical Pearls

➤ Depression is very common in the general population, but patients often seek care for other symptoms, such as fatigue or nonspecific pains.

➤ The clinician must distinguish depression from uncomplicated grief reaction, substance abuse, dementia, and medical illnesses such as hypothyroidism and vitamin B_{12} deficiency.

➤ It is essential to assess suicide risk in depressed patients and to identify those who require psychiatric evaluation. Patients with the highest risk for suicide are those with a prior suicide attempt and those with active suicidal ideation and a specific plan.

➤ Most depressed patients can be treated as outpatients with antidepressant medications, which are chosen based on side-effect profile, patient preference, and drug interactions, because all are about equally efficacious.

REFERENCES

Mann JJ. Drug therapy: the medical management of depression. *N Engl J Med.* 2005;353:1819-1834.

Reus VI. Mental disorders. In: Kasper DL, Braunwald E, Fauci AS, et al, eds. *Harrison's Principles of Internal Medicine.* 17th ed. New York, NY: McGraw-Hill; 2008: 2710-2723.

Case 60

A 42-year-old Hispanic factory worker presents with complaints of dizziness. When asked to describe what "dizzy" means to her, she relates a feeling of movement, even though she is standing still. The first time it happened, she also felt a little nauseated, but she did not vomit. Since then, she has not felt nauseated. In her job, she has to look down to fold cloths coming off the line, and the dizziness occurs if she looks down too quickly. It only lasts about a minute, but it is disruptive to her work. The symptom has also occurred when she is lying down and rolls over in bed. She has no medical history or related family history. Her vital signs and heart, lung, and gastrointestinal (GI) examinations are normal. Her pupils are equal, round, and reactive to light and accommodation. Extraocular movements are intact, and no nystagmus is noted. Cranial nerve examination was normal. Strength, deep tendon reflexes, and gait are normal.

➤ What is your diagnosis?

➤ What is the best therapy for the condition?

ANSWERS TO CASE 60:

Dizziness/Benign Positional Vertigo

Summary: A previously healthy 42-year-old woman presents with intermittent positional vertigo and a normal physical examination.

➤ **Most likely diagnosis:** Benign positional vertigo.

➤ **Best treatment:** A maneuver to dislodge the loose otolith from the affected semicircular canal can be performed in the office, or medications such as meclizine can be prescribed to treat the symptoms. For severe symptoms, diazepam (Valium) or transdermal scopolamine patches can be prescribed.

ANALYSIS

Objectives

1. Understand how to categorize types of dizziness.
2. Distinguish "benign" positional vertigo from more serious central causes of vertigo.
3. Recognize the symptoms and signs related to positional vertigo.
4. Understand the treatment options for vertigo.

Considerations

This previously healthy 42-year-old woman complains of acute onset of "dizziness," especially when moving her head quickly. Upon further questioning, the symptom of vertigo is established, that is, the perception of movement when she is stationary. She has no neurologic symptoms such as cranial nerve dysfunction, headache, or history of head trauma. The normal neurologic examination similarly suggests a benign process. The patient most likely has benign positional vertigo, which is the most common cause of acute vertigo. The pathophysiology likely is debris in the semicircular canals of the middle ear. Anticholinergic medications and positional maneuvers are often useful in therapy.

APPROACH TO

Dizziness and Vertigo

DEFINITIONS

BENIGN POSITIONAL VERTIGO: Most common cause of vertigo caused by debris in the semicircular canals of the inner ear.

DIX-HALLPIKE MANEUVER: Positional maneuver used to diagnose benign positional paroxysmal vertigo.

VERTIGO: Illusory sensation of movement or spinning. **Peripheral vertigo** is caused by the labyrinthine apparatus or vestibular nerve, whereas **central vertigo** is caused by a brainstem or cerebellar process (Table 60–1).

CLINICAL APPROACH

The complaint of dizziness is one of the most common reasons for patients to seek medical attention, and one of the most common reasons for the clinician to throw up his or her hands in exasperation because of the vagueness of the complaint. "Dizziness" is a word that can encompass a myriad of symptoms, including lightheadedness, vertigo, "feeling out of sorts," and even gait instability. **The first step in evaluating patients with this complaint is to ask open-ended questions about the sensation ("What do you mean by dizzy?")** and to listen to the patient's history. Asking leading questions ("Did you feel like the room was spinning?") can cause one to go down the wrong diagnostic path. **The majority of patients who complain of dizziness are suffering from a distinctive symptom—presyncope, dysequilibrium, or vertigo—which can be elucidated by history or physical examination.**

Presyncope is the sensation associated with near-fainting. Patients may describe feeling lightheaded, a graying of vision, or "nearly blacking out." This sensation typically is brief, lasting seconds or minutes, and is self-resolving. The causes of this symptom are the same as those for syncope: most often vasovagal attacks, orthostatic hypotension, or cardiac arrhythmias. The evaluation of these patients is the same as for those with syncope (see Case 15).

Dysequilibrium is a sense of imbalance, usually while walking. It is a multifactorial disorder, commonly seen in elderly patients with impaired vision,

Table 60–1 CHARACTERISTICS OF CENTRAL VERSUS PERIPHERAL CAUSES OF VERTIGO

	PERIPHERAL ETIOLOGY	CENTRAL ETIOLOGY
Duration of vertigo	Intermittent (minutes, hours) but recurrent	Chronic
Associated tinnitus, hearing loss	Often present	Usually not present
Other neurologic deficits (cranial nerve palsies, dysarthria, extremity weakness)	Not present	Often present

peripheral neuropathy and decreased proprioception, and musculoskeletal problems causing gait instability. It may also be one of the presenting symptoms of patients with primary movement disorders such as parkinsonism. These symptoms may be exacerbated by medications, particularly in the elderly; examples include antihypertensives, antidepressants, and anticholinergic agents that can cause orthostatic hypotension or dizziness as a side effect.

Vertigo is the illusory sensation of movement or spinning, and usually arises from a disorder in the vestibular system. Our spatial orientation system is composed of three primary components. In the inner ear, the **semicircular canals** transduce angular acceleration, while the otoliths conduct linear acceleration and fixed gravity. This system sends information through projections to the cerebellum, spinal cord, and cerebral cortex, cranial nerves III, IV, and VI. The **vestibular ocular reflex** maintains visual stability during head movements through these same cranial nerves, as well as projections through the medial longitudinal fasciculus. This integration of the inner ear, brain, and eyes explains why **nystagmus** is observed in patients during bouts of vertigo. Peripheral sensation and visual input are also important in spatial orientation. It is the conflict between the inputs from these various systems that cause the sensation of vertigo. Physiologic vertigo includes motion sickness, or the sensation of movement that may occur when watching motion pictures.

Pathologic vertigo occurs when there are lesions in one of these systems. The first task in evaluating a patient with vertigo is to try to distinguish **peripheral** (labyrinthine apparatus or vestibular nerve) from **central** (brainstem or cerebellum) causes of vertigo. **Central causes, such as cerebellar hemorrhage or infarction, can be immediately life-threatening or signify serious underlying disease and require urgent investigation.** Peripheral causes typically signify less serious diseases and can be managed comfortably on an outpatient basis. Thus, the presence of other neurologic abnormalities, headache, or evidence of increased intracranial pressure is critical to address!

The most common type of vertigo seen is termed "benign" paroxysmal positional vertigo (BPPV), although the symptoms can be far from benign. Typically, this type of vertigo is precipitated by changes in head position, as in rolling over in bed, bending over, or looking upward. Patients may not have all of the typical symptoms at the same time; however, the first bout usually is abrupt in onset and associated with nausea. Subsequent occurrences may be less severe. BPPV is thought to be caused by loose, floating debris in the semicircular canals that causes an increase in neurologic discharge from the vestibular system on that side.

Nystagmus during episodes of vertigo is characteristic of BPPV. To confirm the diagnosis of BPPV in the office, the **Dix-Hallpike maneuver** (Figure 60–1) can be performed to elicit the nystagmus and vertigo. Patients turn their head toward the examiner and lay down quickly with their head hanging somewhat lower than the body. The eyes are kept open. The typical nystagmus is a mix of rotational and vertical eye movements. There is a lag of 5–10 seconds for

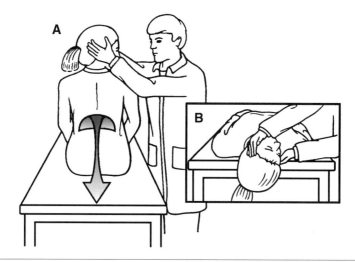

Figure 60–1. Dix-Hallpike maneuver. The clinician holds the patient's head and moves the patient rapidly from a sitting to a head-hanging position, first with the head facing one side and then facing the other side. Individuals with benign positional vertigo will demonstrate nystagmus after a delay of a few seconds.

the nystagmus to occur, and it is accompanied by the sensation of vertigo. A positive **Dix-Hallpike test**, along with the absence of other otologic or neurologic findings, makes the diagnosis of BPPV very likely.

BPPV is a self-limited disorder that may recur at some point in the patient's future. Anticholinergic agents, such as meclizine or diphenhydramine, or benzodiazepines may help lessen symptoms. Alternatively one may attempt positional maneuvers in the office to displace the otolith from the semicircular canal back into the utricle or saccule, such as **the Epley maneuver** (Figure 60–2, see page 536). Table 60–2 lists other causes of vertigo and their associated clinical features.

Finally, approximately 10% to 15% of patients have **nonspecific dizziness**, which cannot be classified as vertigo, presyncope, or dysequilibrium. Patients cannot clearly describe one of these syndromes, can report only that they feel "dizzy," have vague or unusual sensations, and have normal neurologic and vestibular examinations. The majority of these patients have some underlying **psychiatric disorder**, such as major depression, generalized anxiety, or panic disorder. Often the dizziness is associated with **hyperventilation** and can be reproduced in the office by purposeful hyperventilation. Treatment should be aimed at **reassurance** regarding the lack of pathologic causes of dizziness and at therapy for the underlying disorder with medication, such as serotonin specific reuptake inhibitors or benzodiazepines for anxiety disorders.

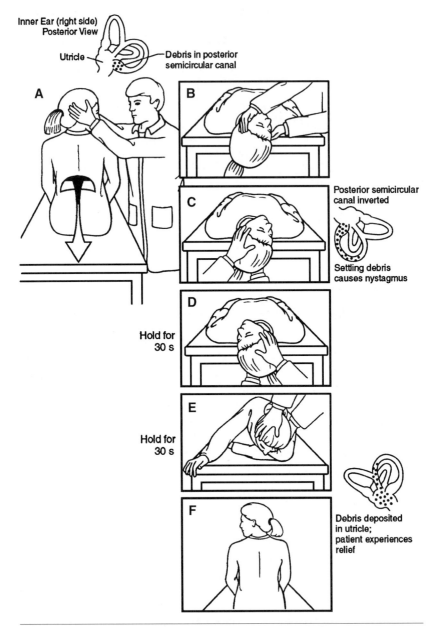

Figure 60–2. Modified Epley maneuver. First the Dix-Hallpike maneuver is performed to identify the affected ear. Then the patient's head is systematically rotated so that the loose particles slide out of the posterior semicircular canal into the utricle.

Table 60–2 COMMON CAUSES OF VERTIGO	
Benign positional paroxysmal vertigo	Nausea associated with nystagmus and vertigo with positional change, improves with time, absence of other otologic or neurologic findings, and a positive Dix-Hallpike test
Ménière disease	Intermittent attacks of severe vertigo are associated with tinnitus and hearing loss, sensation of ear fullness
Acoustic neuroma	Slow-growing tumor, so system compensates and often there is no nystagmus; usually with hearing loss and tinnitus
Vertebrobasilar insufficiency	Vertigo occurs in association with brainstem symptoms such as diplopia, dysarthria, or with numbness.

Comprehension Questions

60.1   A young woman presents to your office complaining of dizziness. When asked to describe the feeling, she gives a vague story of just feeling like "her head is too big." The feeling is associated with palpitations, sweating, and nervousness, and is almost constant. Her examination, including neurologic evaluation, is completely normal. Which of the following is the best next step?

A. Magnetic resonance imaging (MRI) brain scan
B. Obtaining a thorough psychosocial history
C. Dix-Hallpike maneuver
D. Prescribe meclizine
E. Referral to neurology department

60.2   A 75-year-old man presents to the emergency room with the sudden onset of nausea and vomiting. His medical history is notable for coronary artery disease and well-controlled hypertension. On examination he refuses to open his eyes or move his head, but when finally coaxed to sit up, he immediately starts to retch and vomit. Rotational nystagmus is noted. He cannot walk because of the dizziness and nausea that walking evokes. His noncontrast brain CT scan is read as normal for age. Which of the following is the best next step?

A. MRI/magnetic resonance angiography (MRA).
B. Obtain a thorough psychosocial history.
C. Dix-Hallpike maneuver.
D. Prescribe meclizine.
E. Referral to neurology.

60.3   A 65-year-old woman with a history of benign positional vertigo
        returns to your office for follow-up. Although manageable, the symp-
        toms of vertigo continue to recur periodically. Between episodes she
        generally feels normal but occasionally somewhat "off-balance." Today,
        her neurologic examination is completely normal, except that the
        thresholds of both air and bone conduction of a vibrating 256-Hz tun-
        ing fork are elevated on the left side. Which of the following is the
        most likely diagnosis?
        A. Intermittent benign positional vertigo
        B. Otosclerosis
        C. Acoustic neuroma
        D. Acute basilar artery infarct
        E. Panic disorder

60.4   Which of the following is the best next step for the patient described
        in Question 60.3?
        A. Prescription for a selective serotonin reuptake inhibitor
        B. Referral for a hearing aid
        C. Lumbar puncture and serology for syphilis
        D. Referral for an MRI
        E. Reassurance

ANSWERS

60.1   **B.** This young woman is not describing vertigo. The word "dizzy" can
        mean several different things, so it is extremely important when
        obtaining the history to have the patient describe, as best he or she
        can, what is meant by "dizzy." Patients with vertigo often use descrip-
        tors indicating movement, such as "the room is moving around me"
        or "I'm on a roller coaster." Feelings of dysequilibrium, or "out-of-
        body" experiences such as this young woman describes, are not typi-
        cal of vertigo and indicate another problem. It would be important
        to know what the symptoms are associated with; for example, is there
        increased stress in her job or intimate relationship? Is this panic dis-
        order or anxiety disorder?

60.2   **A.** This patient has symptoms of central vertigo. The onset of symp-
        toms was abrupt and severe. His gait is affected. If he were able to
        cooperate with an examination of his cerebellar functions, it would
        most likely be abnormal. His age and history of hypertension and
        coronary artery disease place him at elevated risk for cerebellar
        infarction or hemorrhage. CT is not the appropriate test for examin-
        ing the brainstem; MRI is much more accurate. MRA may be useful
        for delineating the exact vascular cause of the symptoms.

60.3 **C.** Acoustic neuromas are slow-growing tumors of the eighth cranial nerve. Because of the slow growth of the tumor, the neurologic system often is able to accommodate, so patients may have only subtle symptoms that at first may be confused with benign positional vertigo. The keys in this patient's history are the persistent low-grade feelings of dysequilibrium and the finding of probable sensorineural hearing loss on the left side. This finding indicates a possible problem with the eighth nerve, and an MRI would best delineate the anatomy.

60.4 **D.** MRI is the diagnostic test of choice. See answer to Question 60.3.

Clinical Pearls

➤ Patients use the term "dizziness" to describe several sensations: vertigo, presyncope, dysequilibrium, and nonspecific dizziness often associated with psychiatric disorders.

➤ Central causes of vertigo, such as cerebellar hemorrhage or infarction, can be immediately life-threatening and require urgent investigation.

➤ Peripheral causes of vertigo typically produce intermittent but severe attacks of vertigo; they may have associated tinnitus or hearing loss but should not be associated with other neurologic abnormalities.

➤ Benign paroxysmal positional vertigo is the most common cause of vertigo and can be diagnosed by the history of intermittent positional symptoms, absence of other otologic or neurologic findings, and a positive Dix-Hallpike test.

➤ Benign positional vertigo can be treated with maneuvers to reposition the abnormal otolith from the semicircular canal or by anticholinergic medications such as meclizine.

REFERENCES

Balch RB. Vestibular neuritis. *N Engl J Med.* 2003;348:1027-1032.

Daroff RB. Dizziness, and vertigo. In: Kasper DL, Braunwald E, Fauci AS, et al, eds. *Harrison's Principles of Internal Medicine*, 17th ed. New York, NY: McGraw-Hill; 2008:144-147.

Drachman D, Hart CW. An approach to the dizzy patient. *Neurology.* 1972;22:323-334.

Listing of Cases

Listing by Case Number

Listing by Disorder (Alphabetical)

Page numbers followed by *f* or *t* indicate figures or tables, respectively.